HEALTH FIRST!

HEALTH FIRST!

The Black Woman's Wellness Guide

ELEANOR HINTON HOYTT

and

HILARY BEARD

SMILEYBOOKS

Distributed by Hay House, Inc.
Carlsbad, California • New York City
London • Sydney • Johannesburg
Vancouver • Hong Kong • New Delhi

Published in the United States by:
SmileyBooks, 250 Park Avenue South, Suite #201, New York, NY 10003 • www.SmileyBooks.com

The authors of this book do not dispense medical advice or prescribe the use of any technique as a form of treatment for physical, mental, or medical problems without the advice of a physician, either directly or indirectly. The intent of the authors is only to offer information of a general nature to help you in your quest for well being in body, mind and spirit. In the event you use any of the information in this book for yourself, which is your constitutional right, the authors and the publisher assume no responsibility for your actions.

Distributed in the United States by: Hay House, Inc.: www.hayhouse.com • **Published and distributed in Australia by:** Hay House Australia Pty. Ltd.: www.hayhouse.com.au • **Published and distributed in the United Kingdom by:** Hay House UK, Ltd.: www.hayhouse.co.uk • **Published and distributed in the Republic of South Africa by:** Hay House SA (Pty), Ltd.: www.hayhouse.co.za • **Distributed in Canada by:** Raincoast: www.raincoast.com • **Published and Distributed in India by:** Hay House Publishers India: www.hayhouse.co.in

Design: Cindy Shaw, CreativeDetails.net

Grateful acknowledgment is made to the following for their permission to reprint previously published material:
American Obesity Association for the AOA Fact Sheet, Health Effects of Obesity.
Bertice Berry, Ph.D.: Excerpt from *A Year to Wellness and Other Weight Loss Secrets,* Freeman House Publishing 2011.
Gloria Wade-Gayles, Ph.D.: Excerpt from *My Soul Is A Witness: African American Women's Spirituality,* Boston: Beacon Press 2002.
Terrie Williams: Excerpt "From Stressed to Depressed." Reprinted with permission of Scribner, a Division of Simon & Schuster, Inc., from *BLACK PAIN: It Just Looks like We're Not Hurting.* Copyright ©2008 by Terri Williams. All rights reserved.
Iyanla Vanzant: Excerpt from "Saying Yes To Your Life." Copyright ©2005 by Iyanla Vanzant. All rights reserved.
Excerpt from "10 Contemplations." Copyright ©2002 by Iyanla Vanzant. All rights reserved.

The opinions set forth herein are those of the author, and do not necessarily express the views of the publisher or Hay House, Inc. or any of its affiliates.

Library of Congress Control Number: 2011942988

Tradepaper ISBN: 978-1-4019-3695-2
Digital ISBN: 978-1-4019-3696-9

15 14 13 12   4 3 2 1
1st edition, January 2012

Printed in the United States of America

*To the fearless and faithful Black women
who started the National Black Women's
Health Project in 1983.*

*You taught us that the health and wellness
of Black Women—MATTERS.*

Authors' Note

Some names in this book have been changed to protect the privacy of those who graciously consented to share their experiences and life stories. We are grateful for their willingness to participate.

CONTENTS

FOREWORD
By Byllye Y. Avery
Founder, Black Women's Health Imperative

"Magic." That's how I've come to describe that First National Conference on Black Women's Health at Spelman College that launched the National Black Women's Health Project in June 1983. When we put the word "Black" in front of "Women's Health" in the call to come together, something amazing happened. Over two thousand Black women came together to start conversations about topics previously thought unspeakable: emotional and sexual abuse, domestic violence, and abortion. We talked about becoming pregnant as teenagers and how being mothers too early meant being mothers for too long. We knew we had to take the risk of talking openly and honestly about things we'd never talked about before. We simply knew that, in Fannie Lou Hamer's famous words, we were "sick and tired of being sick and tired." We knew that those words described our frustrations, our anguish, and our need to connect with other Black women who felt the same urgent drive to find the tools that would engage us in changing our lives.

This gathering—the start of what would become the National Black Women's Health Project—grew out of the collective consciousness of a nation itself in the grip of change: forced by the civil rights movement to face up to racial discrimination, by the women's movement to challenge gender discrimination, and by the women's health movement to push back against a medical system that treated its patients like children. Across the nation, women were moving from being passive receivers of care to being active participants, demanding reproductive rights, a demystification of medical care, and access to information about their own health.

In my work in Florida at the Gainesville Women's Health Center and Birthplace, a freestanding birthing center, I noted that while most white women used the preventative care services, few Black women did. Health conferences and meetings lacked Black women's perspectives, because we were not present in significant numbers. It occurred to me that we, Black women, had never had an opportunity to talk among ourselves about our health, our issues and concerns. We lived in isolation, not talking about the struggles we faced.

Back then most of us were unaware that we were snared in a conspiracy of silence, keeping ourselves victims of the oppression that racism, sexism, classism and homophobia fueled. Mistakenly believing that we somehow brought about the bad things—rape, molestation, other forms of violence—that happened to us, we kept secrets and thought it was our "business." What we did not understand was that our silence allowed the oppression not only to continue in our lives, but to persist into future generations. We needed a space where we could break the silence, a place to talk about our lives and learn about the lives of others in order to find the tools that would engage us in changing our lives.

Many of us confessed that chronic conditions were plaguing our bodies and that we had watched our families struggle to survive with diseases that access to good care could have prevented. Single mothers talked about the financial burden of rearing children alone—some due to absent fathers, some to incarceration by an unjust justice system, and others to low self esteem compounded by their community's low expectations. We explored our relationships with our own mothers and fathers. Lesbians talked about being outcasts in their families, many choosing to live a closeted life, others taking the risk of being "out." We worried about the examples we were setting for our children by remaining in dysfunctional marriages supposedly for their sake.

We confronted these burdens and fears head on, long before they became popular topics on daytime television. We learned that these issues were not "our business"—they revealed our community's systemic sexism and disregard for the lives of women. Many of us were angry at the world for slavery and other injustices. Some of us were angry at our families and many of us were angry at ourselves. These were difficult issues to grapple with. We persevered and made some of the changes we sought.

For the first ten years, hundreds of women met monthly in self-help groups to plan a path to a healthier existence in body, mind, and spirit. As groups became stronger, they extended their learning to others through conferences, retreats, and sister circles. Health information contextualized by the lived experiences of Black women led to understanding that was meaningful and lasting. Ultimately we were able to make a difference in mainstream public health strategy.

Now, almost 30 years later, our world has changed, yet we still face some of the same conditions that challenged us then. Only now we live in an even more polarized political climate exacerbated by a global financial recession and high unemployment rates that render us all vulnerable. Some insurance companies leave us without coverage when we need it the most, forcing us to put off getting care that compromises our health and drives up costs when we finally are treated.

The good news, however, is that we have a new health-care law—an institutional path that will give us access to better care and put us more in charge of our own health. We will no longer have to make copayments for preventive services such as mammograms, Pap tests, and testing for STDs—it's up to us to get the screenings. If we get sick, we'll no longer need to worry about our policies being cancelled or unreasonable limits set on the amount of care that's covered—it is our right to be covered. Our sick children cannot be denied coverage, and starting in 2014 no one with a preexisting condition will be denied health insurance— we deserve health insurance across the lifespan, at all times. Adult children will be able to remain on their families' policies until their 26th birthdays—our young adults can now get the care they need. Seniors who are on Medicare Part D will pay less for medications and have better access to primary and preventive care—we must oppose all attempts to take away safety nets for our seniors.

Health First! gives us a way to look at our health and our lives in stages and across the life span, starting with the uncertainties of adolescence, continuing through the unpredictable challenges of adulthood, and ending with the time when we are experiencing our greatest losses in our senior years. Taking care of ourselves over a lifetime requires that we adopt a holistic approach: healthy eating habits and preventative care started early can ensure a healthier life, and we learn that it is never too late to start. Access to high-quality care is essential to gaining and maintaining optimal health. A healthy mind fosters good relationships and makes us receptive to loving and being loved. And developing our spirituality enables us to recognize that we can draw on power and strength beyond ourselves.

As we discovered in 1983, when we listen to the stories of women's lives, we understand the factors that influence our decisions, shape our lives, and ultimately provide a path to empowerment and good health—and *Health First!* is filled with women's stories. I encourage you to read them, celebrate them, and learn from them. Use this book and share it with your family and friends. Let them know that you have made a commitment to living your best life. Continue to be a powerful force by putting your *Health First!*

INTRODUCTION

Michelle Obama may be our nation's first Black First Lady, and Oprah Winfrey may have been crowned as the most powerful female force in the American media and among the wealthiest women in the world, but the average Black woman struggles. She struggles to get a decent education, earn a living wage, and sustain meaningful relationships. She struggles to gain the social support she needs, fight society's negative perceptions of her, and deal with her own low self-esteem. She struggles to take care of her children and loved ones, and she struggles even more to take care of her physical, emotional, mental, and spiritual well-being.

The economic downturn that's still unfolding around the globe has intensified Black women's challenges, especially our health challenges, even more than it has for other Americans. Why? Because Black women have grappled with hazardous health conditions for generations. A combination of structural racism, cultural conditioning, environmental factors beyond our control, and—let's face it—our own choices has caused over 70 percent of us to become overweight or obese, limiting our ability to enjoy our lives and increasing our risk of developing chronic and debilitating diseases, such as high blood pressure, diabetes, heart disease, and some cancers. In 2010, Black women's mortality rate was 33 percent higher than White women's.

Truth is, Black women's lives play out within a "perfect storm" of distress, oppression, and misguided optimism. We pay a heavy price for this inconvenient truth. Yet in spite of the odds stacked against us, we continue to function as the defiant backbone of our nuclear and extended families: as single moms; caregivers to elders; and health gatekeepers for our doctor-avoiding men. So when our well-being wanes, it rocks the foundation of the whole Black community. The health crisis we're facing—not least the rapid spread of HIV in places like Harlem, Bedford-Stuyvesant, and Southeast Washington, D.C.—has placed us at a tipping point where Black American survival is on the line.

Over the decades, the Black Women's Health Imperative's focus groups, roundtables, and surveys have confirmed that when you ask a Black woman about the state of her health, she will find a way to tell you she's healthy even if she's not. That's why we developed this book. We know that deep in our spirits, Black women long to be well.

Although Black history is riddled with pain and loss, it is equally shot through with overwhelming triumphs accomplished against all odds when a critical mass of people challenged the status quo and stepped forward to galvanize meaningful change. Black women continue to "beat the odds" and claim success in American life in ways that few would have ever predicted. Attaining good health and quality health care may be formidable challenges, but these are challenges that we believe Black women can meet. The fact that others often don't really "see us," or "don't think much of us," doesn't mean that we can't affirm our value and dare to love ourselves.

> When you ask a Black woman about the state of her health, she will find a way to tell you she's healthy even if she's not.

It's time for Black women to kick old dysfunctional behaviors to the curb no matter where or who we come from. It's time to adopt a new attitude of uncompromised commitment to our own well-being. We must move forward—sister by sister and one woman at a time!

As we educate ourselves about our health, we can break through our denial and discover that it is never too late to put our health first.

Because, as elder-sister Maya Angelou says, "When you know better, you do better."

Our deep desire to do better is what the Imperative has learned from Black women over the past three decades. Black women have told us loud and clear that they want to improve their personal health. No one with a chronic condition that ran in her family said she wasn't concerned for her own health too. We believe that this understanding of the need to change and "do better" is rooted in the core belief that we, as Black women, can take charge of our own lives, our own wellness, and our own self-care.

How to Use This Book

Our lives unfold in a continuous process, with growth marked by changes in our bodies that are reinforced by cultural milestones such as high-school graduation and life transitions such as marriage, childbearing, and divorce. Yet many of us don't see this big picture; we're too busy living from problem to problem and from paycheck to paycheck.

When you think of your life and your health as a process, not just a series of disconnected events, you begin to understand the implications of the changes you need to make for your own health. Decisions you make in one moment have consequences not just for that moment, but in the next moment and the next. At any point in your life, your health is whatever you have made it, building or eroding it in small increments over time, depending upon how you've loved and treated yourself.

> Decisions you make in one moment have consequences not just for that moment, but in the next moment and the next.

In *Health First!* we look at Black women's lives through the life cycle, starting with adolescence and ending with our senior years, paying particular attention to our health as we develop and mature. We look at typical life decisions many Black women make, against the backdrop of the social and cultural factors that shape our circumstances, and show how the consequences of these decisions play out in our health. We also look at the choices we face in caring for ourselves at every level, in body, mind, and spirit. We hope to help you understand how the choices you make build on themselves, helping you to look good and feel strong or causing you to decline into poor health and even debilitating illness.

The information that we draw on in this book to paint a credible portrait of Black women's health comes from experts, researchers, current data published by the federal government, and, most importantly, Black women themselves. It's also informed by the results of almost three decades of the Imperative working with women, conducting polls and surveys, and holding roundtables and focus groups. And for the first time, we are releasing some of the findings from a 2007 Harris survey on the Health Attitudes and Behavior of Black Women, commissioned by the Black Women's Health Imperative.

Quite honestly, some of what we learned in the survey alarmed us. For one thing, we learned that Black women have a very narrow definition of health—over half of us believe that being healthy merely means not having any chronic diseases, disabilities, or injuries. By this definition, a woman can be medically unhealthy, experiencing obesity, pre-diabetes, pre-hypertension, depression, and unsustainable levels of stress, but still believe she's well.

Denial, misunderstandings, and outright naiveté: this deadly combination keeps many of us unaware of impending danger to our well-being, so that we respond far too slowly—or don't respond at all—to some very real threats. Because Black women tend to form the backbone of our families, our denial jeopardizes our health and our life but also our children and communities.

So what do we say stands between us and good health? Some women in the survey said they couldn't afford medical treatment or preventive care; some said they didn't have access to good care (or to a gym); some said they didn't have the time; and others admitted that they weren't motivated to maintain or improve their well-being.

It's never too early to start learning how your actions today affect your health tomorrow. The good news is that it's never too late to learn how to care for yourself the way you need and deserve. The really good news is that it's never too late to shed the fear, to reconnect, to take that bold and courageous step toward wellness.

The book is organized into three distinct sections. *Part I: Your Journey through Life's Stages* examines Black women's lives as they unfold through the life cycle, from adolescence, young adulthood, and adulthood into elderhood. Each life stage describes the unique issues that Black women often face during that time of life and how the choices we make (or don't make) to take care of ourselves during one life stage set us up to experience either good health or health problems in later stages.

We encourage you to read all the chapters in Part I, not just the one about the stage of life you're in right now. If you're an older woman, be willing to start at the beginning: the chapter on adolescents may give you deeper insight into your own formative years, or provide some good ideas for helping a young girl in your life lay a foundation of good self-care, or offer encouragement to turn your health around now. If you're younger, read ahead: the voices of your older sisters and elders can inspire and teach you to make prevention one of your top priorities. A solid prevention plan can help you take control of your well-being and shape the vibrant, healthy life you want to live.

Part II: Beating the Odds zeros in on the Top Ten Health Risks that Black women face. You'll learn why these risks need to be on your personal health radar so that you can avoid becoming another sad statistic. Armed with new facts about Black women's health challenges and resources specific to Black women's health-care, you'll be empowered and more prepared than ever to deal with any health condition that places you at risk.

While we've included a wide variety of Black women's perspectives throughout the book, here we've intentionally shared the thoughts and experiences of women who have beat the odds and made choices to manage their disease, change their behavior, and inspire others along the way. Each entry in this section opens with a story of one woman's health challenge and how she was able to turn the tide. We hope that by reading about the challenges faced, the decisions these women have made, and the lifestyle changes that got them there, that you'll discover some answers to questions

> What makes it
> so difficult
> to be healthy,
> Black, and female
> in America?

that you may not even know you had. Our contributors' willingness to share their stories in order to shine a light on a new path and support you in transforming your own situation makes us very proud.

In *Part III: Self-Care Is Imperative,* we examine Black women's health through a different lens, taking a close look at what it means to be healthy in body, mind, and spirit. We explore what makes it so difficult to be healthy, Black, and female in America. Our hope is that once you understand what you're up against, you won't internalize your struggles so deeply or wrongly take them for personal failings. Rather, we hope you'll feel empowered not only to make a change, but to make the kind of change that places your health first.

This section encourages you to explore what living in health would look like in your life, so that you know what to aim for as you redefine your goals and commitments. We outline the elements of self-care that can lay the foundation for your personal transformation: from your physical health (including eating and exercise) to your mental and emotional well-being to your spiritual fulfillment or peace of mind. We also offer practical guidelines for working with your doctor and taking an active part in your own treatment—one of the most critical steps in self-care.

Putting Yourself First

Today more than at any other time over the past three decades, it is imperative that we commit to taking good care of ourselves. If we are to survive the challenges facing Black people—if we are to protect our children from being left behind in American society and defend our communities against the threats of joblessness, financial crisis, violence, HIV/AIDS, homelessness—we must place our self-care above all the other responsibilities in our life. We need to end the cultural legacy

> We must place our
> self-care above
> all the other
> responsibilities
> in our life.

of slavery that demanded that we attend to the needs of others and give our own health first priority. If we don't, in time we won't be able to attend to anyone's needs at all.

This may be the most troubling aspect of a culture in which Black women's health is devalued: we continue to place the health needs of others above our own. In providing care to our at-risk children, our undervalued, constantly impugned men, and our often sickly elders, we simply find no time for ourselves. Or perhaps it is more accurate to say we find no love for ourselves that inspires us to find the time for ourselves. Why? The reasons are legion and vary from woman to woman, but most of us are saddled with societal expectations of virtue and beauty that slander or cheapen our gifts, and many of us are haunted by negative family dynamics that have crippled our capacity to see ourselves as worthy of the same love and attention that we lavish on others.

In the process of caring for everyone else, we—as well as the people around us— often lose sight of the reality that we need nurturing too. So we rarely pay enough attention to our own selves, our own needs, and our own growth and development to know what we want out of life, or what makes us happy, or how to achieve it. Behind our "strong Black woman" facades, we are slow to admit when something's wrong in our lives and even slower to get around to taking care of it, even to the point of waiting years to make a doctor's appointment.

In these pages, we will ask you to expect more. We'll ask the question of what it means to take that giant step to be a healthy Black woman, we'll explore many answers, and we'll propose some of the decisions you must make to get there. As you read, you will encounter new and challenging ideas that will support your desire to make healthy choices. You will also hear the frank and inspiring voices of Black women as they share their experiences, responses, and stories—some that testify with an all-too-familiar weariness to painful truths, others that speak of incredible resilience and offer fresh perspectives on new ways of being. Most of the time we will encourage you, but every now and then, we may have to put you in touch with harsh realities. Even then, we promise that it will be an honest intervention, rooted in love and respect for all that you are.

We will share with you also insights from several well-known women who eloquently bring us face to face with some of these same truths. In an excerpt from

A Year to Wellness, author Bertice Berry implores us to learn to forgive ourselves for not having fully accepted who we are, how we look, and the mistakes we've made along the way. Mental-health advocate and author Terri Williams challenges us to unmask the secret depression that can be as deadly to our emotional well-being as cancer; in *Black Pain,* she advises us to remove our personal and collective "game face" and take a giant step toward truth and gratitude. *New York Times* best-selling author and motivational guru Iyanla Vanzant challenges us to "Say Yes To Life" and, with that embrace, to make the commitment to stop, take a deep breath, and reflect on what is really going on in our lives.

First and foremost, *Health First!* is for and about Black women seeing ourselves with new eyes. It's about learning to love ourselves enough to take care of ourselves, and caring enough about others to encourage them to do the same. Self-love is not an indulgence: it is a commitment to care for oneself in the highest possible manner. Self-love is not wrong, neither is it selfish. In fact, self-love is an acknowledgment that seeing ourselves as worthy of love is a prerequisite for loving others. And, unlike some other kinds of love, self-love is unconditional.

> We must learn to forgive ourselves for not having fully accepted who we are, how we look, and the mistakes we've made...

This idea of self-love through self-care came into being some 30 years ago when a group of 25 Black women from all across the country answered Byllye Avery's call to come together in Atlanta. For the next two years, we planned, plotted, and were completely outrageous in our passionately determined quest to break the "hold" that White, well-educated, middle-class women had on women's health. In 1983, the first-ever National Conference on Black Women's Health was held at Spelman College under the famous banner—"I'm Sick and Tired of Being Sick and Tired." To this day, as we travel around the country, women, old and young, remember those very first proclamations to make Black women's health matter.

And so here we are again, asking you to plan and plot and imagine with us: what would it be like if you felt healthy, vibrant, alert, motivated, encouraged, and joyful? What would it look like if you could shed those fears of going for your mammogram, if you were the weight you wanted to be, with the energy you wanted to have, if you forgave your mother for not protecting you as she should have, if you began to have positive thoughts and feelings about yourself and others? What if you took the chance and laughed more often, even at yourself? And what if you took the chance as we did in 1983 to put Black women's health—*your* health—first?

It can happen. Living as a Health-Wise woman can become your reality. It's a choice that only you can make—and we hope that you will.

> What would it be like
> if you felt
> healthy,
> vibrant,
> alert,
> motivated,
> encouraged,
> and joyful?

your journey
THROUGH
LIFE'S
STAGES

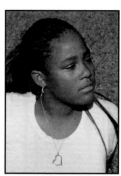

Chapter 1:
Adolescents
(10 to 19)

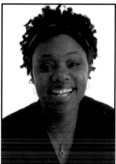

Chapter 2:
Young Adults
(20 to 39)

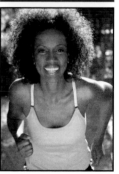

Chapter 3:
Midlife Adults
(40 to 64)

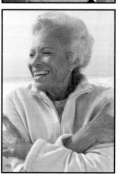

Chapter 4:
Mature Adults
(65+)

Chapter 1

Adolescents

(10 to 19)

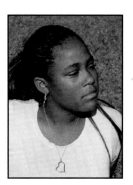

---■---

They get up before dawn, iron their own clothes, feed their younger siblings, and hop two buses cross-town to school. They sing in the youth choir at church, run "suicide drills" on the basketball court, and attend every meeting of their Girl Scout troops. You won't see any of this on the evening news, though; the media prefer to show them as promiscuous teen moms, hair-pulling YouTube pugilists, and out-of-control members of "flash mobs."

Clearly there's far more to the lives of Black adolescent girls than plays out in the press. Black girls live determined, complicated, and resilient lives in the vortex of cultural, economic, and societal forces that propel some of them to great accomplishments, challenge some others' ability to get a foothold in life, and crush some of them outright. They face the inadequate educational systems, high crime rates, and crumbling infrastructure that challenge all urban and inner-ring suburban residents and that disproportionately affect Black youth. But they also inhale the intoxicating promise of a world where a Black President and First Lady and two girls who look like them live at 1600 Pennsylvania Avenue; where they interact with the most diverse peer group in the history of humanity; and where their creativity, souped up on GarageBand, iMovie, a Facebook page, or a YouTube channel, lets them express their wildest imaginings to the entire world.

During the adolescent years of 10 through 19, Black girls metamorphose from bright-eyed children in colorful hairclips and church dresses to sometimes surly, often provocatively dressed, creative and opinionated adults determined to make their mark on the world, with the tools to do so at their fingertips. But they are not always as savvy as they'd like others to

---

believe. They're not always as healthy as they look or aware of how the care they take of themselves at this age—in body, mind, and spirit—can set the course for the rest of their lives.

Adolescence is a uniquely vulnerable time in a Black girl's life. She's becoming susceptible to the media's efforts to shape her delicate psyche into that of the consummate consumer, and for all of her street- and technology-smarts, she may easily fall for the pitches of the fast-food giants and soda companies—and even cigarette and liquor manufacturers—that count on young people to consume products that undermine their well-being. She's also vulnerable to the media's oversexualized portrayal of Black girls, which can not only wreak havoc with her self-image, but also can set up a dangerous model for the way she should be.

It's also a time of opportunity for her to build a strong sense of self and begin to chart a safe path through the world; for the people around her, it's a crucial window of possibility. "Ten to 15 is a critical age range," when girls are most open to adult input, says Dr. Faye Z. Belgrave, social psychology professor at Virginia Commonwealth University and author of *African American Girls: Reframing Perceptions and Changing Experiences.* "Once they get older—say 16 or 17—lots of times their life-course trajectory has changed."[1]

Not only their parents, but also the other adults in their lives—their grandmoms and pop-pops, their aunties and play aunties, their teachers and their youth program directors—are instrumental in helping them both to birth their potential and to protect themselves from the perils around them. Adults encircle their children with positive peers. They offer role models of positive friendships and romantic relationships as well as set an expectation of healthy eating. Adults help young people establish healthy patterns of behavior that can positively influence their lives for years to come. Adults can help teenagers avoid habits that could lead to illness and premature death, such as cigarette smoking and substance abuse; prepare them to make difficult decisions for their well-being, such as insisting that their sexual partners use condoms even when they don't want to; and incorporate the basics of self-care into their daily lives.

In this section we will examine the lives and the health of Black adolescent girls as they progress through early adolescence (ages 10–14), when they tend to be more highly supervised and waver between wanting independence and needing to know that their caregivers are close by; and late adolescence (15–19), when they have greater autonomy, are more influenced by their peers and increasingly likely to be sexually active, may have their driver's license, and should be preparing to graduate from high school. Even at this early stage, they begin grappling with serious health matters, so we will suggest ways for the adults who love them to help prepare them to live healthy lives—physically, emotionally, mentally, and spiritually. Throughout this chapter, adults can also reflect on the wise or not-so-wise choices

JUST THE FACTS:
BLACK TEEN GIRLS

Population:

3.4 million	
16 percent of Black females	

Family structure:

Single mother:	51%
Married couple:	35 %
Single Father:	8 %
Other:	3 %
Siblings:	1 or 2
Family income:	$40,698
Median household:	$34,445

Top causes of death (ages 10–14):

1. Unintentional injuries:	26%
2. Cancer:	10%
3. Homicide:	9%
4. Heart disease:	7%
5. Birth defects:	6%

Top causes of death (ages 15–19)

1. Unintentional injuries:	27%
2. Homicide:	21%
3. Heart disease:	7%
4. Cancer:	6%
5. Suicide:	3%

Source: Leading Causes of Death by Age Group, Black Females – United States, 2006. Department of Health and Human Services, Centers for Disease Control and Prevention; 2010.

they made as adolescents that are affecting their lives today. The chapters ahead will illuminate these connections and show how we can take decisive steps to shift our health in a positive direction.

The picture we're painting of Black adolescent girls' lives is done in broad strokes. Most of the data on them describe urban and low-income girls, including an important 2009 study, *Black Girls in New York City: Untold Strength and Resilience*, published by the Institute for Women's Policy Research (IWPR). Not all Black girls face the grimmest of these realities in their own daily lives, but their lives play out against the backdrop of the bigger societal picture, with its trends toward risky behaviors and dangerous consequences.

Girls to Women:
The First "Change of Life"

Many traditional societies celebrate a girl's first period and welcome it as a signal of her transition into adulthood. In the United States, different groups mark the passage from childhood[2] to adulthood in many different ways. Ritual celebrations include bat mitzvahs, weeklong overnight camps, class trips abroad, European vacations, "Sweet-16" parties, getting a driver's license (and maybe even a first car), and college tours. For many Black young women, no such rituals exist. Rites of passage common to older generations, such as visiting a department store at age 12 to get "fitted" for a training bra, being allowed to wear pink nail polish and getting ears pierced at 13, wearing lipstick, and attending social teas where older women show them which fork to use at 16—have gone the way of the boom box.

Adolescence describes a roughly 10-year period during which children experience a social, psychological and biological transition between puberty and legal adulthood[3]. Our girls develop into distinct individuals, along the way working out a wide range of issues related to who they are and who they will become.

These teens also make their first tentative choices toward what they want to do, where they want to go, and how they want to live. For some this may include their first jobs; for others it may be where to go to college. As they gain independence, it is at this life stage that they also are likely to develop an interest in romantic relationships, become sexually active, and pursue activities that don't involve their family. For all girls, no matter their race or background, some points on the path are sure to be rocky. Black teen girls face many of the same forces and stressors that other girls do—the pressure to be attractive, to dress well, to conform and be well-liked. One 12-year-old in a mentoring program wrote affirmations on Post-it notes: "Be a lawyer," said one; "Be smart but popular!" read another.

Like other girls and women, Black girls define their lives largely through their relationships with their immediate and extended family members as well as their same-aged friends. "For Black adolescent girls, so much is around identity issues: fitting in, belonging, and relationships, especially," Dr. Belgrave says. And like most people of African descent, they tend to have a communal, rather than an individualistic perspective on the world—which might translate into forming strong bonds, but also being influenced by what others are doing.[4]

At the same time, Black girls are taught to be independent: to take care of themselves and to provide for themselves. "What it means to be a woman and be a good woman or strong or ideal woman is very different culturally for us," says Dr. Belgrave. "In our minds, we don't need to be married or have a stable mate or partner to fulfill the cultural roles we've prescribed for ourselves, and we are conveying these norms to our young sisters."

Whether she checks in on her diabetic grandmother, supervises younger siblings and cousins after school, or tends to her own mom when she comes home exhausted, a Black teen often demonstrates the customary feminine traits of nurturing, care-giving, and emotional expressiveness. She's also likely to hold a job after school and on weekends; buy her own clothes and contribute materially to her household; problem-solve when she loses her keys or chart her own course on public transportation around town; stand up for herself if her teachers put her down or she gets harassed on the street—assertive, self-confident, independent, and strong behaviors that mainstream society often associates with males.[5]

In fact, not only do Black girls feel equal to boys, they expect to be treated that way. Unlike other girls of other races, who typically have more traditional notions of femininity, Black girls learn an identity that will help them flourish in a world where Black women have historically filled traditional women's as well as men's gender roles, and often parent alone.

The truth is that for today's Black girl, the storied "village" in which her grandmother and perhaps even her mother grew up no longer exists. Her parents may have moved across town or across the country and away from other family members. Her father or other male relatives may be incarcerated; other family members may be missing because of substance abuse or mental illness.

During the 1960s, 67 percent of Black households contained two parents, but thanks to a combination of forces—among them the decline of the industrial economy, social welfare programs that discouraged Black family formation, the proliferation of crack cocaine, and a war on drugs that targets Black men—almost half of Black girls today are raised by single mothers.[6] In 2009, 37 percent grew up living with both their mother and father; 3 percent were raised by single fathers and grandparents; and 9 percent grow up in non-family contexts, including foster care.[7] But regardless of a Black girl's socioeconomic status or whether she lives in a two-parent or a one-parent home, her life is likely to be stabilized by the presence of a grandmother living in her home or nearby. She probably lives with a sibling or two, as well, and she may have half-siblings in the community.

In Their Image and Likeness

By and large, Black teen girls admire their mothers and seek to model themselves after them. Like adolescents of any race, they come into conflict from time to time, but Black adolescent girls tend to experience less conflict with their parents than girls of other backgrounds. They feel close enough to their moms that they want to share intimate and important topics.[8] They want their conversations to be straight not watered down. They want their mothers to be real with them.

In addition to what they tell their daughters and the behavior (both nurturing and independent) that they model, Black mothers also impart their values indirectly. For better and for worse, we often forget that it's not just what we say: our girls are watching what we *do*. For example, many children of teen mothers end up bearing children at an age close to the age that their mothers birthed them.

"One of the big issues I've seen a lot of the girls deal with is negative influences in their families. If they're not getting positive messages at home, then where are they supposed to get them from?" asks Carla Stokes, Ph.D., founder of HOTGIRLS in Atlanta. "That's not the case for all of the girls. Parents need to be aware of how they're carrying themselves, what they're saying, what their daughters are being exposed to, and how that's affecting them," she continued.

Adolescent girls also tend to mimic their mothers' choices in romantic partners and adopt similar expectations of relationships. For example, if a mother values a man's ability to provide for her materially more than she values his treating her with kindness and respect, her daughter may well internalize her values and play out similar patterns.[9]

GREATEST INFLUENCE ON LIFE, 2009	
Mother	48%
Friend	15%
Sister	11%
Brother	9%
Father	8%
Grandparent	8%
Higher Power	8%

Note: Sum may exceed 100 percent as respondents were asked to select all that apply.

Source: Institute for Women's Policy Research Survey of Black Girls in New York City, 2009.

Daddy's Little Girl

Although they're more likely to live with their moms, adolescent girls strongly value their dads. A young Black teen enjoys her relationship with her father and wants to spend more time with him, whether he lives in her home or not. Research shows that she needs her father's protection and feels protective of him as well. Her father's presence in her life makes her happier, increases her self-esteem, reduces her stress and her fear of intimacy, and helps her to develop a standard of beauty that's based on her own views rather than external standards. A present father may help a daughter internalize his love and values in ways that later help her make positive relationship choices; for example, she benefits from his role modeling and indirect messages about what constitutes appropriate male behavior and what to expect when she is dating. Importantly, girls who live with their fathers tend to start having sex later than girls who don't. And girls who have positive relationships with their fathers tend to have a better body image.[10]

"My dad was my best friend—we did everything together," says Brenda, 45. "I went with him on his Saturday errands and he was my tennis coach. I always tell people that my relationship with him has made all the difference in my life. My life is so much better than many of my friends' because my father sowed into my spirit, but many of their fathers didn't sow into theirs. To give you an example, I don't get treated poorly in romantic relationships because I know what unconditional love and a man who is capable of offering it looks like— a lot of my girlfriends do not."

Of course, when a girl has no relationship with her father—or, worse, when the relationship is hurtful—the opposite is true: her sense of self suffers greatly.

"I have always struggled with self-confidence," admits Sylvia, now 60 years old. "When I was a girl my father wasn't interested in me for me, for who I was; he was interested in me in more of a sexual way because he molested me. Even today and after all the work I've done on myself, there are times when I struggle to find my voice, to feel worthy to say what I want to say."

Girls in the 'Hood

Black girls raised in the inner city tend to grow up in neighborhoods with poor school systems; high dropout rates; low literacy; high unemployment and underemployment; substantial crime, including open-air drug dealing; an epidemic of substance abuse; and high incarceration rates, particularly among men. They often fear for their physical safety; many become victims of crime or other violence. Many Black girls feel unsafe in their neighborhoods, on their journeys to and from school, and even in their own homes.

Black girls experience more street harassment and verbal disrespect than girls of any other background. Sometimes that disrespect includes unwanted touching by boys, catcalls and ogling from older men, and other forms of intimidation. This problem isn't limited to the inner city, but it is most pervasive there. Black girls raised in inner-ring suburbs tend to feel safer, though some say they also feel invisible, particularly in the education system.[11]

The poverty rate among Black teens far exceeds the rate among other youth. One-third of Black children live below the poverty level—roughly three times as many as White children (10 percent), and the consequences are devastating. Black girls in poverty are forced to grow up faster than girls whose financial security helps shelter them from poor school systems, dangerous housing, decrepit recreational facilities, joblessness, street crime, and other urban challenges to a girl's health and safety. They're less likely to have health insurance and have less access to health-care than their White peers. They are less likely to form a long-lasting romantic relationship than other girls and more likely to stay poor in adulthood.[12]

Caring adults can help vunerable Black girls stay on the right path, show them how to stay safe without using violence, and let them know that someone has their backs. For example, signs were posted all over one Baltimore neighborhood when mothers and community leaders learned of threats Black girls faced on their streets: "Leave our daughters alone!" [13]

To protect themselves, Black adolescent girls often turn to aggression. For them it's a survival tool[14], though others may see them merely as violent and lacking self control. Because of the inequities in a justice system that treats Black girls and young women differently than White girls, for many a misstep here is the first step on a real downward path—what women's studies professor Meda Chesney-Lind, Ph.D., calls the "school-to-prison pipeline." [15]

Making the Grade

Most Black adolescent girls understand that education is important; they want to do well in school and to prepare themselves for their future. But in the public-school system, some teachers actually stand in their way: they hold low expectations of their Black students, discourage them from having high hopes for themselves, and even mock their plans to attend college. And sometimes their work with the girls focuses more on regulating behavior than on cultivating minds.[16]

Black girls' desires to excel may also clash with the reality of their lives: underfunded school systems, long early morning commutes, and insufficient support from their parents and extended family, as well as their responsibilities to hold jobs, cook, clean, and help care for their siblings and aging family members. By the time they reach 10th grade, many Black teen girls lower their career goals and expectations for the level of success they can hope to achieve. From this perspective, that 12-year-old's note to self—"Be a lawyer"—seems poignant indeed.

They often lower their expectations still more and graduate at a low 62 percent from high school. Even when Black girls do graduate, particularly if they attend school in a large urban school district, the quality of their education may leave much to be desired.

Not surprisingly, Black girls in other socioeconomic situations don't usually experience

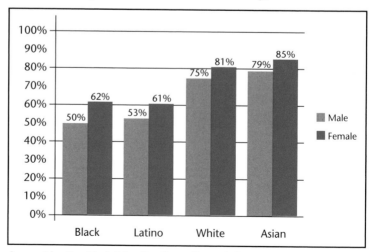

**High School Graduation Rates
By Gender And Race/Ethnicity, 2008**

Source: Education Week. Education Counts Research Center, 2008.

all the drama and trauma of inner-city girls' lives. Their education tends to follow a smoother course. Black girls in middle-income families often benefit from resources similar to those of their White peers. Many even become super-achievers, excelling academically, getting involved in social and civic life, and becoming leaders in their community and society at large.[17]

Image and Identity

No matter where they grow up, Black girls will inherit an increasingly diverse world in which overt racism is less common than it was in their grandparents' time, but in which systemic racism, sexism, color bias, and classism are still going strong. And the "isms" that Black girls encounter still do them harm, reducing the expectations that others have for their lives and, in turn, the expectations they have for themselves—unless their caregivers explicitly teach them to appreciate their ethnic identity and gender and show them survival skills to cope with a society that often does not respect them.

If the adults in Black girls' lives aren't giving them this support, then—absent the traditional "village" and rites that reflect and reinforce Black cultural values—music videos and TV reality shows fill the gap. They invite Black adolescents to join an American popular culture that encourages them to dress and behave hyper-sexually, disrespect themselves and each other, and engage in other modern-day buffoonery that corporate America then markets as entertainment.

"There's just so much media exploitation around sex that so many people are also misinformed by the media," says sex therapist Gail Wyatt, Ph.D., a psychology professor at UCLA. "Teenagers are very vulnerable and see horrendous messages of promiscuity."

The media also expose them to dysfunctional dynamics well beyond their years, encouraging them to behave in adult ways before they are mature enough to understand what they are doing or handle the consequences. So-called reality shows give Black girls "the message that they should be causing drama with each other and that this is a positive thing," says Dr. Stokes. "They see a lot of drama and divorce and get a lot of mixed messages—and negative messages about Black women."

Many Black girls struggle with trusting each other, and they often learn this mistrust from their mothers—an issue that may flow from the gender imbalance in the Black community. When there are too many women for the number of available men, it's not hard to see how young girls are encouraged to compete with each other and to not trust other girls.

"Girls feel more comfortable having guy friends, and they seek out friendships with boys because they feel that other girls cause drama," says Dr. Stokes. "These girls have really adversarial relationships with each other and at really young ages. It's scary—the competition, the constant 'She's hating on me.'"

"I don't really have girlfriends," says 16-year-old Lenisha. "Girls, you can't trust them."

Some of the competition—and sexual pressure—is fueled by the shortage of desirable boys: the gender imbalance already at work. "At younger ages, they're competing so much with each other that if they like a guy and these other girls are willing to do different things for and with him, they feel the pressure to do things that they wouldn't otherwise," Dr. Stokes observes. "Other girls have lowered the bar." Social media such as Facebook give some girls platforms from which to bully each other and refer to each other as "bitches" and "'ho's." There's even a cohort of girls who sexualize themselves on social media, posting provocative pictures, calling themselves "freaks." Too many girls don't see role modeling at home to show them what a healthy relationship, sexuality, or self-image looks like.

In this environment, girls may tend to build their sense of self on superficial values, for lack of a stronger foundation. "I see a lot of Black girls with high self-esteem, but it tends to be derived from their appearance," Dr. Stokes points out. "They tend to get validated by others, but they're not getting, as a whole, positive reinforcement about who they are as a person." Like other American teens, Black teens are ensnared by materialism and highly susceptible to the media's messages about how they should look, act, and be—and they suffer when the ideal is beyond their means: "They strive to have expensive clothes, fancy labels, and cars; and feel stress when they are unable to afford or keep up with what peers have and what they see on TV." Who hasn't heard a child ridiculed for not wearing the right shoes or having the right clothes?

It's an uphill battle, no question about it. Yet many researchers believe that Black women and girls have greater resilience and/or tap into a wider array of resources for support— family members, neighborhood ties, friends, religious community—than do Whites who, research shows, are generally connected just to friends. For a Black girl growing up, whether she is in a proud but poor family or is being raised in a struggling middle-class family, having an extensive and protective world around her lessens the impact of the mainstream society's rejections.[18] Her strong family ties may keep her from becoming depressed by the overwhelming circumstances that she faces and allow her to achieve success despite the odds.

Setting the Stage for Good Health

During adolescence, Black girls unknowingly make choices that set the stage for health and well-being throughout their lives. But how well-equipped are they to make the right choices, given the challenges they face? Many of them don't really know what good health is: like their mothers, Black girls tend to judge health on the basis of appearance.[19]

"Being healthy to them means looking good," says Dr. Belgrave. "This is sometimes a problem with HIV prevention messages, because you can look very good but still be HIV-positive." You can also look good and be poorly nourished or overweight, have an anxiety disorder, be in an abusive relationship, or have high blood sugar or hypertension. For many Black girls, such assaults against their well-being begin during adolescence. When we adults assume that their youthful excitement and energy are expressions of genuine health and vitality, we're often wrong.

Adolescence is famously a time of risk taking, and American teenagers of all backgrounds engage in behavior that increases their risk of accident and injury: the number-one cause of adolescent deaths. What teens and the adults who love them often don't realize is that the things they do without a thought—spurning healthy dinner in favor of fast foods, skipping meals, communicating via social media instead of being active—can morph into habits that are heartbreakingly difficult to reverse later in life. Other, more obviously risky choices, such as smoking cigarettes or marijuana, drinking deadly sweet alcoholic beverages, driving recklessly, fighting, and having unprotected sex, can bring swifter, more devastating consequences than their parents ever imagined. This is particularly true for Black children, whose safety net, if they have one at all, is often tenuous.

This may be part of the reason why many Black teen girls, as other teens, say that they feel they're under more stress than they can handle, experiencing stress-related symptoms and behaviors such as anxiety, physical illness, aggressive behavior, withdrawing from friends, or abusing substances in order to cope. Black adolescents develop diseases, suffer injuries and disability, and die earlier than their White counterparts. This is in large part due to the consequences of poverty—including, poor diet, unsafe neighborhoods, environmental pollution, and limited access to health-care. On the other hand, behaviors and habits that support their well-being—running on the track team, finding a mentor, singing in a choir—can improve the quality of their life today and tomorrow, and now is the time to start.

In the rest of this chapter we'll discuss what we know about the health of Black adolescent girls, and how understanding their health patterns can help our daughters live better. We'll draw primarily upon the extensive data collected by the Youth Risk Behavior and Surveillance System (YRBSS), conducted by the Centers for Disease Control and Prevention (CDC). It surveys young people about their behavior in six areas that contribute to the top causes of teen chronic conditions, disability, and death. The data reported here are from the survey conducted in 2009.

Dangerous Curves: Overweight and Obesity

Black girls tend to live in less than healthy food environments—with more access to fast and fatty foods than to whole foods, too few options, and too little role modeling. A Black girl who keeps her weight in the recommended range during adolescence will be much better able to withstand the temptation of junk foods and avoid the debilitating effects of excess weight. Obesity is now the most common chronic health problem among children in the United States, and low-income teens and Black girls have the highest rates. Having obese parents, as many Black girls do, more than doubles their chance of becoming obese. Black girls from families with a low level of education are far more likely than young women from families with a high level of education to grow into adulthood obese. These realities make carrying excess weight the "new normal" for Black girls, and maintaining a healthy weight a lot like swimming upstream.[20]

Thirteen percent of Black teen girls in the YRBSS study reported being overweight or obese, compared to six percent of White and 11 percent of Hispanic teens.[21] Girls who carry excess weight at a young age when they tend to be more active are likely to have a more difficult time maintaining their weight as they move into adulthood, and the reality is that almost three-quarters of Black women become overweight or obese.

"Most black girls are overweight from pre-pubescence," says Dr. Wyatt. "They go into puberty chunky, chubby, overweight, obese and they never get to see what they're supposed to look like. So when they make a decision later in life that they want to lose weight, they can't even imagine what they want to get to." Compounding matters, Black girls, like their mothers, think less about the relationship between their weight and their health and more about the relationship between their weight and their looks, so when they do pay attention to their weight, they're not going about it in a way that's good for them.

"Girls want to look like Beyoncé or Kim Kardashian," observes Dr. Stokes. "Even Black girls want to starve themselves to lose weight and look like them. If a girl is working out, it's more likely that she's doing it because she wants to look a certain way than to achieve a healthy way of life."

Experts now forecast that half of Black children will develop diabetes because so many are overweight in their youth. Other studies suggest that high blood pressure, another condition related to excess weight, may also be increasing among the young.[22]

But even with these risks, Black mothers tend to underestimate their children's body size, question whether mainstream weight standards should apply to them, and express confusion about how much their children are supposed to weigh. These mothers often haven't made health a priority in their own lives, so it's hard for them to set a good example. With the best of intentions, they are often at a loss for what to do.

We Are What We Eat

Young people of all backgrounds tend to eat less healthily as they gain independence and start making their own food choices. But many Black girls' families aren't eating healthy to begin with, so when the girls miss meals and their food quality declines, the situation goes from bad to worse.

Consequently, Black teen girls tend to eat a lower-quality diet than teen girls of other races and ethnic groups,[23] including more high-fat, high-calorie foods (think: fast foods, fried foods, and processed foods, like lunch meats and sweet and salty snacks). Eating foods that provide lots of calories but little nutrition leaves them inadequately nourished, making it more difficult for them to concentrate, think clearly, and learn; they can even lead to problems like weak fingernails and hair loss. These foods also set them up to experience problems with managing their weight and enjoying good health later in life.

Physical Activity

Physical activity doesn't just make it easier to run for the bus; it also helps to stabilize weight. Nevertheless, during their teens, 70 percent of Black girls are not active enough—not surprising when considering that physical education is no longer offered in many urban schools. What's more, Black girls often live in neighborhoods that lack safe, appealing recreational facilities, and their downtime activities tend to be more sedentary—watching TV, talking on the phone, and hanging out with friends, rather than going for a walk or run through the (unsafe) park.

Only 21 percent of Black adolescent girls are as physically active as experts recommend, compared to 28 percent of White girls. The percentage of Black teens who exercise to lose or maintain their weight (51 percent) is lower than the percentages of White girls (72 percent) and Hispanic girls (66 percent) who do the same.[24] By the time they are 16 years old, 56 percent of African American girls say that they don't participate in any physical activity at all during their free time, as compared to just 31 percent of White girls who are physically inactive.[25]

Melicia Whitt-Glover, Ph.D., president and CEO of Gramercy Research Group, cites one study, following girls from kindergarten through high school, that painted an even bleaker picture: "They showed a 100 percent physical-activity decline in Black girls. By high school Black girls were doing no physical activity at all versus a 50 percent decline among White girls." We can step in here, if we're aware of the patterns and the risks, and instill in young girls the habits that will keep them active and prevent their becoming obese adults.

Sexual and Reproductive Health

Adolescents have unique reproductive and sexual health needs, but often these needs are ignored or labeled abnormal by the adults around them—or worse, the girls are made to feel abnormal for having the needs in the first place. We, as a community, have just begun to address the challenges a girl faces in being a "girl," when she feels sexual attraction for the first time towards boys (or, for that matter, towards other girls).

This is the time of puberty when girls become sexually mature, occurring between ages 10 and 14. You will see the physical changes: they are growing taller, getting acne, growing underarm and pubic hair, developing breasts, and beginning their menstrual periods. But most of all, this is a time of enormous change in a girl's relationships, experiences and emotions. One 14-year-old in a youth leadership session commented, "I used to be such a goody-goody and always did well in school and paid attention in class and followed all the rules; now all I can think about is my boyfriend."

When societal norms and cultural taboos collide with the realities of wanting to be liked and attractive to boys, that's when Black girls today, like their mothers and grandmothers before them, get the message: "Keep your legs closed." So what is a girl to do? She knows it's not that easy; as one 13-year-old confessed, "It's like somebody put up a big flashing neon-light sign in my head that said SEX. It's scary." What's more, this narrow focus on preventing early sexual activity overlooks the real complexities and variations in Black teens' experiences, and the message can be confusing and devaluing for them. In one Imperative community forum with mothers and daughters in Washington, D.C., one girl remarked, "Everybody thinks everybody is doing it, and that's not true."

What is true is that many Black adolescent girls start having sex long before they are able to protect themselves from the downside: unintended pregnancy, sexually transmitted diseases (STDs), HIV, intimate partner violence, and potential emotional abandonment.

Sexual mistakes can devastate Black teen girls' lives, causing them humiliation and mental and emotional distress. They can also derail their education; confine them and their children to a lifetime of poverty and compromise their ability to conceive when they are older and better able to support a child.

Further, they could increase their risk of developing cervical cancer during their 20s; and put them at risk for STDs such as genital herpes, which they carry forever and can pass on to their newborn, or HIV, which can emotionally and financially devastate and eventually kill them.

The more sexual partners a woman has—particularly if she does not know their HIV status and if either she or a partner is not monogamous—the greater her risk for STDs (including

HIV), which travel through social networks of sexually active friends and acquaintances. STD rates among Black Americans are higher than among other groups, so the risk in our network is greater.[26] A study published in 2008 by the CDC showed that 48 percent of sexually active Black teens, ages 14 to 19, had at least one active STD, compared to 20 percent among White and Mexican-American girls.[27] Black girls ages 15 to 19 had the highest rates of chlamydia and gonorrhea among women, followed by black women ages 20 to 24.[28]

Even more worrisome: though Black teens represent only 17 percent of the U.S. population, they accounted for 68 percent of new AIDS cases reported among teens in 2009. AIDS is among the top six leading causes of death for Black women ages 15 to 54. But because it can take 10 years for HIV to progress to full-blown AIDS, experts suspect that many young women who die of AIDS during their 20s and 30s became infected with HIV during their teens. If current trends hold, 1 in 16 Black men and 1 in 30 Black women are likely to become infected with HIV during their lifetime.[29]

Black adolescents know a lot about HIV/AIDS; in some communities, they accept HIV/AIDS as very common. However, our girls want and need more information about their overall sexual health—hygiene, self-care, and the way their bodies work. The adults in their lives are not doing enough to help girls prepare and protect themselves or delay sexual initiation and prevent early pregnancy and STDs. Dr. Belgrave remembers participating in a focus group that brought a communications gap to light: "The moms were saying, 'We're talking about sex,' or 'We're telling them not to get pregnant.' But the daughters were saying, 'Nope, I did not hear that from my mom!'"

"An unintended pregnancy or an abortion can derail a woman. But womanhood is not when we have the biggest problem, it's in early adolescence," Dr. Wyatt explains. "Mothers simply are not working with their daughters enough to help them to define who they are. So girls are doing it by themselves. They're using their bodies to define themselves rather than finding out who they really are." Knowing this, we shouldn't be surprised to learn that 37 percent of Black girls become pregnant as adolescents, the highest rate reported among any racial or ethnic group.[30] While the statistics remain unacceptably high, the mot recent sharpest declines in unintended pregnancies are occurring among Black teens.

Violence and Abuse

Shockingly, a number of unintended pregnancies among Black teens aren't truly accidental; the girls are victims of birth control sabotage, a form of intimate partner violence (IPV) that the National Domestic Violence Hotline defines as "threats or acts of violence against a partner's reproductive health or reproductive decision-making. It includes forced sex, a male partner pressuring a woman to become pregnant against her will and interference with the use of birth control." The Hotline reports that 25 percent of callers say that their partners have engaged in coercive behavior that includes discouraging them from using birth control, hiding their contraception, poking holes in condoms, or flushing their birth control pills down the toilet.[31] In a Chicago study of young women ages 11 to 21, of whom 95 percent were Black, 48 percent of the black ones said they'd experienced verbal birth control sabotage and 14 percent reported that their boyfriends exhibited sabotaging behavior.[32] Another study showed that 40 percent of abused women experienced unintended pregnancies, compared to 8 percent of women who were not being abused.[33]

IPV takes many forms, and far too many girls begin to experience it early on in the form of verbal, emotional, and physical abuse. While Black women are believed to experience rates of IPV similar to those among White women, homicide at the hands of a current or former intimate partner is the number-one form of homicide against young Black women ages 15 through.[34]

Black teen girls are more likely to have been threatened or injured with a weapon, have been raped, or have experienced IPV than girls of other ethnicities and backgrounds. Fourteen percent have experienced dating violence and 12 percent have been raped versus White girls (8 and 10 percent, respectively) and Hispanic girls (12 and 11 percent, respectively).[35] They're also less likely to report it. The 2009 YRBSS found that 14 percent of Black teen girls and boys had been hit, slapped, or physically hurt on purpose by their boyfriend or girlfriend, significantly higher than White (8 percent) and Hispanic (12 percent) teens. Black students (both genders) are less likely to have been bullied on school property (14 percent) than White (22 percent) or Hispanic (19 percent) students, but they are far more likely to have been in a physical fight in the past 12 months or to have come to blows on school property.[36]

Still, because violence against women has become part of American culture, IPV sometimes stays under the radar—even for the girls who are its victims. "Unless it's blatant and it's physical and somebody hits them or throws them on the ground, they don't always recognize it as violence," Dr. Stokes observes. And exposure to violence during adolescence sets them up for violent relationships later.

Yet there's reason to hope for better: more awareness, more options, a better start. Some Black girls, like the 121 adolescent girls in the Imperative's Straight Talk Intergenerational HIV prevention program in Washington, D.C., very much want to know about healthy relationships and expect to have them in their own lives. Because these girls have adult women in their lives to show them the big picture, and a program that focuses on their needs, they're able to see the unhealthy relationships between adults in their lives for what they are and know that they want something better for themselves.

Emotional Well-Being

Similar to their mothers, Black girls tend to "soldier" through their emotional pain. While they are just as likely to experience depression as girls from other racial and ethnic groups, they are less likely to get treatment or even admit there's anything wrong. Instead, they attempt to balance schoolwork with taking care of others and helping run the household, always with threats to their physical safety lurking in the background (or the foreground). Not surprisingly, the stress can be enormous.

Dr. Stokes observes that many of the Black adolescent girls she works with are taking care of their own caregivers. "A lot of girls seem to have parents who are sick at home," she says. "I've had girls lose their mothers. That issue can be extremely difficult to deal with at any age."

"My mother had a stroke and was in a wheelchair," says 17-year-old Mira. "My grandmother and I helped her a lot, and she could do a lot of things for herself. She is still a great mom, but sometimes when I was growing up, it was like, oh my God! I just couldn't take it anymore."

In spite of the stress, eating disorders—the plague of many teen girls—pose less of a problem for Black girls: they're less likely to vomit their food or take laxatives (4 percent), compared to White (7 percent) and Hispanic (17 percent) girls. Black adolescent girls consider and even attempt suicide in increasing numbers. Ten percent of Black teen girls have tried to kill themselves—almost 3 percent more than White girls, though 1 percent less than Hispanic adolescent girls. Increasingly we are finding this to be a growing problem as 18 percent of Black girls in the YRBSS study had considered suicide; another 13 percent had actually made a plan.[37]

It's hard to protect our children from stress when our own lives are so often filled with it—but we can do a lot to ease their worries and set a good example if we're open and honest with them about their problems and ours. "My mom, she has to take medicine for high blood pressure and diabetes," says 12-year-old Ling Mae. "Last week she had surgery for some lady thing she won't tell me."

Keeping pain hidden and keeping health a mystery only encourages our girls to do the same—just at the time when they're beginning to experiment with risky behaviors, such as smoking and drinking and facing some of their greatest challenges to staying safe and well.

In the Black community, we are quite aware that tobacco companies are persistent in their efforts to lure young Black smokers. What you don't know is that Black teen girls are actually more likely to say no to cigarettes than girls of other backgrounds. While a little less than half of Black girls reported that they had tried cigarettes (44 percent), less than 2 percent of Black girls frequently smoke cigarettes versus 9 percent of White girls.[38]

Black adolescent girls also tend to avoid binge drinking more than young women of other backgrounds. Just 12 percent of Black teen girls reported consuming more than five drinks in a row at least once within the past year, whereas 28 percent of White and 22 percent of Hispanic girls had done so.[39] Black, White, and Hispanic girls use drugs at about the same rate—roughly 17 percent; however, Black girls generally don't use cocaine, injection drugs, or heroin. When they do get high—after alcohol, marijuana is their drug of choice. They often get high to please others or go along with the crowd, and they usually obtain drugs from older boyfriends, siblings, friends, and relatives.[40]

As independent and self-assured as many Black adolescent girls seem to be in saying no to drugs and alcohol, Black adolescent girls who do become involved with drugs and alcohol often experience serious unwanted consequences, such as unplanned pregnancy, intimate partner violence, or STD infection—and even HIV. Black girls need adults, the church, and the community to help steer the way; they need systems of support to lean on in times of distress; they need information; and they need a relationship with the health-care system. Most of all, they want to be understood and listened to more. Our girls need us. They deserve more—and better. This is the time to help them make the transition to young adulthood feeling good about who they are.

Why Prevention Is Better Than Cure: Recommended Adolescent Screenings

Although we have seen many positive trends in the lives of Black youth in recent years, including decreases in substance abuse, high school dropout rates, and teen pregnancy, having good health is not a priority for many Black girls. And while they know the basic facts about healthy eating and being physically fit, they do not necessarily put this knowledge into practice. How do they look? What clothes do they wear? Do boys like them? Do they fit in with the right crowd? These concerns have become the norm, and it's not one that necessarily encourages healthy behaviors.

Many Black teen girls have a regular health provider, but some rely upon the emergency room for care; and so emergency care is all they get. For these girls, it's more likely that health problems that begin during their teen years will go undetected, setting them up for more serious problems down the road. It also sets a precedent for them to remain outside the health-care system for their health problems to be diagnosed late or not at all; and for their own children to inherit a legacy of poor health and nonexistent care.

For these girls and all girls, adolescence is the time to begin connecting the dots and laying out how being overweight puts their health at risk now and in the future. This is the right time to let Black girls know that they don't have to live in fear of violence. This is the time to help them reject risky sex behavior. And this is the time for them to know and begin valuing their health. The following recommended screenings and vaccinations, though not all of them are for all girls, establish a baseline for marking health milestones, such as noting in her annual exam when a girl starts her period or when she develops breasts.

Let's make that commitment now for every Black girl to be a "well girl."

RECOMMENDED HEALTH SCREENINGS AND VACCINATIONS
ADOLESCENTS AGES 10–19

SCREENING TESTS	WHEN TO GET THE TEST
GENERAL HEALTH	
Well-Girl physical exam	Yearly
Ob/Gyn baseline exam	Prior to the onset of sexual activity to establish baseline and monitor STDs; discuss with your health- care provider
Sexual Assault, Drug Use, Alcohol Abuse	Depends on individual teen
REPRODUCTIVE HEALTH	
Chlamydia test	Yearly until age 25 if sexually active
Sexually transmitted infection (STI) test	Both partners should get tested for STIs, before initiating sexual intercourse
ORAL HEALTH	
Dental exam	Routinely
IMMUNIZATIONS	
Tetanus, Diphtheria, Pertussis	11–18 years old Every 10 years
Human papillomavirus (HPV) vaccine	Three doses up to age 18, if not already completed vaccine series; discuss with your health-care provider
Meningococcal vaccine	11–18 years old; college students

Chapter 2

Young Adults
(20 to 39)

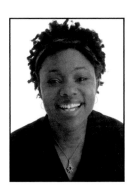

Black girls transition from adolescence into adulthood with the glow of promise. Between the years of 20 and 29, young women typically start to work full-time, move out on their own, date and then seek serious partners in love, and begin forming a family. Some of us complete college, often times embarking on exciting and possibly lucrative careers. But the road of life, sunny with youthful optimism and hope, which leads Black girls into adulthood, often grows bumpy with challenges. If such issues are left unattended, they can undermine our quest to live joyful, healthy, and productive lives.

The health stakes climb during this stage for a young Black woman. During adolescence, her body is still developing and forgiving when it is mistreated; ideally, she is insulated from the outside world by her caregivers and their health insurance plans. Once she is out on her own, however, and free to fend for herself, she begins to suffer the real world's sharp stings: the obvious forces of racism, sexism, and economic classism, as well as other more subtle forces such as societal pressure to succeed.

No matter what the state of her health is as she exits her teen years or graduates from her 20s to her 30s, a young woman is far more capable of recovering from youthful excesses and neglect than she will be as she ages. Young adulthood is the perfect time to make lifestyle changes that will support her health: before her metabolism slows, her estrogen levels decline, and the demands of family and career place her personal time at a premium, making self-improvement changes beyond her reach.

In this chapter we explore health issues affecting Black women during early adulthood, in two stages: emerging adulthood, ages 20 through 29, and young adulthood, ages 30 through 39.

During these years, young Black women suffer health problems whose seeds may have been planted in adolescence. Many of us continue to gain weight, leading to overweight and even obesity, setting ourselves up to experience conditions such as pre-diabetes and pre-hypertension, precursors to serious problems. Others experience a range of sexual and reproductive health issues—HIV, STDs, and fibroids. Emotional challenges such as stress, depression, and intimate partner violence also begin to appear on the health scorecard. If these problems aren't addressed they can snowball and overtake a young woman's ability to live her dreams. In fact, late in this part of the life cycle, heart disease, cancer, diabetes and stroke become leading causes of death.

The Millennial Generation

Most young Black women's lives during these two decades don't follow the path our mothers and grandmothers traveled; nor do they follow our female peers of other races and ethnicities. The generation represented in this life stage—categorized by demographers as "Millenials" or "Echo Boomers"—is unique, with a mix of traditional values, the progressive beliefs of its Baby Boomer parents, and the unlimited horizons that technology and globalism give to its thinking.

JUST THE FACTS:
YOUNG ADULTS (20–39)

Population:

6.2 million

28.7 percent of Black females

Leading Causes of Death ages 20–24:

1. Unintentional injuries (accidents)
2. Assault (homicide)
3. Heart disease
4. Cancer
5. HIV disease
6. Suicide
7. Diabetes
8. Pregnancy complications
9. Chronic lower respiratory disease
10. Stroke

Leading Causes of Death ages 25–39:

1. Unintentional injuries
2. Heart disease
3. Cancer
4. HIV disease
5. Homicide
6. Pregnancy complications
7. Diabetes
8. Stroke
9. Anemias
10. Suicide

Source: Leading Causes of Death by Age Group, Black Females – United States, 2006. Department of Health and Human Services, Centers for Disease Control and Prevention; 2010.

Not so long ago, as young adults, women completed their education, found their first jobs, embarked upon a career, started a family, and bought a house—usually in that order. But the lives of the Millennial generation are unfolding quite differently from those of their parents. No matter their race or ethnic background, today's 20-somethings take longer to start a career, move out of their parents' house, graduate from college, stand on their own two feet, and start a family of their own. This reality is leading researchers to identify a stage of development they're calling the "odyssey years," when young adults meander through their 20s toward maturity.[1]

Yet Millenials' unprecedented opportunities are coupled with challenges unfathomable to earlier generations. Black women Millenials have to blaze trails where there are no historical paths. We have to face the imbalance between the numbers of eligible Black women and men, exacerbated by the high rates of joblessness and incarceration among Black men. Moreover, we must confront our inability to gain a solid foothold in life because a college education costs so much that it can be prohibitive to finish—or even start. We may not be able to afford medical care when we need it, even though we can now stay on our parents' insurance until age 26. Young Black women are also unable to count on parental financial support, which young adult women of other backgrounds often enjoy well into their 20s, 30s, and even longer.

Black Millenials are also delinking other traditional rites of passage, such as getting married first and having children second. But we are reconnecting to some beliefs even more traditional than our parents'. In the process we are creating a mixture of values, some of which belong to older generations and some of which are unique to Millenials and are being seen for the first time.

Education

Millenials are on track to become the most educated generation in the history of the United States.[2] Young women of all races are slightly more likely to be college educated than men of their race. In 2008, more women were enrolled in college than men, and women of all races earned more bachelor's and master's degrees than men of the same background. This educational gap was even more pronounced among young people of color: among Blacks and Hispanics, women earned more than 60 percent of bachelor's and master's degrees. Today two out of three Black undergraduates in colleges and universities are women.[3]

Yet pursuing a higher education creates stress for many young Black women, much of it centered on finances. The competition for scholarships and financial aid is fierce, and it will intensify as more students compete for scarce resources. What's more, many Black women come to campus with challenges that the average undergrad may not face. "A lot of students are first-generation college students," says Dr. Belgrave, a professor at Virginia Commonwealth University. "They're dealing with schoolwork, and some have children. So they're dealing with being a mother, working, and going to school."

Consequently, while the number of Black women who have enrolled in college is comparable to women of other backgrounds (except Asian women, who enroll in greater numbers), Black women are significantly less likely to earn a degree, even by as late as age 50.[4] Twenty-two percent of young Whites finish college versus 10 percent of Blacks. Black Millenials are more likely than Whites to say that they want to earn a diploma, yet they face multiple economic barriers to achieving their goals.[5]

College Enrollment Status of Recent High School Graduates 16 to 24 Years Old, by Sex and Race/Ethnicity: October 2009 and 2010

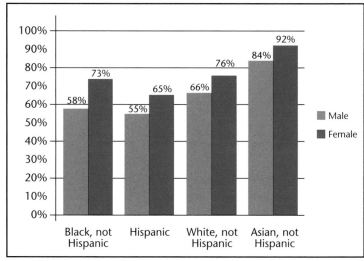

Source: IWPR analysis of Current Population Survey School Supplements, October 2011

Employment and Economic Realities

Less individualistic than Gen Xers and their parents, the Millenials are more of a "we" generation. We value spending face-to-face time with family and friends, doing meaningful work that helps others, being creative, and surrounding ourselves with idealistic co-workers who are committed to a cause.[6]

Nevertheless, for Millenials, coming of age during a major economic downturn has been a painful reality. In 2010, 41 percent were employed full-time, 24 percent worked part-time, 13 percent were students, and 22 percent remained unemployed. Blacks in this age group fared much more poorly than Whites, with just 34 percent employed full-time.[7] These unemployment data reflect people looking for work; actual unemployment rates are much higher because many of the unemployed have stopped looking for work.

Women have generally fared better than men, as they are often protected by jobs in less cyclical and more rapidly growing occupations such as health-care. However, they are increasingly affected on the back end, as teaching and public service jobs are cut and the retail sector recovers slowly.[8]

Women are generally more likely to work in administrative-support jobs within professional offices and in lower-paying jobs in education and health-care. But women of color are twice as likely as White women to be employed in the low-paying service segment of the economy, with few benefits, no health insurance, and few opportunities for advancement. We have difficulty transitioning to professional jobs even if we have the education and training.[9]

Less-educated Black women are not the only Millenials grappling for a foothold in the labor market. Many recent college graduates "spend years trying to find a job," says Dr. Carla Stokes. "Not like I remember when I graduated back in the late 1990s, when all my friends had a job after college or grad school. I'm seeing discouragement because things are not working out the way they wanted them to.

"I also see a lot of girls who feel that they're supposed to know what they're supposed to do, but if they don't know they feel bad about it," she adds. "They don't always realize that they're not supposed to know everything, that it's okay not to have a perfect plan. I tend to see it from families where expectations are higher—expectations that they're going to college and be a doctor or whatever. It's a lot to live up to."

Today, the unemployment rate—even among college-educated Blacks—is at Great Depression–era levels.[10] Unquestionably, Millenials are living in difficult times, and especially young Black women. Before the downturn in the late 2000s, young women ages 18 to 35, whatever their background, were beginning their adult years with a median wealth of zero. This means that at least half the women in this age group had no assets, or worse, had debts greater than the value of their assets.[11]

Black women's earnings lag far behind their peers: in 2010, for every dollar a man earned, a woman earned 77 cents; this wage gap is wider for women of color, with Black women earning only 62.3 percent as much as White men.[12] To demonstrate the dire conditions that a lot of younger Black women face, one in four women ages 18 to 24 of all races is so poor that she does not always have enough food, worries that her food will run out, skips meals, or cuts serving sizes so that there will be enough to go around.[13]

When asked about their parents' marital status during most of their childhood, 63 percent of Millenials say they grew up with both parents, while 20 percent had parents who married but divorced, and 12 percent were born to parents who never married at all.[14] Their values about marriage, family, and parenthood are different than previous generations. A study of 18- to 29-year-olds found that more than half believe being a good parent is one of the most important things in life, but less than one-third said the same about having a successful marriage. No surprise, then, that fewer Millenials are marrying and that they're more likely to live together without being married than any other generation at their age.[15]

Adults under age 30 are also less likely than their elders to believe that a child needs both a mother and a father in the home to grow up happy. To them, being a single parent or bearing children outside marriage does not come under the heading of "choices that undermine society." Marriage itself is optional. Almost half believe that it's becoming obsolete; one-quarter aren't sure that they ever want to get married. Many believe that you do not need to be married to be happy or even that you should get married in order to have children—a strong reflection of what they have seen in the media and in their own homes.[16]

When the link between marriage and parenting is severed, the burden falls disproportionately upon young women. While 30 percent of millennial women have children and live with them, only 13 percent of men have children and live with them.[17]

The values shift in the millennial generation has particularly affected young Black women's expectations for their lives. "I'm not against marriage, but I think it's an oppressive atmosphere for people to be in," says 20-year-old Lola. "That's based on the images that I see in real life and in media—they never really end well. I feel like if you're on your own, you don't have to depend on somebody else."

Black women are significantly less likely to marry than their peers of other races, in large part because there are so few marriage-ready Black men, "They are celibate, or they put up with a lot of bullshit because it seems like there are 40 women for every one guy," says Pamela Freeman, a Philadelphia-based therapist. "Young women are despondent because they have no one to date. A lot of the depression I see among young women is, 'I'm getting these skills, but for what? Are we going to live in female-based societies all of our lives? Are we ever going to have kids?' These are things that the younger women are bringing to me."

When we do marry, our wedding bells ring later than others—on average, at age 31, compared to age 27 for White and Hispanic women.[18]

Yet we start having babies at an average age of 23—three years earlier than White women begin their families, and a full *eight* years earlier than we are likely to marry—if we marry at all. For us, the disconnect between marriage and motherhood seems, if anything, more pronounced. "I think Black women's expectations about marriage are not quite the same as the expectations of other women," says Dr. Belgrave. "Marriage is no longer normative in our community. It's better to be married or partnered and have a child than to be single, but they don't quite get that," so Dr. Belgrave thinks.

The way young Black women form families isn't just a point of sociological interest. It has significant implications for our well-being. Not only do we enter adulthood with fewer resources, more tenuous family and community support systems, and weaker romantic relationships than do our peers of other races; we also fight the headwinds of racism, sexism, and classism. The decision about when to bear children is important. It can bring great joy and give our children the opportunity to excel in life. Or it can become the proverbial straw that overloads our ability to provide for them and traps our children in a lifetime of struggle.

Studies show that single mothers experience significantly higher levels of stress than other women do.[19] For all of Black women's bravado about how we don't need a man and how we can raise our children by ourselves, in reality many of us desperately want to be loved and appreciated and raise a healthy family. But the fathers of our children are often ill equipped to succeed in life, a relationship, or parenthood. "I have all these women in my practice in their 20s and 30s who are so depressed because their friends are having kids and they're not, and they don't know what to do about it," says Pamela Freeman. "They know it's really hard being on your own and raising a child in a healthy way."

Setting the Stage for Good Health

Since the health promises or challenges young Black women experience often have their roots in the issues they faced as teens, their ability to make conscious choices about how they take care of themselves in this stage of life will resonate far into their future. This chapter examines some of what is known about the health of Black Millenials as they transition from emerging adulthood to young adulthood. We use the findings from the Black Women's Health Imperative Harris survey on health attitudes and behavior and results from roundtable discussions and polls, interviews with experts, and other research studies that measure the well-being trends of younger Black women.

Overweight and Obesity

In adolescence, 23 percent of Black women are overweight and 13 percent are obese, and during the young-adult years these figures continue to rise. According to the Harris health survey commissioned by the Imperative in 2007, women who are younger than 35 (and single women of any age) are more likely than women of other ages to keep two or more sizes of clothes in their closets—"fat clothes" and the clothes they used to, or hope to, fit into. This reflects the reality that, absent an intervention—which almost never takes place—Black women in their early 20s are beginning the steady march from being "phat," "thick," and "curvaceous" toward being obese before they reach midlife. There is nothing in American culture or Black culture to stop us—certainly not neighborhood restaurants, college cafeterias, or the food court at work or at the mall—so change has to be up to us.

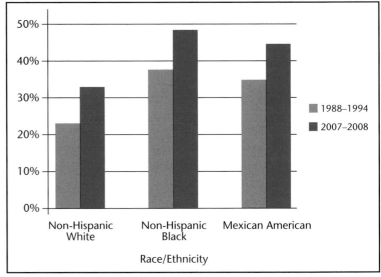

Prevalence of Obesity Among Women Aged 20 years and Over, by Race/Ethnicity: United States, 1988–1994 and 2007–2008

Note: Obesity is defined as a body mass index (BMI) greater than or equal to 30.

Source: CDC/NCHS, National Health and Nutrition Examination Survey III 1988–1994 and 2007–2008

Research also shows that Black women do not perceive themselves to be as big as they are—and they certainly don't take it kindly when doctors tell them that their children need to lose weight. Perhaps this is because we are in denial. Perhaps it's because being overweight has always been the norm in the Black community and among Black women. Or maybe it's a bit of both.

In either case, emerging adulthood provides an important opportunity to help young women bring their weight under control. Aside from the obvious goal of preventing chronic diseases later in life, if we are a healthy weight, we will always have a baseline perception of ourselves as healthy people. This offers young women a target to shoot for should they later need to become physically fit, and a way to avoid depression, shame, and many of the chronic diseases that young Black women are experiencing today.

As happens with many young adults, Black women in this age group rely upon fast foods and convenience food. Fast-food companies market dollar menus to us, and we eat these foods because we are broke, the foods are cheap, and we have developed a taste for them at home because we were raised on them. Unlike earlier generations, many young Black women never learned how to cook, and because our mothers were often too busy or overwhelmed to prepare meals—relying on takeout instead. Many did not learn healthy eating habits at home. Combine these facts with the reality that Black women are very sedentary by the time they outgrow adolescence, and you have the makings of an obesity epidemic. It is an epidemic that we have failed to come to grips with due to our focus on weight, rather than improving access to adequate nutrition and fitness.

Tobacco and Substance Use

Only about 16 percent of Black women smoke cigarettes. In general the likelihood that a person will smoke decreases as the level of income increases. Among all races, women with higher incomes were more likely to never have smoked. Fifty percent of Black women smokers ages 18 to 44 have tried to quit at least once—the highest of any age range.[20] The earlier you start using tobacco, the harder it becomes to quit.

The amazingly low incidence of smoking among Black teenage girls and young adults has led to research interest in the reasons why. According to one qualitative study at the Tobacco Use Prevention Program at the Center for Health Promotion and Disease Prevention, University of North Carolina–Chapel Hill, the researchers found that White women smoked to feel glamorous, empowered and equal to men, and attractive and sexy. These are the same themes promoted through tobacco advertising, which means that these girls have been influenced by advertising. Black girls and women felt differently. Rather than seeing cigarettes as glamorous, these young women thought that smoking was unfeminine, marred their image, and was too closely linked with other sinful behaviors involving sex and drugs.[21]

Like Black adolescents, young Black women are less likely to use or binge on alcoholic beverages than the national average.[22] About 28 percent of Black women drink alcohol, and women with higher incomes are more likely to drink than women with lower incomes. Over three-quarters of women consider themselves light or infrequent drinkers, with women consuming two drinks, on average, when they do drink.[23]

Young Black women are slightly more likely than other women to use illegal drugs. Among the 18 to 34-year-old profile, almost 14 percent of Black women ages 18 to 25 get high. They are most likely to smoke marijuana and less likely to abuse prescription drugs.[24] "If you took all the weed away, you'd see a lot of mental illness," says Dr. Gail Wyatt, a psychologist.

Substance Use among Black Females Aged 18 or Older Compared with the National Average, by Age Group: 2004–2008

Age Group	Alcohol Use: Blacks	Alcohol Use: National Average	Binge Alcohol Use: Blacks	Binge Alcohol Use: National Average	Illicit Drug Use: Blacks	Illicit Drug Use: National Average
Total	36.6%*	48.5%	14.4%*	15.9%	6.2%*	5.7%
Aged 18 to 25	44.9%*	56.9%	18.6%*	33.1%	13.9%*	15.7%
Aged 26 to 49	43.9%*	53.7%	17.7%*	18.9%	6.7%	6.2%
Aged 50 to 64	27.3%*	46.7%	10.4%	8.9%	2.5%	2.8%
Aged 65 or Older	14.4%*	31.5%	3.5%	3.7%	0.7%	0.5%

*The difference between blacks and the national average is statistically significant at $p < .05$

Source: 2004 to 2008 SAMHSA National Surveys on Drug Use and Health (NSDUHs).

"Some who are at home and not doing anything—they're not necessarily irresponsible and idle people. Some have undiagnosed mental health problems and really need a lot more than our society is offering them."

Drug use tends to taper off as Black women age, with just 7 percent of women ages 26 and older still using illegal drugs. However, as women age they are more likely to get hooked on prescription drugs. About 4 percent of Black women report abusing these.

It goes without saying that staying away from a fast lifestyle is in the interest of Black women's health. "Smoking, drinking, partying—those kinds of things can bring on early aging," says Dr. Wyatt. Other people's behavior can impact us directly, too: for example, in about one-third of domestic violence cases the batterer is drunk.[25]

Sexual and Reproductive Health

Sexual and reproductive health is intimately tied to every woman's quality of life. Women spend most of their young life into midlife—over 30 years—trying to manage their reproductive health needs, mostly related to pregnancy and childbirth, contraception, or preventing STDs. Reproductive health requires women to navigate hormonal changes in their bodies, from menstruation to menopause. It is about choosing whether and when to become pregnant, about having a safe and healthy pregnancy. It also includes understanding and weighing the risks, responsibilities, outcomes, and impacts of sexual activities and practicing abstinence when appropriate. Because our health affects pregnancy outcomes, we must become fully aware of our sexual and reproductive health and know our bodies and our menstrual cycles.

Sexual and reproductive health includes freedom from sexual abuse and discrimination and the ability to integrate sexuality into our lives, derive pleasure from it, and reproduce if we so choose.

A woman's ability to express her sexuality is an essential part of her health. She must be well in mind, body, and spirit. "You can't have great sexuality if you're sick," says Dr. Wyatt.

These realties highlight the fact that young Black women must learn to assert their positive sexual health. Negotiating condom and contraceptive use, feeling comfortable with our partners to talk about our own sexual needs and expectations are all integral parts of sexual and overall health.

This is the real world: many adolescents do not receive comprehensive sexual education—information about birth control—in school, so they enter young adulthood ill-equipped to take charge of their reproductive health. They are not aware of the many forms of birth control that could protect them from an unintended pregnancy or an unwanted STD. "My parents only wanted me to know about how to avoid getting pregnant. I wish they had told me more about STDs," said one young woman in an Imperative roundtable on contraceptive use.

What's more, the man shortage leads some women to fear losing their relationships if they insist on using contraceptives; they may experience birth control sabotage, in which partners manipulate or coerce them, sometimes violently, into making choices they do not want.

Furthermore, many people with low incomes and without health insurance may not have regular health-care providers. Perhaps they cannot afford follow-up visits to fine-tune their method of contraception. They just stop using it; or perhaps they relocate or have an unstable life situation and cannot keep a consistent connection with a doctor. Typically young women use an ob/gyn as their primary care provider. Men, though, don't have such a natural next step, so they often go without care after graduating from their pediatrician. Many seek out a doctor only if they are having significant problems, so they are much less likely than women to be tested for STDs and HIV. This reality underscores a critical point,

Percentage of Black Women Using Various Contraceptive Methods

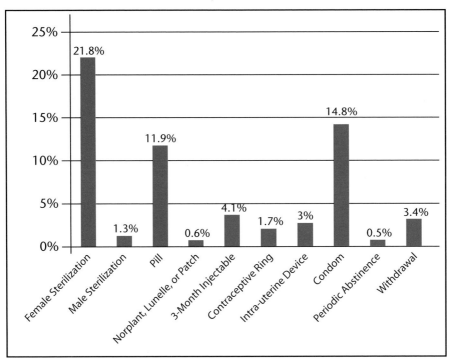

Source: Use of Contraception in the United States: 1982–2008. Centers for Disease Control and Prevention, Vital Health and Statistics, August 2010.

putting Black women at risk for sexual health problems that can lead to compromised fertility, HPV, cervical cancer, and HIV, to name a few. These challenges can prevent women from using their birth control consistently and correctly.

Only 14 percent of Black women use condoms, one of the most effective forms of pregnancy and STD prevention. Not having effective long-term contraceptives is among the many factors that contribute to high rates of unplanned pregnancies during early adulthood, and approximately half of all pregnancies in the United States *are* unplanned. Among young women ages 18 to 29, 70 percent of pregnancies are unintended, according to the National Campaign to Prevent Teen and Unplanned Pregnancy, and Black women are three times as likely as White women to get pregnant by accident.[26] Women with unintended pregnancies are more likely to develop complications, according to the CDC.[27]

FORMS OF CONTRACEPTION

Method	What is it?	Prevents STDs: Yes or No	Advantages	Effectiveness
Abstinence	Eliminating any intimate sexual behavior involving skin to genital, genital to genital, or body fluid to genital contact.	Yes	✓ Guaranteed safety ✓ Completely eliminates the risk of STI or un-planned pregnancy.	100% in preventing pregnancy and STDs
Female Condom	The female condom is a non-reusable tube-like synthetic pouch that fits inside a woman's vagina. It catches semen and stops sperm from fertil-izing an egg.	Yes	✓ Made of polyurethane which is non-aller-genic ✓ Provides female-initiat-ed protection against unplanned pregnancy and STDs	79–95%
Male Condom	A condom is thin latex or synthetic, non-reusable covering that fits over the erect penis. It catches the semen and stops sperm from entering the woman's body.	Yes	✓ Available in various sizes, colors, and flavors ✓ Often free at clinics and health centers	85–98%
Diaphragm Cervical Cap	A diaphragm is made of latex and is shaped like a saucer with a flexible rim. It fits over the cervix (opening to the uterus) to stop sperm from enter-ing. It must be inserted before intercourse and removed and cleaned after.	No	✓ If inserted correctly, neither you or your partner will feel it ✓ Is reusable ✓ Uniquely designed by your doctor to fit your cervix	84–94%

FORMS OF CONTRACEPTION (CONT)

Method	What is it?	Prevents STDs: Yes or No	Advantages	Effectiveness
Emergency Contraception (EC)	EC is a hormone pill that can prevent pregnancy by stopping the release of an egg, changing the lining of the uterus, or changing the movement of the egg and sperm. EC can be used after unprotected sex, or failure of a birth control method such as a broken condom.	No	✓ Can be taken up to 72 hours after unprotected sex and prevent an unplanned pregnancy ✓ Available at local pharmacies without a prescription ✓ Available at family planning and university clinics at reduced rate	95%
Intrauterine Contraceptive Device (IUD	An IUD is a small soft piece of plastic shaped like a "T" with a nylon string on it. There are two types of IUDs. One type of IUD has a thin copper wire wrapped around it and another type of IUD releases a small amount of hormone. A doctor must insert the IUD. It mainly works by preventing fertilization. It may also stop a fertilized egg from growing inside the uterus (womb).	No	✓ Convenient ✓ Does not interrupt sex ✓ Can stay in place for 3-5 years but can be removed by a doctor at any time	99.2–99.9%

Method	What is it?	Prevents STDs: Yes or No	Advantages	Effectiveness
Patch	The birth control patch looks like a large, thin, beige bandage. The sticky side contains hormones (similar to the hormones in a woman's body). The hormones are released continuously through the skin and stop the release of an egg from the ovaries. Pregnancy cannot occur if the body does not release an egg. The patch is changed weekly for three weeks, followed by a one-week break from the patch.	No	✓ Does not interrupt sex ✓ Convenient	92–99.7%
The Pill	The combined hormone birth control pill contains small amounts of two natural hormones (estrogen and progestin) that stop the release of an egg. Pregnancy cannot occur if the body does not release an egg.	No	✓ Does not interrupt sex ✓ Can be a part of your daily routine	92–99.7%

FORMS OF CONTRACEPTION (CONT)

Method	What is it?	Prevents STDs: Yes or No	Advantages	Effectiveness
The Shot	Injected into the arm or buttock every 12 weeks. It stops the release of an egg and makes the mucus in the cervix (opening to the uterus) thicker so that sperm cannot enter the uterus. Pregnancy cannot occur if the body does not release an egg.	No	✓ Convenient ✓ Does not interrupt sex ✓ The hormonal injection lasts for 12 weeks	97–99.7%
Sponge	The sponge is a non-reusable piece of soft foam that is filled with spermicidal and must be inserted inside the vagina before intercourse and must remain in place for six hours after intercourse.	No	✓ As long as sponge stays in place for six hours after sex, you can be protected for multiple rounds of intercourse. ✓ Can be purchased at drugstores for low price	88–91%
Tubal Ligation Female Sterilization	Surgical sterilizing that cuts or ties your fallopian tubes and prevents your eggs from traveling and getting fertilized by sperm. Can be reversed only on occasion.	No	✓ Highly effective ✓ Immediately effective ✓ Does not interrupt or reduce sex drive	99.5%
Vaginal Spermicidal	There are different types of spermicides available: contraceptive foam; contraceptive jelly; and vaginal contraceptive film. A spermicide must be inserted into the vagina before each act of intercourse. It contains an active ingredient (Nonoxynol-9) that kills sperm.	No	✓ Can be purchased at a drugstore ✓ Neither partner can feel it	71–82%

FORMS OF CONTRACEPTION (CONT)

Method	What is it?	Prevents STDs: Yes or No	Advantages	Effectiveness
Vaginal Ring	Soft, flexible, clear plastic ring that is inserted into the vagina, where it slowly releases hormones. These hormones are similar to a woman's natural hormones and stop the release of an egg from the ovaries. Pregnancy cannot occur if the body does not release an egg. A woman inserts and removes the ring herself. It is left in place for 21 days. A new ring is inserted after a 7-day break.	No	✓ Convenient ✓ Does not interrupt sex ✓ You can insert the ring into your vagina once a month without a doctor.	92–99.7%
Vasectomy	Vasectomy is a permanent method of birth control that sterilizes the man. A surgical procedure closes the vas deferens (tubes) that carry sperm. Occasionally this method can be reversed, but you need to talk to your doctor. Vasectomy reversals can be expensive.	No	✓ Local anesthetic (freezing) is used during procedure ✓ Brief 15–30 minute process ✓ Highly effective ✓ Does not interrupt, affect, or lower sex drive	99.9%
Withdrawal	Withdrawal is when a man pulls his penis out of the vagina prior to ejaculation.	No	✓ Does not cost money ✓ Does not require additional birth control devices or hormones	73–96%

Source: Adapted from the World Health Organization Family Planning Fact Sheet, April 2011 and Planned Parenthood, Comparing Effectiveness of Birth Control Methods, online.

Pregnancy

In an ideal world, every woman would consciously plan for her reproductive choices, proactively deciding, for example, when she's going to get pregnant and readying her relationship, her finances, and her support system beforehand.

"I believe in a woman's right to choose when and under what conditions she bears a child—so I'm pro-choice, in theory," says Alexis, age 36. "But in reality I probably wouldn't have an abortion. After I made a certain amount of money and was able to support a child myself, I really couldn't justify having an abortion. But I also don't want to be a single mom—it's just too hard—so I'm very careful about contraception."

In reality, few women possess Alexis's clarity, and conversations about the whens, whys, and what-ifs are all too rare. Ideally, women would discuss these issues openly, and early, with potential partners—and reflect on them honestly within themselves.

"If you've thought through who you are and just how you want to express your sexuality and with whom, all these decisions can help you to avoid an abortion or unintended pregnancy," suggests Dr. Wyatt. "If you say, 'I'm a woman who's on my way to the top. I'm going to school, and I've got 10 more years before I can actually make any money,' then you know that you are not prepared to have children. You ought to be using a form of contraception along with condoms if you are sexually active and not allow yourself to get caught in the heat of the moment. Something like that can derail a woman."

Family planning is essential, not only to avoid derailing the plans for our lives, but also so that when we do begin to have babies, we are prepared to avoid pregnancy-related complications. Ideally we would also engage in preconception self-care—before we conceive— to prepare our bodies to have a healthy pregnancy and to increase the odds of delivering a healthy baby. In this way, pregnancy presents an important opportunity to improve our own well-being: when we are pregnant, we are often more open to messages to improve our baby's chances for good health, as well as our own health. Getting pregnant can often be a catalyst for us to eat more healthily, exercise, and kick habits like drinking wine with dinner every night.

When a baby is just a glimmer in a woman's imagination, she should meet with her doctors so that they can help her take steps to eliminate any problems, such as high blood pressure and diabetes that could interfere with the pregnancy and reduce the risk of having a child with birth defects.[28] She should educate herself about prenatal care technology, such as ultrasonography and amniocentesis, and know what tests to ask for to assess or monitor the baby's health in the womb.

She should make sure that she has enough support, knows her health insurance benefits, and has established a relationship with a health-care provider. Vanessa Cullins, M.D., vice president for medical affairs at Planned Parenthood Federation of America (PPFA), suggests that women should ask themselves: "Are you really prepared to support and to nurture a child or children? Your relationship needs to be decent before you bring children into it. The child tends not to cause someone to stay in a relationship; it places stressors on the relationship."

Childbirth

Just as it is important to create the conditions for a family to thrive, women can and should have a plan for the birth itself, including choice of a care provider. While most American women opt to have an ob/gyn deliver their babies, this isn't the only available choice. Many Black women are beginning to turn to midwives for their prenatal care and delivery. Though natural childbirth seems like a foreign concept to many Black women today, Black midwives have a long history of providing women with holistic care during childbirth.

Until the 1950s, natural childbirth was the rule rather than the exception in the Deep South, and we Black women were the ones catching the babies. Like ob/gyns, midwives are trained experts in providing care during labor and delivery and after birth. The main difference is their outlook on the childbirth experience: midwives focus on keeping the process as natural as possible. They try to avoid medical interventions that can disrupt the normal pattern of labor, such as the use of unneeded drugs and forceps to pull the baby out. Shafia Monroe, a certified midwife and president of the International Center for Traditional Childbearing, puts it this way: "Black women should consider midwifery services because they will receive more personalized care, a better birth outcome, and a decreased risk of having a caesarean section. With the abnormal amount of stress that Black women experience in general, midwifery care is a good step in ensuring quality care to reduce pregnancy complications and infant mortality."

These are the same reasons Thomasina, age 38, opted to use a midwife for the birth of her two youngest children. She says her midwife helped her feel safer and more empowered. "She was also more sensitive to my needs," Thomasina explains. "For example, she asked before she touched me and described what she was doing. There was a great difference and I felt much more comfortable."

Just as ob/gyns aren't the only people able to deliver a baby, a hospital isn't the only place to have a child. Many Black women don't know about other options they have: dedicated birthing centers and their very own homes. Either place may prove beneficial unless there is a high-risk pregnancy likely to need emergency care.

Abortion

Today's 20-somethings dip in and out of school, the workforce, relationships, live-in situations, and their parents' homes. They don't marry until later than previous generations did, creating challenges in managing their sexual behavior. During their "odyssey years," young adults have an extremely high risk of having an unplanned pregnancy and abortion. In fact, 20-somethings' abortion rates are considerably higher than those among teens, whose pregnancy rates have been declining.[29] Compared to older women, young women are more fertile and likely to be sexually active. And because a lot of them do not have health insurance,[30] they are also more likely not to have a doctor or ready access to contraceptives or family planning services. Prior to the passage of the Patient Protection and Affordable Care Act (ACA) of 2010, 30 percent of women ages 20 to 24 did not have health insurance. Not surprisingly, young women's unplanned pregnancy rate is twice that of women overall and twice that of married women.[31] The abortion rate among Black women is almost five times that among White women, and at every income level Black women have higher abortion rates than Whites.[32]

Or at least we have higher *reported* abortion rates. We will never actually know how the numbers stack up, because Black women, young women, and low-income women tend to get abortions from government-funded providers that are required to report certain data to the government. "Those are data that are collected from public hospitals and guess who goes there? Black women," Dr. Wyatt answers. "White women go to private doctors and private clinics, and those entities don't report abortions. So it makes it look as if black women and Latinas are disproportionately seeking abortion services, when researchers are not getting the same data from private facilities as they get from the public clinics where poor people go."

Even so, the numbers are high. "I don't know if they're higher than anybody else's but it really doesn't matter," says Dr. Wyatt. "The point is they are higher than they need to be because women are not educated about what their choices are before they have sex. So it ends up being a matter of 'Are you going to have an abortion or not?' when the decision should have been made much further up the pike."

Sexually Transmitted Diseases

Sexually transmitted diseases are very common among young people in their teens and early 20s. Although 15-to-24-year-olds represent only one-quarter of the sexually active population, they account for nearly half (9.1 million) of the 18.9 million new cases of STDs each year.[33]

STDs are even more common among young Black women. In 2008, the chlamydia rate among Blacks was more than eight times higher than that of Whites (1,519 cases per

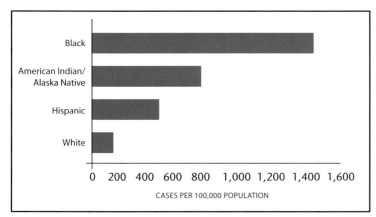

Rates of Reported Cases of Chlamydia, 2008, by Race/Ethnicity

CASES PER 100,000 POPULATION

Source: CDC. Sexually Transmitted Disease in the United States, 2008.

100,000 versus 174).[34] Black girls and women ages 15 to 24 had the highest chlamydia rate of any group. Over 40 percent of the cases of chlamydia and gonorrhea in the United States occur among Black people; Blacks are five times as likely as people of other races to contract syphilis.[35] How STDs affect Black women will be discussed in more detail in Chapter 5, "Top Ten Health Risks for Black Women."

"STDs are shared among people in sexual networks," explains Dr. Irene Doherty in an article by Sherri Crute published by *TheRoot.com*. Dr. Doherty, who is part of a team of researchers at the University of North Carolina exploring how STDs spread, says, "The theory of sexual networks is simple: it's not what you do; it's what your partners do and what your partner's partners do. Our data show that Black women do not have more sex or more high-risk sex than other women. They select partners from a small pool that has a high rate of STDs."

While many people dismiss STDs as something they can just take some pills or get a shot for, the fact is that these infections have a significant impact by making women more vulnerable to emotional stigma and insecurities. "When I was 22 I got genital herpes from the third guy I'd had sex with," says Jackie, now 35. "I had been careful about using condoms; I couldn't believe it had happened to me. Back then the stigma related to getting herpes was like getting HIV today. I was so ashamed, and I thought no one would ever want to be with me. That turned out not to be true at all—but it follows me from relationship to relationship. At just the point that I fall in love, I am terrified that I'm going to be rejected."

Having herpes or another STD also increases a woman's risk of being infected with HIV. Not only can STDs create microscopic tears in the vaginal tissue through which the virus can enter the bloodstream, they also weaken the immune system, leaving a woman more vulnerable to other types of disease. When STDs go untreated, it can also become more difficult—if not impossible—for a woman to get pregnant. "One of the goals of preventive health-care—using protection and using condoms—is protection of fertility so that when you decide you want to become pregnant, you can easily become pregnant," says Dr. Cullins.

Clearly, stressing the importance of safe sexual practices, nonviolent social environments, and regular reproductive health screenings can greatly enhance the health and social well-being of young adult Black women.

Violence and Sexual Abuse

Intimate-partner violence includes a pattern of mental, physical, emotional, or sexual abuse in which one partner makes the other partner feel scared, weak, isolated, hurt, or sad. It is a major problem in the United States. Each year, women experience about 4.8 million related physical and sexual assaults, according to a 2009 fact sheet from the Centers for Disease Control and Prevention (CDC). For young Black women, the statistics are most grim. This issue will be discussed in more detail in Chapter 5, "Top Ten Health Risks for Black Women," since violence is a major health risk that many of us face.

Low-income tends to be an indicator for abuse, though violence is not confined to any one social class. The difference is having options and resources to escape—options not always enjoyed by those struggling to survive day-to-day. Feeling trapped leads many women to stay put—and in peril. According to a 2008 study of 2006 data by the national nonprofit Violence Policy Center, Black women are killed at a rate nearly three times higher than that of White women. The reasons for the higher death rate among Black women are still unknown, but according to the CDC and other studies, being exposed to violence as a child can increase the risk that someone will hurt his or her partner.

Indeed, exposure to violence as a young child was an impetus for Harold L. Turley II, a former abuser who wrote a memoir about his healing, *My Darkest Hour: The Day I Realized I Was Abusive.* "I had pent-up aggression," the Washington, D.C.-based author and performance poet told *The Root.* "I had problems dealing with and channeling my anger. My breaking point came when I put my hands on a woman with whom I had been in a two-and-a-half-year relationship. I did not want to become what I hated most, which was my stepfather, who was abusive toward my mother. That wasn't the man my mother raised me to be. That's when I decided to get help."

Turley says that in his experience, women become involved with abusive men because they see the man's potential instead of his flaws. Helping him reach his potential is like a project. But more often than not, the flaws outweigh the potential, and then the abuse sets in when both parties become frustrated. "A lot is happening when you are dealing with love," he says. "The woman can see the potential within that man and the things he can be, versus the reality of who he really is."

Intimate Partner Violence

Women ages 20 to 24 are at greatest risk of domestic violence (except for incidents of violence that result in a woman's death).[36] The poorer a woman's household, the greater the risk that she will experience domestic violence.[37] According to a U.S. Justice Department study, nearly 30 percent of Black women report having experienced violence at least once at the hands of an intimate partner.[38] And the rate of domestic violence perpetrated upon Black women increased by 75 percent between 2003 and 2004.[39]

"Some of it has to do with not having enough eligible men within the community," says Dr. Cullins. "Certain men feel entitled to treat women however they want, and some women feel that they have to take it or risk being alone."

A growing concern being heard from young Black women is that they have little understanding of what a healthy relationship is in the first place. How do we know what a healthy relationship looks like if we have never seen one modeled in our home or community and can't find a rerun of *The Cosby Show*?

"A healthy relationship is a give and take. You're being respected, what you say is being respected, and you also respect what you're hearing from the other person," describes Dr. Cullins. "While you all are never going to agree on everything 100 percent, at a certain point you have to either kind of walk away from the issue, agree to disagree, or decide that the issue is so important that you won't actually walk from the relationship. The relationship is not one of property and control: I don't own you; you don't own me. We're coming to this thing as equals; we've got different areas of skill or expertise, and we're trying to work together as a team."

Homicide

Homicide is the second-leading cause of death among young Black women between the ages of 15 to 24 and the fifth leading cause of death among Black women ages 25 to 34. Young adults ages 18 to 24 are more likely to be victims of homicide than any other demographic group. Though killings of Black women have declined by almost two-thirds since 1976, Black women are murdered by their partners disproportionately—more than any other group, and most often by a boyfriend or husband. In fact, in 2005 Black women made up just 8 percent of the U.S. population but 22 percent of the victims of intimate partner homicides.[40]

Women are not the only victims of crimes, either. Between 1990 and 2008 the share of women arrested for committing violent crimes rose from 10 to 18 percent. Young women ages 18 to 24 had the highest arrest rate: about 31 percent of women convicted were Black.

What's the one time that Black women are more likely to be killed than at any other time? When they're pregnant and vulnerable, killed by their intimate partner.[41]

Rape

One out of every six women will be a victim of a rape or attempted rape during her lifetime, according to the Rape, Abuse and Incest National Network.[42] Almost half of those women are under 18; 80 percent are under 30. One in five women will be raped while she is in college; fewer than five percent of those sexual assaults will be reported. Only seven percent of rapists are strangers to the victims.

Being raped has a debilitating effect on women well beyond the immediate trauma. Victims of sexual assault are:

- 3 times more likely to suffer from depression

- 6 times more likely to suffer from post-traumatic stress syndrome

- 13 times more likely to abuse alcohol

- 26 times more likely to abuse drugs

- 4 times more likely to contemplate suicide.[43]

"The sobering reality is that women alone can't prevent rape," says Aishah Sahidah Simmons, award-winning activist filmmaker, and incest and rape survivor, who was raped during her sophomore year in college. She later wrote, produced, and directed, *"NO! THE RAPE DOCUMENTARY."* As Simmons commented, "We should not fool ourselves into thinking that if we dress properly, whatever that means, or only go on a date with someone we know, it will make us immune from rape." But there are things that women can do to reduce their risk, she advises. "If we go to a party, we go with friends and we leave with friends. We don't leave our drinks unattended, even if we're just drinking water—if you have to go to the bathroom, you either pour it out or take it with you—because the date-rape drug is clear: you can't even see it."

Reproductive Coercion

About 20 percent of women experience reproductive coercion, or reproductive control, a situation in which a partner is "pushing someone to keep a pregnancy, become pregnant or to have an abortion. Pulling off patches, throwing away pills, putting holes in condoms: they are all additional forms of control being forced upon, really being perpetrated upon, a woman partner," says Planned Parenthood's Dr. Cullins. But where do we draw the line in an emotional conversation about, say, keeping or ending a pregnancy? "When one partner is feeling very uncomfortable about the way the conversation is going or the behavior the other partner is exhibiting; when they have the feeling of being forced or cornered.

"Sometimes it starts out being very flattering: 'I want you to have my baby,'" Dr. Cullins mimics. "And then she might begin to be thinking about it. 'Do I want a baby now? Do I want a baby from this partner?' If there's a difference in will, it might escalate."

The Emotional Tightrope

During early adulthood Black women are more vulnerable to stress and depression—and more likely to commit suicide—than at any other time in our lives. All the factors examined so far come into play: we are negotiating a number of important life transitions, graduating high school, starting full-time jobs, starting college, embarking upon our careers, contemplating serious relationships, and trying to maintain our foundation. We are living in an extremely complicated world and often doing so without adequate emotional, financial, or familial support.

As in their teen years, many young Black women also lack female friends, keeping other women at arm's length. "I hear that there's too much drama. They're friends with men and are 'associated' with women," says Dr. Belgrave. "It is an issue of trust. It's not how Black people have survived in this country, which has been because of collectivism, and helping each other and trusting each other."

"The root of a lot of it is jealousy. She's dating that guy and I like him, or she took my boyfriend," says Dr. Stokes. "They see it on TV and think that's how you're supposed to be. They don't see any healthy friendships among women."

For women of all races, but particularly for Black women, seeing highly sexualized, overly dramatic women who meet narrow and unrealistic standards of beauty and behave in overly dramatic ways has become the norm.[44] "The image of a Black woman in the media is not who a Black woman is," observes sex therapist Wyatt. "You see women who are very physical and very sexualized, so women will pick that piece up and sexualize themselves."

Experts do say, though, that many Millenials and younger people are able to think critically about media rather than simply buying into those images. Young adults are more tech-savvy than any other age group, with 90 percent of them online, including 91 percent of Blacks, highlighting the significant amount of access Blacks have in consuming popular media.

The Internet places the world at our fingertips, but it also shuts it down. "You can't develop a social life until you can relate to people. So you can imagine what kind of relationships people like that are gonna have. They're gonna resonate with people who are like that as well," says Dr. Wyatt. "They don't have a sense of relatedness. Their sense of relatedness is Tweeting."

In this subculture of social isolation, as well as of trauma and violence, too many young Black women experience severe depression or other mental illness during this phase. As members of the Internet generation and targets of consumer culture, Millennials still struggle to find peace—and themselves—amid the noise. "I'm really trying to get young women to learn how to be still and get quiet and become aware of their own thoughts," Dr. Stokes says of the young women with whom she works. "There's just so much stimulation going on. Everything comes from an outside source, and it's hard for them to hear their own inner voice." Overall, young Black women are struggling to find a space that nourishes their inner selves and become more in tune with their values so that they can engage in putting their health first.

Spirituality

Although those of us who attend church hold traditional religious values, in other ways our values reflect greater acceptance of differences than earlier generations. This means that young Black women are rethinking the way we express and engage their spirituality.

"I go to church pretty often but I also dibble and dabble in other stuff," says Latisha, 32, who participates in an Eastern meditation group with spiritual underpinnings in addition to attending her family's AME church.

Another young Black woman expresses her confidence in communing with the Spirit outside of the traditional meeting place: "I still believe in God, but I'm not going to a church that tells me that something is wrong with me," says Amanda, 33, who identifies as "queer." "I'm definitely religious; I'm definitely spiritual; I'm definitely blessed; I just don't go to church."

"I spent much of my teens and early 20s feeling lost in a way I can't really describe—I was searching for something, but I didn't know what, and I wasn't finding it in the club," laughs Kenya, 30, an aspiring artist."I'd been raised Catholic, but there was a point where my parents couldn't even fake it anymore—it wasn't working, even for them, so they let me stop going. Hallelujah, praise Jesus! Then when I was 27, I found this great Baptist church filled with everyone from health professionals and government workers, to prostitutes coming in off the stroll. They encouraged you to come as you are, which was a revelation to me. That's when I stopped feeling like everything I did was going to send me to hell, which was my basic take-away from growing up Catholic. Now I *love* going to church. I don't miss it for the world!"

Overall, young Black women are struggling to find a space that nourishes their inner selves in one place because there is a growing recognition that there are myriad ways that they can engage their spirituality.

Why Prevention Is Better Than Cure: Recommended Young Adult Screenings

From ages 18 to 24, as we graduate from high school and our parents' health insurance plans, the percentage of us who are insured declines to 66 percent, and the uninsured percentage triples. When we do not have insurance, we are almost twice as likely to go without seeing a doctor, getting medical tests, keeping up with treatments, visiting a specialist, or filling a prescription for a medical problem than are our insured peers. Among low-income young adults, however, women are more likely to be insured than men[45]. Experts estimate that in 2011 1.2 million young adults will receive coverage through the Affordable Care Act under a provision allowing people under age 26 to remain on their parents' health plans.[46]

Throughout their reproductive years, women's reproductive health has repercussions for every aspect of their lives, and it, too, is woven in with their total well-being. Many barriers exist for younger Black women in accessing essential preventative services such as contraception and prenatal care. As young adult Black women, we should insist on full and accurate information from our health-care provider about all screenings, options, medications (including side effects, health risks, and benefits), costs to obtain and discontinue a contraceptive method, and procedures involved. By ensuring that women have lifelong access to preventive health-care, including reproductive health services, we can safeguard the health of families and communities, too. Younger Black women will benefit greatly from the recommended screenings below to ensure that they can enjoy their reproductive years and beyond in good health.

RECOMMENDED HEALTH SCREENINGS AND VACCINATIONS
YOUNG ADULT WOMEN AGES 20–39

HEALTH SCREENING TESTS	WHEN TO GET THE TEST
GENERAL HEALTH	
Well-woman care—a full health checkup, including weight and height	Yearly
Thyroid (TSH) test	Discuss with your health-care provider.
HIV test	Get this test at least once to find out your HIV status. Ask your health-care provider if and when you need the test again.
HEART HEALTH	
Blood pressure test	At least every two years
Cholesterol test	Start at age 20; discuss with your health-care provider.
DIABETES	
Blood glucose or A1c test	Discuss with your health-care provider.
BREAST HEALTH	
Clinical breast exam	At least every three years starting in your 20s
Breast self-examination	Perform breast self-examinations at the same time each month.
REPRODUCTIVE HEALTH	
Pap test	All women should begin cervical cancer screening within three years after they start having sex and no later than age 21. Screening should be done every year with a regular Pap test. Beginning at age 30, women who have had three normal Pap test results in a row may get screened every two to three years.
Pelvic exam	Yearly beginning at age 21. Younger than 21 and sexually active, discuss with health-care provider.

Chlamydia test	Yearly until age 25 if sexually active. Age 26 and older, get this test if you have new or multiple partners
Sexually transmitted infection (STI) tests	Both partners should get tested for STIs, including HIV, before initiating sexual intercourse.
MENTAL HEALTH SCREENING	Discuss with your health-care provider.
EYE AND EAR HEALTH	
Comprehensive eye exam	Discuss with your health-care provider
Hearing test	Starting at age 18, then every 10 years
SKIN HEALTH	
Mole exam	Monthly mole self-exam by a health-care provider as part of a routine full checkup, starting at age 20.
ORAL HEALTH	
Dental exam	Routinely; discuss with your dentist.
IMMUNIZATIONS	
Influenza vaccine	Discuss with your health-care provider.
Tetanus-diphtheria-pertussis booster vaccine	Every 10 years
Human papillomavirus (HPV) vaccine	Up to age 26, if not already completed vaccine series; discuss with your health-care provider.
Meningococcal vaccine	Discuss with your health-care provider if you are a college student or military recruit.

Chapter 3

Midlife Adults

(40 to 64)

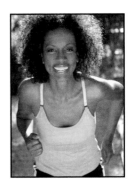

Black women who have taken good care of themselves in the young adult years often look and feel fabulous during midlife. Our energy levels are high, our spirits remain joyful, and we look youthful—without Botox, nips, or tucks. We come to know and accept ourselves and we feel freer than ever before to be who we truly are.

We dare to free ourselves for travel and adventure, to reconnect with old friends, and to begin contemplating the next book to read or movie to see. This is when we really see and feel the tangible benefits of stepping away from the box of donuts at work or actually going to the gym as well as to accept that a massage is not an indulgence but a necessity. We bravely take out our compass and set sail for new destinations in the adventure of midlife.

If a woman has taken care of herself all along, or if she's now jumping onto the health bandwagon with enthusiasm, the 40s can be a "wonderful phase—the best time of a woman's life," says UCLA professor Gail Wyatt, Ph.D. She laughs as she describes the 40s as the gift of having survived your 20s and 30s, but also as a phase when most women have finished childbearing and know enough about themselves to get what they want out of life. The 50s can be an invigorating time of life, too—"but only for those women who really understand their bodies," she says. "With the ending of menstruation and hormonal changes—with all that stuff that they had taken for granted, fading—women have to do a lot of work on how they feel about themselves. All the rules change."

Those of us who have taken care of everyone but ourselves or have let our health go to hell in a hand-basket need to act quickly now. As we move through our 40s, we start running out of time to take charge of our health while we have estrogen— which also helps to build bone and regulate cholesterol[1]—in relatively high levels in our bodies. During middle age, we must take control of our health or risk finding ourselves stuck in a body we never imagined, trapped in health circumstances that we cannot back out of, or even dying earlier than expected.

By their 40s most Black women are struggling with their weight, and many develop chronic diseases, such as heart disease and diabetes. It's not uncommon to feel fearful because our health is declining and we do not understand what is happening to us; angry when the people we've sacrificed for take us for granted and don't help us; embarrassed that we've lost the shapely figure of our youth; sad that we're paying the high price of self-neglect and are not living up to our own potential. "I think about the years that are gone and the things I could have done, and I mean it's just too late," says Denise, age 45. "Last year I was taking like two or three pills and now they've got me taking nine pills. I'm like what is going on?"

Even though it's harder to change once our habits have become ingrained, especially in a phase when we're often experiencing the very real time constraints that accompany (often single) parenthood, being middle aged need not mean becoming set in our ways or stuck in behaviors

JUST THE FACTS

Population:

7.9 million
36.6 percent of Black females

Top causes of death (ages 35–44):

1.	Cancer	21%
2.	Heart disease	16%
3.	HIV	11%
4.	Unintentional injuries	9%
5.	Stroke	5%

Top causes of death (ages 45–54)

1.	Cancer	33%
2.	Heart disease	23%
3.	Diabetes	6%
4.	Stroke	6%
5.	Kidney disease	3%

Top causes of death (ages 55–64)

1.	Cancer	33%
2.	Heart disease	23%
3.	Diabetes	6%
4.	Stroke	5%
5.	Kidney disease	3%

Source: CDC. Office of Women's Health, Accessed, April 2011.

that no longer serve us. At any age, we can free ourselves from patterns that are not working for us and open up exciting new approaches to living that enliven our spirits, enhance our health, and improve our quality of life.

This chapter discusses the health of adult women, ages 40 to 64—a span that encompasses two phases of life: the premenopausal years of 40 until roughly 49, an age when many women experience menopause, the end of their menstrual period; and 50 through 64, as they transition into their new post-menopausal identity and prepare for their senior years. Because so little qualitative research is conducted on Black women in midlife, this section relies heavily on data from (1) the health survey of over 600 Black women's attitudes and behaviors commissioned by the Black Women's Health Imperative;[2] (2) a series of Imperative focus groups and roundtables held in Chicago, Los Angeles, New Orleans, Philadelphia, and Washington, D.C., in which middle-aged and older Black women with chronic diseases talked about their health; and (3) a 10-city focus group study of Black women in midlife commissioned by the National Council of Negro Women (NCNW).[3] We will share what Black women continue to tell us in our ongoing conversations and what we have discovered about Black women in our monthly polls in the decades since the Imperative was founded in 1983.

Black Women In Midlife

Traditionally during midlife we focus on raising a family, creating an environment that feels like home for our children, and becoming grandparents, as well as taking care of our own aging parents, worrying about our finances, and wondering how we are going to be able to retire.

For many, the dream of slowing down during their 40s and 50s now seems like a fairy tale from a long ago and far-away time. Women of all races and socioeconomic backgrounds—even the ones who have done all the right things financially—can no longer count on the same resources and lifestyles that sustained previous generations.

Many middle- and working-class women are struggling to pay their mortgages; millions of Americans have been foreclosed upon or otherwise priced out of their homes; and homeownership is near its lowest point since World War II. As a result, homeowner equity—historically a source of cash during retirement—has declined sharply.[4] Many women have been forced to raid their financial futures by taking out loans against their 401(k)s to keep their families afloat.

Health-wise, these same women are under a great deal of stress, and high stress leads to poor health. Those who have health insurance are paying more money for less coverage; many reasonable health insurance claims are being routinely denied. Many illnesses begin to occur during this life stage—particularly for women who have not cared for themselves well until now. More than ever women simply cannot afford to become ill.

Because of the unique circumstances of our lives, the economic downturn has hit midlife Black women particularly hard. As the economic gap between the haves and the have-nots grows, Black women and children are in danger of slipping into a deeper and more intractable poverty than America has witnessed for generations.

"A middle-class woman may be back to the lifestyle of a poor woman, not in terms of where she's living or the type of job she's doing," notes Dr. Wyatt. "She may be college-educated, but she's very much at risk for falling out of the middle class."

Education, Employment, and Economic Realities

Black women who focused on their education during their 20s tend to do relatively well professionally. However, many of us enter adulthood with less education than our White peers, so we tend to end up in lower-paying and less-secure jobs and have fewer career prospects—all realities that leave us more vulnerable during difficult times. And as much as we love our children, for those who become mothers young, before going to college or investing in technical or professional training, the everyday economic price can be high.

With their families shifting—their children out of the house, perhaps their marriages entering a new phase or ending—many women take this time to focus on educational dreams that they had to leave behind. Some women reach significant educational milestones during this phase, either graduating from a program they began during their 30s or 40s or returning to school to upgrade or acquire new skills now that their children are older.

Consider Jasmine, who graduated high school and went to technical school, where she was trained as a home health aide but never bothered getting her state certification. "I've had to take jobs under the table and they 'short' me a lot—there's always some reason I have to prove my time sheet. About a year ago I lost my job and had to go live with my daughter in a shelter," she adds. "It took me 11 months to get a new job—at Chick-fil-A—but then I got hit by a car on the first day of work. Now my ankle's in a cast and I can't work for three months. It seems like every time I try to go forward, I go backwards."

The unemployment rate among Black women has skyrocketed to 14 percent,[5] but in reality it's probably higher; that figure doesn't include women who are no longer looking for work. Many women who do have jobs are working on less favorable terms than in the past. More are underemployed, have settled for lower-paying jobs, are working part-time, or are cobbling together several jobs to make ends meet. Increasingly, Black women work jobs that don't offer adequate—or any—health insurance. And very few Black women in midlife are financially situated to enter their senior years; only 25 percent of Black female elders have pension income, and in the generations coming after them, the number will be lower still.[6]

"Many Black women won't be able to retire, though they want to," says Dr. Wyatt. "Because maybe they've just had jobs but not careers—the majority of Black women have jobs. For that reason they want to stop, and that's not possible."

The stark reality is that the average Black woman earns about 63 cents on the dollar compared to the average White man.[7] While women's earnings relative to men's have been climbing over the years, prior to age 50, women of color have virtually no wealth. What is wealth? The value of what we own outright (personal property, savings, and income-generating assets, such as stocks) minus the debt we owe to creditors. Wealth is a personal safety net: if something happens, we can sell your assets for emergency funds. It also allows us to leave an inheritance to our children. In Black families the reality is that each generation must pull its entire weight, while in many White families, the economic assets held by family elders help to lighten the load through inheritance.

What's more, debt levels have been rising among people ages 55 to 64—the age just before retirement. In 2007, over 60 percent of American households headed by a person aged 55 or older had debt—an increase of seven percent since 2001. The average total debt increased to $70,000. Debt levels among upper-middle-income families reached new highs as people refinanced their homes, cashed out equity, and purchased homes during the real-estate bubble.[8] In the foreclosure crisis that followed, disproportionate numbers of Black women lost their homes. One study reported that Black women were 256 percent more likely than White men to receive subprime loans.[9] Perhaps not surprisingly, in the 10-city focus groups on midlife women, nearly 30 percent of midlife Black women identified their finances as their greatest source of stress.

A Black woman's upbringing, which often requires her to take on significant responsibility in the family and play more than a stereotypical feminine role, leads others to see her as independent, competent, and demanding of respect—classic leadership traits—and this may work to her professional advantage.

"African American women may not be seen as prototypical Blacks, and they may not be seen as prototypical women," Dr. Kathleen Phillips says. "That invisibility might end up being something that's helpful in allowing [them] to take on behaviors that otherwise would not be allowed. Black women may be in a unique position to, in fact, step into leadership positions, to be embraced in leadership positions." [10]

That's not the whole workplace picture, though: "The complexity of how race and gender interact is not as simple as we typically thought," says Stanford University visiting organizational behavior professor Kathleen Phillips, Ph.D.

Marriage and Family

"Blacks have the lowest rate of marriage of all groups in the United States; when they do marry or cohabit, they have the highest rates of disruption; and when they divorce, they have the lowest rates of remarriage," Dr. Patterson wrote in an editorial[11] in the *Washington Post*. Even our dating relationships are less stable than others'.

"By 40 a woman is acutely concerned about the fact that she is or is not in a happy relationship, if that's what she wants," says Dr. Wyatt. "It's a considerable source of stress and dissatisfaction if you haven't been able to accomplish your goals in terms of relationship-building, much of which begins in the 30s."

Women who do not have partners often start to be blamed during this age range for the fact that they are alone. As if pressure from parents and family members to get married or have grandchildren is not enough, people begin to assume that single women are gay, particularly if they opt not to bear children.

As society has become more accepting of differences, some women have become clear that they are lesbian, although that doesn't necessarily make life easier. "You gotta be really strong," says Helen, 38, a key account manager for a major corporation. "If I could choose, I would. It can be so stressful that you would rather not be bothered. Some people end up by themselves forever because they're torn by religion or family, and they can never be happy or comfortable."

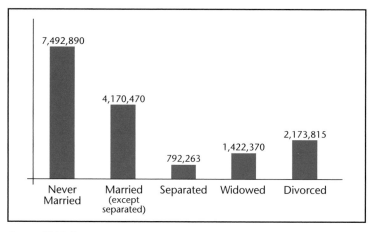

Marital Status: Black Women in America 2010 Census

Never Married: 7,492,890
Married (except separated): 4,170,470
Separated: 792,263
Widowed: 1,422,370
Divorced: 2,173,815

Source: 2010 Census

BLACK FAMILY STRUCTURE BY HOUSEHOLD TYPE (ADULTS)

Household Type	Number	Percent
Married Couple	4,274	46%
Single Father	939	10%
Single Mother	4,145	44%

Source: U.S. Census Bureau, Current Population Survey, Annual Social and Economic Supplement, 2010.

About 53 percent of American women are married and living with their spouses, as compared to 44 percent of Black women, who are more likely to be single heads of household.[12]

Single mothers of color are more likely to be poor than any other women. Even prior to the economic downturn, women of all races experienced what's known as a "motherhood wealth penalty"—the financial price paid for becoming moms that accumulates when we take time out of the workforce or work part-time. Single moms typically pay a higher penalty, carrying the financial burden of groceries, school books and uniforms, and basketball camp—not to mention sick days and mornings off for parent-teacher conferences. The price of being the custodial parent is particularly high when you do not receive child support. The motherhood penalty for women of any color is tough, as race and gender discrimination make the uphill climb of single parenthood even more difficult.

It shouldn't surprise anyone to know that the average Black single mother has no assets; she has a median—that is, half have less and half have more—net worth of zero dollars, compared to $6,000 for a White single mom.

Single mothers have tremendous difficulty saving money and building wealth. From child-care to health-care expenses, they tend to shoulder disproportionate costs. They also earn less, tend to be segregated into lower-paying occupations, disproportionately do not have health insurance, do not have pension and retirement plans, experience individual and institutional racism and sexism—the list goes on.

Homeownership

Traditionally homeownership has been the dream of Black women in this age group. Large numbers of Black women successfully achieved their vision; however, disproportionate numbers of Black women and children have been thrown out of their homes during the foreclosure crisis. While FOX News correspondents are quick to blame the victim, one needs only to scratch the surface of the issue to understand some of the structural reasons why.

"The gender disparities in mortgage lending are consistent across race and ethnicity lines. All women are more likely to receive subprime mortgages than their male counterparts of the same racial or ethnic group," wrote Avis Jones DeWeever, Ph.D., executive director of the National Council of Negro Women, in an article about the impact of the foreclosure crisis on women.

"Most disadvantaged have been African American women, who stunningly are 256 percent more likely than White men to receive subprime loans," Dr. DeWeever wrote. "Upper-income Black women fare even worse: they are nearly five times more likely than White men to be saddled with high-cost mortgages." [13]

A story published in *The New York Times* described how the foreclosure crisis was affecting single Black mothers living in the working-class Belair-Edison neighborhood in Baltimore, which prior to the recession had been composed primarily of homeowners.[14] Even in January 2008, when the story was written, one in 35 houses in the neighborhood of 6,400 homes already had been foreclosed upon. The article states that nearly half of the mortgages sold to women in 2006 had been subprime.

"When I bought my house, it was the American Dream," said Deborah, 33, a single mother of three who is scrambling to avoid losing her row house, on which she defaulted after losing her job. "Now I need to save it for my boys. If it was just me, OK, I'd have to give up my first home. But it's different when you have it for the kids. When they turn 18, I want this to be theirs." [15]

Setting the Stage for Good Health

While almost 95 percent of Black women in the Harris survey characterized themselves between somewhat healthy to very healthy, many Black women are well on the way to developing poor health by midlife. Some of us deceived ourselves, pretending that the cultural use of the word "healthy," meaning overweight, can be a stand-in for the medical definition of the word "healthy."

Research shows that we define health in a very disconnected way. We also express ambivalence about achieving good health. This lack of understanding of what good health is and what it takes to attain it keeps our expectations low; we settle for a poorer quality of life than we deserve and stop short of reaching our promise.

For example, over 55 percent of Black women believe that being healthy means not having any chronic diseases, disabilities, or injuries. But by that definition, our lives could be miserable; we could be spiritually disconnected and out of touch with our children, family, and friends, and our bodies could be one day away from having several chronic diseases. Is that really good health?

Without the self-esteem, knowledge, and willpower to do something about it, far too many Black women during these years give up any notions of being in good health and settle for good looks instead. "We always take care of our bodies around the margins—our hair, our nails, our shoes. Black women buy a lot of shoes," Dr. Wyatt notes. "It's not the core of our bodies that we're fixing."

These are the years in which Black women develop chronic diseases in shockingly high numbers, including obesity, diabetes, hypertension, heart disease, and cancer.

"I always had a blood pressure problem, but I never thought it would really get out of hand. At age 38, 39, my blood pressure got real bad, and I couldn't afford the medications; my blood pressure killed my kidney. So they put me on dialysis at age 39 and I was on dialysis ever since then," says Theresa, a Nashville-area single mother of four. Theresa stayed on dialysis for five years until she had a kidney transplant.

Participants in 10-city focus groups on midlife Black women say they are "extremely" or "very" concerned about being affected by diseases for which they have a family history, including heart disease (39 percent), cancer in general (36 percent), diabetes (35 percent), breast cancer (35 percent), obesity (31 percent), and stroke (29 percent). Many are "scared straight" when faced with the prospect of illness and make dramatic changes quickly.

"It turned out that I am a diabetic," says Evelyn, 52. "That's what changed my whole eating habit, the fact that I had to realize, 'You're not taking care of yourself, and you are taking care of everybody else.'"

It took being confronted with a debilitating disease whose prospects include blindness, heart attack, stroke, and the loss of her limbs for Evelyn to finally get it. Midlife is a prime time to stop ignoring the danger signs and get serious about learning to care for self before the consequences of denial and self-neglect become life-threatening.

For many Black women, valuing strong family connections, along with a sense of personal control in their lives, influences their chances for more positive health outcomes in later life. In a 2004 study on midlife Black women, 60 percent expressed a sense of control and said they felt that what happens with them is a consequence of their own behavior.[16] These can be strong motivating factors for making and maintaining lifestyle changes. "I want to make sure my children grow up in a comfortable home and that I am able to see them grow up and do well," says Donna, 55.

Black women who have not taken care of themselves may experience a different reality. "If women have gone into their 40s overweight, out of shape, and with a lot of maladaptive eating, smoking, drinking, and partying behaviors, the 50s can be very harsh instead of very satisfying," says Dr. Wyatt.

This section explores some of what is known about the health of midlife Black women. It discusses how they perceive their health and how what they value can affect their health. It draws on the Imperative survey, interviews with experts, evidence-based research and other studies that measure the well-being of Black women—and, of course, the experiences of Black women themselves.

Overweight and Obesity

"My health goals really boil down to the fact that I'm trying to stay off of the electric scooter you see people riding around on at the grocery store," laughs 48-year-old Audrey. "I know that's kind of offensive, but what I really mean is obesity and the health issues associated with it and the image of a fat Black woman have become the norm. So 'staying off of the scooter' for me means developing the discipline, getting the information, and eating the types of foods I need to eat to change my definition of what it means to be a middle-aged Black woman."

"What is your normal? For most Black women, that's the question," says Dr. Wyatt, since so many women have been heavy for so many years. "For a woman who makes the decision in her 50s to work out, it's a scary thing. They're unhappy in their size, but if they became obese during their teens and then had kids on top of that, women don't even know what they're supposed to look like anymore."

In the Harris health survey, 85 percent of Black women reported that they were overweight or obese, yet 94 percent of these women described themselves as "somewhat healthy," "healthy," or "very healthy." [17] Clearly there is a disconnect here: we're not getting the message that being overweight and being medically healthy are mutually exclusive states of being. Having new shoes cannot fix this; wearing the latest hairstyle does not change this; spending the morning at the day spa does not make this go away. Using the word "healthy" in an aesthetic sense to describe someone's shape or size does not fit the model of optimal health description of the same person, who would be considered as overweight or obese. This is not a difference in beauty standards; it's a medical reality: carrying extra weight increases a person's risk of disease.

"I guess my consolation prize is the fact that when you're fat, you don't get all those wrinkles," says Shante, a mother of two, who has struggled with weight for most of her adult life but hasn't succeeded in shedding the 75 pounds the doctor says she needs to lose. Constance's blood pressure runs high, and she is terrified that she will develop diabetes, which runs in her family. Yet she delays her doctor visits because she fears what she is going to learn. While the three overweight sisters in her family struggle with their blood sugar and diabetes, their thin sister, a dietitian, does not. "I never really understood that it would come down to this," Constance says of what she now views as a fight to keep from losing fingers and toes to the disease.

For some women, obesity arises from being set in our cultural ways. "Why does a summer gathering have to look like only hamburgers and hot dogs and potato salad?" asks Anna, who is trying to eat more healthily but admits that she overeats sweets. "Why can't we find a different approach to that? Once we know, we can do it."

Some experts think women know what they could do better, but lack the motivation to change. "I don't think it's an issue of not knowing that you're not supposed to eat fried chicken or drink a lot of soda and juice," says Connecticut ob/gyn Natalie Achong. "I think it's a notion of what's the point; everybody else is doing it; and I'm going to die of something anyway. I'm living for today."

Although many of us do need to improve our eating habits, some women overeat to feed a different need.

"I didn't realize I was an emotional eater until I did a checklist that was given to me by a physician. I kept saying 'No, I'm not,' but I am because of stress," says Lana, 48. "Family matters just sent me over the edge and I cured my emotions by eating. Before I knew it, I had tipped the scales to 240, and that's the biggest I have ever been. I just had to say this is ridiculous."

Midlife Black women are not known for being physically active. When we're not working, we tend to value rest over exercise. The Imperative study showed that only 17 percent of Black women engaged in regular physical activity—slightly over half as many as the 31 percent of White women who exercised regularly.

"I don't need exercise, I need rest," says Tiana, a retail salesperson. "I am on my feet all day. I need to take my shoes off, put my feet up, and take a nice bath. The last thing I want is to go to the gym." But some of us are realizing that the way we treat our bodies now will make all the difference in the way we look and feel as we grow older. Pattie, 46, admits that she's usually a little hard-headed—but a conversation with one of her aunts, in which the older woman spoke honestly about the physical and emotional toll that all her illnesses had taken on her, made Pattie start to worry about her own health and to open her mind to other options.

One of her friends had been encouraging her to join her at yoga class. Pattie joined her friend "kicking and screaming—though just for dramatic effect," she laughs. But aside from feeling a little self-conscious, she was surprised that she enjoyed it. "I don't know what I expected—I guess that I'd be humiliated in a class filled with skinny girls who could twist themselves into a pretzel. But there were several Black women in the class, and a couple of women whose bodies looked very 'middle-aged.' So when the teacher said that every stretch can be done at a different level—from the beginning to the most advanced—I said, 'Okay, maybe I can do this!'"

Reproductive and Sexual Health

During these middle years, sexual health is as important as it is during our prime reproductive years. But it can get tricky. Midlife Black women are less likely to marry, we marry late when we do marry, and we are less likely to stay married and to remarry. Consequently, we may have many long- or short-term, serious or casual relationships over the course of our sexual life. A choice in a partner that may seem liberated, innocuous, or fulfilling can become highly problematic from a health standpoint, if we haven't come to grips with what it means to have a positive and respectful sexual relationship. The World Health Organization defines sexual health as follows:

> " . . . a state of physical, emotional, mental, and social well-being related to sexuality. Sexual health requires a positive and respectful approach to sexuality and sexual relationships, as well as the possibility of having pleasurable and safe sexual experiences, free of coercion, discrimination, and violence."

Although many of us may not fully grasp what all of this means—having pleasurable and certainly safe sexual experiences; free of coercion, discrimination, and violence, seems like a good game plan. It's not too late from this day forward to embrace not only sexuality but sexual health, too.

Keep in mind that these are our midlife years—when it depends on what phase we're in as to how our bodies act, look, and need. Women in their early midlife, from 40 to 50, will face different issues than those in their later midlife years. In early midlife, women may run the risk of getting pregnant—believing their chances of getting pregnant are low, and they are—and also thinking that they are done with having children. There are also those who find themselves having difficulties becoming pregnant, having waited until the time was right, or so they thought.

Many well-educated, middle-class Black women are delaying childbirth until their late 30s and early 40s, when all females' fertility decreases. [18] "Unlike men, who produce sperm on a regular basis throughout most of their lives, women are born with a set number of eggs," explains Dr. O'Delle M. Owens, a Black doctor who was Cincinnati's very first board-certified fertility specialist. "Women are born with millions of eggs. But each month, a woman loses 10,000 eggs. The older you get, the fewer eggs you have." In fact, that problem, says Dr. Owens, can affect women as young as 28 years old.

In our later midlife phase, we become more aware of "aging" and all that it means as our body shows us some of its limitations—and as the world around us starts to see us differently in families, on our jobs, and in the wider community. A society that stereotyped us when we were younger now views us as mother figures. As we sweat through the night and feel sad for no reason, we are deeply reminded of this rite of passage.

Going Through "the Change"

During this phase, a woman undergoes many significant transitions: her children move out of the house, her marriage may end, and she may lose confidence that she's still that wonderful, exciting, and desirable person she once knew she was.

Among the most important of these changes is the transition through perimenopause, a time when women's hormone levels decline, just as they rose during the adolescent years. At some point close to age 50, we will experience menopause itself—the so-called "change of life," when our period stops. We haven't reached menopause until our period has not occurred for 12 consecutive months, and until that happens, we still can get pregnant.

Menopause is a stage of life all women share. However, recent studies have shown that the experience of menopause is different among different racial groups. Black women have more estrogen-related symptoms (hot flashes, night sweats, vaginal dryness, urine leakage) than any other women. Additionally, Black women are less likely to have somatic symptoms (headaches, difficulty sleeping, racing heart, stiffness and soreness in joints) than women of other ethnic groups. While many women find the ending of their period to be a relief, freeing them from the fear of becoming pregnant and other burdens such as the heavy bleeding associated with fibroids, other women grieve what they perceive as the loss of their femininity. Society will begin to see menopausal women as "older" now, and sexually less desirable. However, Black women, tend to have a more positive attitude toward menopause and are less likely to experience depression.

According to the findings from the 10-city research study on midlife women, many Black women noted that they were satisfied with aging and looked forward to a better life during this stage. Yet at the same time they were not attuned to their vulnerability to risky sexual behaviors—and misunderstood risk can be deadly. AIDS, which many think of as a young person's problem, is the third-leading cause of death for Black women aged 35–44 and the fourth-leading cause for Black women between 45 and 54.

All sex is risky sex—at any age, with anyone, same sex or not," Dr. Achong reminds us. "When you have sex, you're having sex with all of the people he's having sex with. You only know what you're doing; you don't know what he's doing. I'd even say that sex is risky in a so-called monogamous relationship."

"I didn't use protection with a guy I just met, but he was only 23; it was new and exciting, I was turned on that he was younger and I was in the heat of the moment," said Perry, age 49. "My attitude was, 'Who says I have to use a condom? I'm older and I'm having a good time.'"

No problem with the May–September thing, but Perry and her partner should have used precautions. Denial of this kind is common among Black women, who in the focus groups and the health survey of over 600 Black women, identify HIV/AIDS as the greatest health risk in our community, but not a risk for themselves. The truth is that it is a risk—for any and all women. The epidemic gained its foothold during the 1980s and early 1990s, when our community wrongly believed that AIDS was a disease that affected only White gay men, or the four H's—the homosexuals, hookers, heroin addicts, and hemophiliacs—who public health officials first told us were at risk. People became infected and unknowingly gave it to others. And HIV, like other STDs, spreads throughout people's sexual social networks.

Once an STD is introduced anywhere in a network of people with overlapping sexual partners, any individual's risk of encountering the disease increases dramatically. All it takes is one person not using a condom one time for the disease to begin its spread. And many middle-aged women, like Perry, reenter the dating scene as though it's still the 1970s.

"Of course, reality hit me afterward," Perry continued. "I was angry at myself. I'm a nurse; I should have known better. I didn't know this guy. A long time ago, people didn't use protection; it's too dangerous to roll like that now. It's been on my mind heavily. I'm too afraid to get tested."

Violence and Abuse

Violence is a major problem in the United States and can take many forms, including domestic or intimate partner violence, sexual assault and abuse, dating violence, and elder abuse. It especially affects women, of all backgrounds and ages. Violence can have terrible and costly results for everyone involved: the women themselves, their families, communities, and society. For Black women, the statistics are shocking. According to the National Violence Against Women survey, almost 1 in 3 Black women has been subject to intimate partner violence—rape, physical assault, threats, or emotional abuse. With abuse so pervasive in our community, beginning young and continuing until late in life, it's a wonder that Black women can remain sane while under siege. We do know that many women are known not to get the services they need to protect themselves.

There is little data on violence against women in midlife, unlike on adolescents and young adults. This may be the time when Black women have their armor up, are embarrassed, or have been socialized to be strong and silent. What is known is that unintentional injuries are one of the leading causes of death across the lifespan, including in midlife. What is not known is why Black women are disproportionately affected, but according to the CDC, several factors—drug or alcohol abuse, exposure to violence as a child, and unemployment, with the stress it brings—can increase the risk of violence or abuse.

"I just didn't feel worthy. I was just petrified to open my mouth," says Johnnie Ruth, age 53, of the years after her stepfather molested her in her early teens. "But I always felt that there was something inside of me that I wanted to get out. I was determined to find my voice. For many, many years I would make myself do things to improve myself. At community college I would take public speaking. I would do lots of little things to make myself victorious. I was well into my adulthood—about 40—when I finally found my voice."

Tobacco and Substance Use

Smoking is the #1 cause of preventable death in the United States, causing over 393,000 deaths per year—and Blacks overall are more likely to develop and die from lung cancer than people of any other racial or ethnic group. Compared to White Americans, Black Americans overall are at increased risk for lung cancer, even though they smoke about the same amount; the lung cancer incidence rate for Black women is roughly *equal* to that of White women, despite the fact that they smoke less. [19]

According to the American Lung Association, smoking potentially harms almost every organ in the human body. In addition to lung cancer, it is a main cause of chronic obstructive pulmonary disease (COPD, including chronic bronchitis and emphysema). It is also a cause of coronary heart disease, stroke, and a host of other cancers and diseases.[20] Black people suffer disproportionately from these other deadly and preventable diseases associated with smoking as well.[21]

Young Black women are less likely than their peers of other backgrounds to start lighting up—but for women who began smoking during their youth, the risks are serious. Many start trying to quit at some point during their midlife years, a difficult process that takes on average, many years and multiple attempts before they succeed—if, in fact, they do.

When it comes to alcohol, Black women generally partake in moderation. A large number do not touch the stuff. Research shows that depending upon their age group, between 45 and 60 percent of Black women abstain from drinking altogether; about 35 percent drink infrequently; and between 2 and 8 percent are heavy drinkers. By age 40, the majority of Black women do not drink at all. Some research suggests that religious values and active participation in church communities help protect Black women from alcohol's downside.[22]

"I drank when I was in college and when I went clubbing as a young adult," says 53-year-old Nisa. "But when I turned 35, it was like overnight my body couldn't take it anymore. I'd drag for a couple of days, and who has time for that? Plus I wanted to treat my body like the temple I know that it is. So that was the end of my two-margarita nights."

About 4 percent of American adults smoke marijuana, a rate that has held relatively steady over the years. But one study found that while the percentage of Black females who smoke marijuana decreases between the ages of 30 and 44, as it does in many populations, our use increases significantly between ages 45 and 64—in our middle years—quite possibly as a means of relieving stress, which is not as innocuous as it may sound. Many Black women tend not to think of stress as a health condition or health issue, when in fact it can be one of the most reliable indicators of how healthy we are.

The Emotional Tightrope

In the Imperative surveys and the 10-city focus groups, Black women ages 35 to 54 reported experiencing the most stress of any midlife age group. Those who had the least stress were either 55 or older or earning over $100,000 per year. Of the Black women who reported having experienced a "very stressful" or "extremely stressful" week, only 5 percent felt that they handled stress "well," while two-thirds reported handling stress "somewhat well" or "not well" at all.

Stress plays a significant role in determining our mental and emotional well-being. It can cause us to become angry or depressed, for instance. Unfortunately, we tend not to take care of our emotional needs, even though our state of mind plays such an important role in determining how happy and healthy we are.

"If you're not balanced in your mind and in your emotional state—if you're not whole—it makes it difficult for any health message to penetrate," says Dr. Achong. Chronic health problems can also impact our emotional well-being, making us feel fearful, anxious, and out of control. In fact, research shows that 51- to 61-year-olds with chronic conditions are more likely than the general population in that age range to rate their emotional health as being "fair" or "poor."

At this stage of life, women may be watching their own children come of age in a world that's not always welcoming or even safe. Many women feel unable to protect their children from the disappointments and assaults that accompany racism and sexism. Still others fear losing their children—and particularly their sons—to drugs and street violence.

"You worry every time they leave the house," says Vanessa, a mother of four, including two sons, ages 16 and 19. "No matter how good you train them, you never know who they're gonna run with or what they'll get caught up in. I'm always scared that this could be the night that he's not going to come home."

"I know I am threading a needle trying to get my son to manhood alive," says Nicole, whose home in a middle-class Black neighborhood wracked by the foreclosure crisis now backs up to a drug house that the police ignore. "I will protect him no matter what."

On the positive side, it is during middle-age that some of us begin to work toward healing from the hurts and losses that we suffered in our youth. In the words of best-selling author, Iyanla Vanzant, "At every single moment, we are given the opportunity to choose our future." During midlife, many women are choosing to deal with their losses and define their future.

"I'm seeing that there is some recognition that people have to do something about their own mental health or they're going to lose it," says therapist Pamela Freeman. "There is more recognition that good mental health is desirable and they want it."

"A lot of women are reflecting when they are in their 40s and 50s on things that happened when they were in college," says Dr. Achong. "Women don't have to be imprisoned by that, but women don't believe that women are plagued by past hurts in a lot of ways."

As many Black women reach the upper end of midlife, they experience one benefit of having children younger—the joy of seeing their family tree grow by an additional generation. But these days they also experience a backlash of sorts as many enter into what is now called, not the sandwich, but the "club sandwich" generation: caring for aging parents, their own children, and their children's children.

"Let me say this: I love my grandchildren," says Geraldine, 58, of St. Louis, "but I sure will be glad when my daughter finishes her schooling and I don't have to spend all my evenings and weekends shuttling my grandchildren around to games."

"I am just disgusted that my daughter can't get it together," says Angela, 62, "But she will not be exposing my grandchildren to any more street life than they've already seen. I don't have the money and I hadn't planned on it, but they will never live with her as long as she's in the state she's in." Angela is raising two granddaughters, ages 11 and 13, and a grandson, age 7, all with different fathers and half- and step-siblings, who are in and out of her home. "I worked my way up from the factory floor and into management," she says. "I paid for my little house and put away a little so I could enjoy my retirement—and now this!"

In fact, a disproportionate percentage of Black women during their adult years are challenged by the need to "re-parent," raising their grandchildren as their own, while their children struggle with drugs, alcohol, mental illness, or return to school. Those who expected a more traditional life, perhaps a simpler life, may find themselves working two jobs to meet the financial challenges of re-parenting. Managing this stress has to be part of the plan to be healthy and happy. As one psychiatrist puts it, there is no such thing as a stress-free woman. To be healthy and happy requires managing stress, not expecting to eliminate it, but not allowing it to dominate our lifes either.

Living the Spirit

Although Angela was not in control of her life due to family obligations, many midlife Black women do express a sense of being satisfied generally and being spiritually connected. Sixty percent believe that that their life is meaningful, that it has a purpose, and that they see a bright future ahead of them. Of particular note, yet to no one's surprise, they believe in prayer and are spiritually aware and engaged. Drive through a Black community on a Sunday morning and you'll see middle-aged Black women walking down streets, riding in cars, and standing at bus stops in their Sunday best, going to church.

Middle-aged Black women form the bedrock of the Black church, filling the pews, contributing their tithes, and holding positions of leadership, though not often the pulpit. In addition to being a place in which we praise God, express our appreciation for our lives, and pray for Divine intervention, churches and spiritual communities give many of us the opportunity to experience aspects of ourselves that the outside world may not appreciate: the heart to serve others.

Many Black women attend a traditional church, but as they mature, they often learn to appreciate less traditional ways of worshipping God. "I wake up at 4:00 in the morning to meditate," says music teacher Carolyn, 41. "That early morning time, before anybody's up and the dew is rising, is a powerful time to commune with Spirit."

Erica says, "I go walking in my neighborhood park as often as I can get there. I walk four miles, then go sit down by a stream that runs near my home and just listen to the sound of the water and the birds singing and talk to God. It's amazing when you get away from all the houses and cars and people and just go sit quietly where you can really see God's handiwork and the seasons change."

There are as many ways to manage the stress in our lives, as many places to seek peace and solitude, as there are hours in the day. It is important for each of us to find what works best for us so that we are able to focus on our health. What we all know in our hearts is that in order to succeed, we must have a "plan of action"—and when it comes to our health that means knowing what is happening with and to our bodies.

Why Prevention Is Better Than Cure: Recommended Midlife Screenings

Among women with health insurance, almost 40 percent of Black women have plans that offer a significant number of preventive screenings—Pap smears, breast cancer, cholesterol, diabetes/pre-diabetes, etc. Yet over half of Black women the Imperative polled did not know whether their health insurance covered such screenings. Of the ones who were not certain, over half did not know if HIV/AIDS tests were covered—even though Black women in general say they view it as the number-one threat to the well-being of our community. Almost half did not know if weight-loss counseling was covered, though they say they're concerned about becoming obese and developing weight-related diseases. One-quarter did not know if diabetes or cholesterol screenings were covered. Clearly there's a disconnect between what we say we worry about and our willingness to take responsibility for what we need to do about it. Over 22 percent of the women said they were not motivated to maintain or improve their health, and almost as many said that they did not have time.

When we do know that our insurance plan offers some preventive screenings, we tend not to know exactly which tests are covered. The more negatively we view our health, the less likely we are to know what our health benefits are. Perhaps our fear of what we will learn causes us not to want to know what's happening—like Evilene in the movie *The Wiz*: "Don't nobody bring me no bad news." But if we have some condition or disease, it's in our body whether we have received a formal diagnosis or not. When we know what we're dealing with, we become empowered to care for ourselves in ways that can restore us to health or prevent the condition from progressing.

"I was very stubborn because I wasn't trying to accept the changes they were telling me about and different food-eating and all of that," says Henrietta. "So when I would go to my doctor, he said, 'Ms. Jones, you have to do these things I'm telling you to do.' He said: 'You want to live? You want that son? You want to see those grandchildren?' I said yes. He said, 'Well, you have to do what you've got to do. Diabetes is very serious.' Immediately they put me on insulin."

Taking care of ourselves can contribute greatly to our peace of mind. One focus group member offered the following account of her experience after her diabetes screening (blood-glucose or A1c screening): "So I went to all the classes. I had a very good diabetes teacher. She taught me real well, and I would go see my doctors every three months. They would ask me questions. We'd be asking so many questions and we'd be talking and asking him everything. He always wanted me to try to get my A1c down, and finally I got it all the way down: It was a 12, and I'm now down to an 8. I just went to see him just this Thursday, and he fussed at me because he wanted my A1c to be lower than 8. So I said okay. The last time I had an appointment I got all my pills and everything, so all my doctors are wonderful."

Even as we dye our hair, pamper our skin, shimmy into our Spanx, and otherwise fight back the signs of aging, the way we take care of ourselves—body, mind, and spirit—during midlife largely dictates what our lives will be like as we move into elderhood. Now is the time for midlife women to map their plan for good health. We deserve it!

RECOMMENDED HEALTH SCREENINGS AND VACCINATIONS
MIDLIFE ADULT WOMEN 40–49

SCREENING TEST	WHEN TO GET THE TEST
GENERAL HEALTH	
Full checkup, including weight and height	Discuss with your health-care provider.
Thyroid (TSH) test	Discuss with your health-care provider.
HIV test	Get this test at least once to find out your HIV status. Ask your health-care provider if and when you need the test again.
HEART HEALTH	
Blood pressure test	At least every two years
Cholesterol test	Discuss with your health-care provider.
BONE HEALTH	
Bone density screen	Discuss with your health-care provider.
DIABETES	
Blood glucose or A1c test	Every three years.
BREAST HEALTH	
Mammogram (x-ray of breast or digital mammography)	Every 1–2 years discuss with your health-care provider.
Clinical breast exam	Yearly
Breast self-examination	Perform breast self-examinations at the same time each month.
REPRODUCTIVE HEALTH	
Pap test	Every three years
Pelvic exam	Yearly
Chlamydia test	Get this test if you have new or multiple partners.

Sexually transmitted infection (STI) tests	Both partners should get tested for STIs, including HIV, before initiating sexual intercourse.
MENTAL HEALTH SCREENING	Discuss with your health-care provider.
COLORECTAL HEALTH (USE OF THESE THREE METHODS)	
Fecal occult blood test	Yearly
Flexible sigmoidoscopy (with fecal occult blood test)	Every five years
Colonoscopy	Every 10 years
EYE AND EAR HEALTH	
Comprehensive eye exam	Get a baseline exam at age 40, then every 2–4 years or as your doctor advises.
Hearing test	Every 10 years
SKIN HEALTH	
Mole exam	Monthly mole self-exam and an exam by a health-care provider as part of a routine full checkup.
ORAL HEALTH	
Dental exam	Routinely; discuss with your dentist.
IMMUNIZATIONS	
Influenza vaccine	Discuss with your health-care provider.
Tetanus-diphtheria-pertussis booster vaccine	Every 10 years

RECOMMENDED HEALTH SCREENINGS AND VACCINATIONS
MIDLIFE ADULT WOMEN 50–64

SCREENING TEST	WHEN TO GET THE TEST
GENERAL HEALTH	
Full checkup, including weight and height	Discuss with your health-care provider.
Thyroid (TSH) test	Discuss with your health-care provider.
HIV test	Get this test at least once to find out your HIV status. Ask your health-care provider if and when you need the test again.
HEART HEALTH	
Blood pressure test	At least every two years
Cholesterol test	Start at age 20; discuss with your health-care provider.
BONE HEALTH	
Bone density screen	Discuss with your health-care provider.
DIABETES	
Blood glucose or A1c test	Start at age 45, then every three years.
BREAST HEALTH	
Mammogram (x-ray of breast or digital mammography)	Every 1–2 years discuss with your health-care provider.
Clinical breast exam	Yearly
Breast self-examination	Perform breast self-examinations at the same time each month.
REPRODUCTIVE HEALTH	
Pap test	Every three years
Pelvic exam	Yearly
Chlamydia test	Get this test if you have new or multiple partners.

Sexually transmitted infection (STI) tests	Both partners should get tested for STIs, including HIV, before initiating sexual intercourse.
MENTAL HEALTH SCREENING	Discuss with your health-care provider.
COLORECTAL HEALTH (USE OF THESE THREE METHODS)	
Fecal occult blood test	Yearly beginning at age 45
Flexible sigmoidoscopy (with fecal occult blood test)	Every five years
Colonoscopy	Every 10 years
EYE AND EAR HEALTH	
Comprehensive eye exam	Every 2–4 years until age 55, then every 1–3 years until age 65, or as your doctor advises.
Hearing test	Every three years
SKIN HEALTH	
Mole exam	Monthly mole self-exam and an exam by a health-care provider as part of a routine full checkup.
ORAL HEALTH	
Dental exam	Routinely; discuss with your dentist.
IMMUNIZATIONS	
Influenza vaccine	Discuss with your health-care provider.
Tetanus-diphtheria-pertussis booster vaccine	Every 10 years
Herpes zoster vaccine (to prevent shingles)	Starting at age 60, one time only. Ask your health-care provider if it is okay for you to get it.

Chapter 4

Mature Adults

(65+)

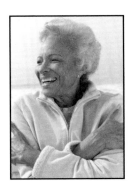

As mature adult Black women journey through their mid-60s and beyond, many begin to joyously reap the benefits of having come into full possession of themselves in midlife—developing new attitudes about life and new relationships, getting their annual checkups, setting new goals, updating their skills. Others face a frustrating and preventable downward spiral physically, emotionally, and spiritually, particularly those of us who ignored the early warning signs and postponed prioritizing our health and well-being. Those who made a deal with the devil by putting off yesterday's wellness goals until tomorrow or making our own legitimate health needs second to the needs of others are now faced with the inevitable bill for our decisions.

During this final stage of life, experiences of unexpected loss and isolation abound. There's the loss of our legendary "can-do," strong-Black-woman superpowers, as well as a loss of self-confidence, especially as our physical appearance and strength start to diminish. Those who were married often lose their spouses. Single heads of households must cope with the loss of being the alpha woman—the one who calls the shots and sets the standards for the family. Whether confronting the end of our work lives, with loss of professional status and influence in the wider community—older Black women sometimes feel like the game is rigged. Our support network may weaken as our peers, too, find themselves ill and alone; or simply hard pressed to manage daily life, let alone make decisions about health.

In times past, as people became elders in their families and communities, they were valued more, not less—respected for their struggles and sacrifices, achievements, the wisdom they had gained and the new generations they had birthed. But in 21st-century America, including Black America, becoming a senior citizen often signals a loss in social value. Older Americans are increasingly becoming throwaways in our society, diminished to stereotypes of incapacity, drains on Social Security, overentitled to Medicare, and irrelevant to the new world order. In Black communities, female elders are no longer revered as the indomitable matriarchs and focal points of extended families; many have been left behind by children who migrate to other cities, or may find themselves overburdened with children and grand-children unable to stand on their own two feet. Although often older Black women remained relatively invisible to mainstream society, they have played critical roles in their families and communities. Consequently, the loss of the authority and influence that have defined their lives hits particularly hard.

In this time of life, far too many of us find ourselves trapped in bodies and circumstances that we never realized we were creating. Health issues such as arthritis, high blood pressure, high cholesterol, diabetes, and heart disease—often associated with carrying excess weight—begin to dictate what we can and cannot do and significantly reduce the quality of our lives. Many women who get sick will need more and more medications and may not have the means to pay for them. At the same time, an increasing number of women in this life stage start to look at health issues with new clarity and candor.

One focus group member voiced her concerns from this insightful perspective: "Physicians give us too many psychiatric referrals when we have health problems, too many operations like hysterectomies and too many drugs for pain."

Another participant put it this way: "What I know is that my health is my responsibility and my illness is, too."

"Truth in good health comes from how we feel about ourselves," said a third.

Of course, there is always another side to the coin. Those fortunate enough to learn self-care early enter the golden years feeling healthy and vibrant, able to live full and exciting lives. "I was walking down the street and this sister came up to me and said, 'I just wanna say, you look amazing!'"says Tammie, age 69, a mother of three and the matriarch of a large extended family. "She probably looked at me and said, 'She has gray hair, she is an old woman who has taken care of herself, her skin looks good.' I get those kind of compliments all the time, so I know that there's power in eating right and taking care of yourself, your mind, your body."

As our culture as a whole redefines aging, mature Black women are becoming an integral part of "igniting the soulful side of 60." This age group is determined to not be shoved into a closet or sentenced to a wheelchair or a nursing home to spend its final days. There is a revolutionary spirit afoot and a determination to embrace the feisty side of 65 by modernizing our notions of what it means to "grow older." In fact, if we have made it to age 65, it is very probable that we will live to enjoy another 18 years on earth, fulfilling the average life expectancy for mature Black women of 83.7 years. Mature Black women recognize that the degree to which we remain in control of our lives as we age depends on our ability to create and activate a new life plan.

"At my age, the only time I have left is time to live the good life. That's only going to happen when I understand that my wealth is not defined by my 401(k) balance—'my true wealth is my health,'" says Victoria, age 66. "Girlfriend, I'm ready to strut my stuff because 65 is the new 45! I refuse to go out with a whimper. I'm going out with a bang!"

As older and wiser Black women get clear about the price we have paid for neglecting ourselves, we often try to warn younger generations not to fall into the traps that waylaid us. "My daughter really pushes herself too hard. Sometimes I have to tell her to relax," says Constance, 71, the mother of two 30-somethings. But the important truth is that we can learn this lesson at any age: it's never too late to start taking care of ourselves. Each spoonful of daily intervention can add up to an overflowing cup of revitalization and well-being restored.

Even if we are already experiencing chronic health problems, taking multiple medications, or sometimes struggling to muster up enough energy to get through a particularly hard day, we can reclaim ownership of our bodies and our health-care. Just as importantly, we can finally rediscover for ourselves the joy in life that emanates directly from self-care.

JUST THE FACTS

Population:

2.1 million

9 percent of Black females

Life expectancy:

83.7 (at age 65)

Top causes of death (ages 65 to 74):

1.	Cancer	30%
2.	Heart disease	26%
3.	Diabetes	7%
4.	Stroke	7%
5.	Kidney disease	3%

Top chronic conditions (ages 65 to 74):

1.	Arthritis
2.	Diabetes
3.	Heart disease
4.	Coronary artery disease
5.	Stroke

Source: CDC. Office of Women's Health, Accessed, April 2011.

This chapter profiles the experiences of older Black Women, ages 65+, those identified as the "hybrid Black Civil Rights generation" of women, as they transition to a new identity. Because so little mainstream, evidence-based research has been done on this special group, we rely largely on unpublished findings from the Imperative's health surveys over the years, along with information gleaned from focus groups on chronic illnesses in Philadelphia, polls, and the Health-Wise Woman programs. Out of these groundbreaking studies, we gain insight into how older women with chronic diseases feel about their health and their health-care. We also share candid conversations with Black women from around the country who talk about the quality of their lives and the range of their health-care needs.

The Civil Rights Generation:
The Silent Generation/Traditionalists and the Early Baby Boomers

The Civil Rights generation in America, like many powerful social movements, reflects the contributions of visionary leaders and fearless young Turks. The "hybrid Black Civil Rights generation" comprises two distinct demographic groups: the vanguard of Silent Generation or Traditionalists, born between 1925 and 1945, and activist Baby Boomers, born between 1946 and 1964. And of course, there are a few prominent older individuals who fall outside these strict demographics who paved the way for the modern Civil Rights movement. [1]

Members of the Civil Rights advance guard included extraordinary men such as Dr. Martin Luther King, Jr., Malcolm X, Harry Belafonte, and James Baldwin, and unsung women like Dr. Dorothy Height, Fannie Lou Hamer, Shirley Chisholm, and Barbara Jordan. These social, political, and cultural pioneers were often born into families that literally had nothing (or had lost whatever they did have in the Depression) and came of age in a society poised to undergo seismic change.

Although the Silent Generation has been known for its relatively low impact on American society compared to its predecessors, the so-called Greatest Generation (World War II), and those who came afterwards—the Baby Boomers—in the Black community, this generation was anything but silent. It was this generation of Blacks that spearheaded the modern Civil Rights movement, a revolution that changed America and established a model for social justice that would be emulated around the world. They pushed open the doors of discrimination, walked through with dignity, and held fast until they caught the first glimpses of equal opportunity that the revolution made possible.

Members of the Silent Generation were the products of traditional values. They were seen as hardworking, disciplined, civic-minded, and self-sacrificing. They believed that marriage was for life and that unions protected their workers; they lived in the shadow of both the Korean and Vietnam conflicts. As this heroic generation confronted the American legal and judicial establishment, individually and collectively, it demonstrated unprecedented amounts of courage and determination. Then, as the movement gained momentum, the Silent Generation was joined on the frontlines of sit-ins, protest marches, and boycotts by the initial wave of Baby Boomers, the first generation raised on TV.

The Silent Generation's activist credentials were established by the creation of the Southern Christian Leadership Conference (SCLC). However, the movement was put on steroids when "why we can't wait" Baby Boomers like Stokely Carmichael and Jesse Jackson of the Student Non-Violent Coordinating Committee (SNCC) and other young radicals challenged the power structure. Optimistic, driven, and team-oriented Black Baby Boomers and the disciplined, self-sacrificing Silent Generation with whom they joined hands believed that they could and should change the world. Today these world changers are the elders of our community.

Black women of the Civil Rights era were the breakthrough generation. They came of age in complicated times and they lived on the cutting edge of the civil rights, Black power, and women's consciousness movements. As race and gender roles and entrenched attitudes were radically transformed, many Black women benefited from the gains won at every level of society. This created a space for Black women's health advocacy in the '80s and the birth of the National Black Women's Health Project, now known as the Black Women's Health Imperative.

Today as we contemplate the health status of our elders, we are more aware that many everyday Black women, those who marched and protested, are today the most vulnerable among us. These women were unable to take care of themselves for many reasons: they were working to fulfill the dream of an integrated society, pursuing unprecedented job opportunities, raising families, tending to their husbands and homes, building and stabilizing our communities, and figuring out how to remain sane and available for all those who depended on them. Their families needed them. Their jobs were essential to their survival and sense of self. The church was their bedrock—it sustained them in good times and in the deepest dark hours. These are the women we focus on in this section—the first generation to be caught up in the cultural myth of being the "Black superwoman."

Economic Realities

When the Civil Rights generation entered the workforce, discrimination was still rampant and opportunities for stable, fair-paying employment were scarce. The disparities that Black people of this generation encountered in the labor market put them at a long-term economic disadvantage, leaving our elders in a relatively powerless position in what ought to be their "golden" years.

Today's Black elders may have once dreamed of the same stress-free retirement that their White peers looked forward to, but for many the reality has been quite different. "It's a big disappointment for some people that they don't have their lives at a point where they can retire," says Gail Wyatt, Ph.D., a UCLA psychology professor. "It's perfectly acceptable not to retire—for very good reasons. But people get resentful if they think they're supposed to be retired and they are not. Black people don't meet the same markers of other groups for a lot of different reasons."

Not least among those reasons: Black women's plans for their elder years are often derailed when they face the necessity of re-parenting, taking on the burdens of supporting children all over again although their own children are grown. "Many times they're taking on more work to deal with the financial challenges," says Dr. Wyatt. The majority of Black women do want to retire, she explains, in part because work for them is often a job, rather than a career that's likely to continue engaging them into old age. When they cannot stop working because they need the paycheck, it's tough: "If your expectation is for a traditional life, it brings on a lot of dissatisfaction and depression."

Most American seniors live on a fixed income, and almost 30 percent live on an income under 200 percent of the poverty line—that is, $20,578 for an individual or $25,964 for a couple. However, the average income of those 65 or older without a high school diploma was $16,471 in 2009 versus $25,000-plus for those with an education ranging from a high school diploma to an associate's degree,[2] almost $43,000 for those with a bachelor's degree, and $62,163 for those with a graduate degree. About 36 percent receive a pension, over half receive interest income, and 22 percent receive dividend income.[3]

The median income in 2009 was a little under $15,000 for Black women, compared to $19,161 for Black men. A distressing 23 percent of Black elders live below the poverty line—a little less than $11,000 in 2011—almost three times as many as Whites.[4] More than 76 percent of Black seniors do not have sufficient financial resources to meet their estimated lifetime expenses. Health-care expenses that balloon as we age, especially on top of a life-time of self-neglect, consume 34 percent of our monthly income—a figure that's rising. Our housing expenses are high, and 44 percent of us either rent our homes or have no equity in homes we own.

For older women, a whopping 17 percent of us in 2009 lived in poverty; more than half of us lived primarily off of our measly Social Security check in 2010.

Fewer than 25 percent of Black seniors receive interest income, compared to over half of their White peers. About 22 percent of White seniors receive dividend income, but less than six percent of Black elders do. And here's a sobering fact to top it off: thanks to the economic downturn in the late 2000s, people who are retired now are actually *better* prepared financially than the generations coming after them are likely to be.[5]

Rocky finances aren't just bad for our peace of mind; they are hazardous to our health. A primary concern for Black women in this age group is that they cannot afford medical plans that are adequate to address their costly health needs. Among many women, there's a sense that insurance companies are running the show and dictating their care. "You've got to have that $20 co-pay, so sometimes that keeps you from going to a doctor," says 71-year-old Mamie.

Wellness and wealth do tend to be closely intertwined, and the connection makes it hard on our elders, says Aisha Young, president and CEO of African American in Gerontology. "Poverty is generational. If you've never known anything else, it's normal. And if you were born during or shortly after the Depression, it's been that way for a long time. For unhealthy black elders, it's often a socioeconomic status thing."

What about older Black women whose lives haven't followed this model—Black women who rose to high levels in corporate America, academic institutions, and the federal government, and had the emotional and social discipline to stay there? These are the small number of women who were able to achieve a higher standard of living, higher incomes, bigger houses, travel, fine clothes, and luxury cars. While we can fairly safely assume that all of them had health insurance and consistent care and got their annual well-woman exams, many of them were not able to put their health and wellness at the top of their priority list either. In fact, during those high-income-producing and connecting years, when life was good and their social status was high, health took a backseat. Now, in their senior years, they may have the resources for a comfortable retirement, but they too often lack a cushion of good health to fall back on.

Marriage and Family

The Silent Generation was raised with time-honored values that it has tended to retain; most of its members married and stayed married. "In my generation they stayed together no matter what," says Anne, age 76. Of course, married couples accumulate financial assets more readily than singles do, and they are known to have better emotional health. The reality is that Black women have a longer life expectancy than Black men—by almost five years— and when widowed, since we generally have fewer assets than White women to support ourselves, many of us are unprepared to face our remaining years alone.[6]

Prepared or not, a substantial number of us will be alone. In 2008, 25 percent of older Black women lived with their spouses, 32 percent lived with other relatives, 2 percent lived with non-relatives, and 42 percent lived by themselves. By contrast, 54 percent of older Black men lived with their spouses, 11 percent lived with other relatives, 4 percent lived with non-relatives, and 30 percent lived alone.[7]

Many older Black women take pride in the ability to stay independent—a stark contrast with our more communal roots, in which multiple generations often lived in one house. "Integration was the best and worst thing to happen to African Americans," Aisha Young declares. "With integration came the desire to assimilate. Before that we generally had multigenerational households and elders had roles in our families. But with assimilation we began to move across country and 'I-live-my-life-and-you-do-your thing; I'll-get-with-you-in-July.'"

Setting the Stage for Good Health

As older Black women, how healthy are we really? Listen to these women from focus groups conducted over the past 15 years:

"I have a bunch of stuff—arthritis, osteoporosis, and scoliosis," says one.

"I have lupus and I've had poliomyelitis, which is a weakness of all your joints," says another.

"I have diabetes and I have some upper respiratory problems that I use an inhaler for," says a third, "but overall I think that I'm basically healthy."

Did that last one surprise you? It's not a fluke. The truth is that nearly all the women who rattled off these diseases and disorders—and there were many more—also said that they thought of themselves as basically healthy.

This disconnect is well documented. In 2008, 61 percent of Black women and men ages 65 and older reported being in good health.[8] In one of the few surveys on Black women ages 50 and older conducted by the National Center on Women and Aging, 60 percent of participants said that they had difficulty or limitations in activities such as housework or exercising and were receiving disability checks. This means that only 40 percent of participants weren't having physical problems—quite a difference from the 61 percent who said they were in good health.

How can so many of us have a positive perception of our health when a reduced quality of life slaps us in the face every day? To put it bluntly, Black women say that we are doing okay, but we are not. Our rates of diabetes, heart disease, and disability are astronomical, but when people poll us, we invariably rank our health as good or excellent. Either doing poorly has become normative for us, or we just don't want to let on.

This section explores the little information we know about the health of the Civil Rights generation. In laying out the issues that face this often invisible group, we will show how the cultural myth of the strong Black woman collided with the reality of our experiences as the decisions we made during middle age follow us into older age.

Denial: Not Just a River in Egypt

When we take a sweeping look at Black women's lives, we see the paradox of Black women perceiving themselves in good health, yet acknowledging their struggles with everything from obesity to chronic pain to autoimmune disorders. The women of the hybrid Civil Rights generation have been mothers, daughters, wives, partners, workers, and now they must face growing old. A large proportion of our elders have at least one chronic health condition, and many are overwhelmed with them. Among the most common: hypertension (84 percent), diagnosed arthritis (53 percent), diabetes (29 percent), all types of heart disease (27 percent), sinusitis (15 percent), and cancer (13 percent). The excess weight that many of us have been carrying for years contributes to our disproportionately high rates of hypertension, arthritis, and diabetes. And once you have diabetes, your risk of dying from heart disease increases dramatically.

This gap between our perception and our reality has a number of possible explanations. To hear some women tell it, doctors do not get the bad news across effectively, whether because they have low expectations of us—perhaps they fear we cannot handle the truth or don't trust us to implement the necessary changes. Or perhaps they do not have the skill or the heart to be the messenger of bad news. It could be that the overall well-being of the Black community has created a "new normal" of compromised or poor health: if we are measuring ourselves against other members of a community in which it seems everyone is sick, we are bound to think we are in pretty good shape by comparison.

It's also possible that a certain level of denial has become embedded in Black culture. According to Aisha Young of Blacks in Gerontology, one of the major health challenges we face is not understanding the severity of certain conditions or thinking that these things don't happen to Black people. "I never thought about diabetes," said one Philadelphia focus group participant in the Imperative's study on improving communications with health-care providers. "I've got glaucoma, and you hear about it, but then after that, you don't think it's going to be you."

The Paradigm Shift

Those of us who come into older age after a lifetime of self-neglect are more likely to develop a disease, suffer its complications, and die from it at a younger age than other women, including those Black women who began early to place their health first. All these changes take an emotional toll that's hard for many of us to handle, especially if we are not in the habit of taking care of our emotional selves either. Ultimately, during what should be our golden years, many of us are struggling, and our dignified, hardworking, self-sacrificing lives have taken a heartbreaking, yet highly preventable, turn.

The reality is that most of our health problems and risk factors could have been prevented, modified, or treated had we had the inclination, information, and resources to tend to them. For example, the National Diabetes Prevention Program has found that 20 minutes of moderate physical activity per day helps program participants lose 5 to 7 percent of their body weight, which lowers the risk of developing Type 2 diabetes by an astonishing 58 percent.[9] According to the Harvard School of Public Health physical activity recommendations walking briskly for even one to two hours a week (15 to 20 minutes a day) starts to decrease the chances of having a heart attack or stroke, developing diabetes, or dying prematurely.

As one focus-group participant put it, though, "You don't know what you don't know." If only someone had communicated this type of information to us with directness we could understand and compassion we could trust. If only someone had taken us by the hand, shown us what to do, walked alongside us, and kept us company as we changed our habits. If only someone had warned us how our lives might turn out if we did not.

But "if only" takes us only so far. What do we do about it now? "Our paradigm for changing is often 'if it's not broke, don't fix it.' But now it's broke, so how are you going to fix it?" asks Aisha Young of Blacks in Gerontology. There needs to be a paradigm shift—one that says "you can start very small and you can start wherever you are." "Say, for instance, you have diabetes," says Young. "Frying potatoes in lard and grease tastes good, but now try baking them."

Black women who took good care of themselves when they were younger are often living a dramatically different reality at this time of life. Their experience flies in the face of the common assumption that the words "Black," "old," and "chronically ill" go together like biscuits and gravy—and it can be a model for those of us who are getting a later start.

"When you eat certain things, you'll have more energy, you'll look better, you'll keep your weight down," says Tammie, the 68-year-old who talked about getting compliments on the street. "Now that I'm getting older, I see the wrinkles and my hair is gray. But I still feel energized and young and alive because I chose the right food throughout most of my life."

Tammie began to educate herself about healthy eating habits during her 20s, and as she learned how to take care of herself, she also taught her friends. "People would say, 'Go over to Tammie's; she knows how to cook. Ask Tammie about the herbs; ask Tammie about meditation.' So I taught a community of people, not even realizing that that's what I was doing. I was just sharing what I was learning and wanted other people to benefit and be healthy, too."

Research confirms that many older Black women like Tammie use herbal products and home remedies as part of their self-care. They are a source of alternate health information for friends and family. "They tell you what to do and what not to do and how to avoid any complications," says Gigi, Tammie's neighbor.

In the Imperative's focus groups, many older women discuss how important it is to "know what they don't know"—to educate themselves about their disorders and diseases so that they can embrace the changes they need to make and take responsibility for their own well-being. "There's no special 'I have to read this book,'" says Roxanne, age 69. "You know what to do and you know why. In this day and age, being in denial is unacceptable. It's not a secret anymore. You know you're supposed to get your yearly checkups; we know a lot more about how to eat. People in my generation know what to do."

"Keep up with yourself," 71-year-old Emily advised her 25-year-old friend. "Because when you're 25, you have so much in life and you don't worry about the things I worry about now. Is my skin clear? Is my skin getting wrinkled? Am I losing my hair? Now I try to keep up on those things—the Pap smear, the mammogram, I'm working on losing the weight. Girl, you need to educate yourself about yourself."

Rounding Those Dangerous Curves: Overweight and Obesity

If you have been carrying 20, 30, or 50 extra pounds for several decades, by the time you hit 60, your body is feeling the strain. Whether it causes diabetes or hypertension, arthritis that leads to a joint replacement, or simple exhaustion, obesity disables or severely limits many Black women, holding them back from participating fully in what could be the "golden" years. Even though we are aware of the price we pay for being so overweight, a good number of us seem not to be able to stop ourselves from almost literally eating ourselves to death.

"I'm unhealthy right now because I'm fighting a losing weight thing, and it's been a while," admits Annie, age 68, who began to lose her hold on her health back in her 30s, when she didn't shed the baby weight she'd gained during her last pregnancy. "It's hard because I have a problem with salt and junk food. I don't know what it is. I have high blood pressure, so I know I shouldn't really eat salt. But I just have this thing for salt."

"My girlfriend knows I love candy and she gives me my favorite kind," says Mae, age 70, who has been diabetic for 23 years. "I take it, but I know it's not good for me, see? We hurt our own selves because we don't do what we should do."

But that doesn't mean we have to give up on ourselves. Many older women are open to making changes. It's just that after a lifetime of living one way, some of us don't know how.

"Putting those things into practice, having the resources—they don't always know what to do," says gerontologist Young. "They'll tell you, 'I know I'm supposed to eat healthy. What do I need to do?' The resources are out there, but it requires self-management. You have to want the change."

Physical activity is an essential part of weight management—but with so many Black women overweight and obese at this age, many of us are not moving around as much as we should. "Right now I'm at the point where I eat well, but that's as far as it goes," one Philadelphia focus group woman shared. "Physically it's hard. If I can just get off the bed, get to work, and get back home, sit down, and then walk up the steps, I'm happy. That's as far as I can go right now."

Still, some women are able to become more active and find that they enjoy it and feel good about themselves even though it can be difficult. "We walk around this park like five times," said one focus group participant. "We started off three times, so we're doing pretty well."

For many women, fitness is a way to spend time with loved ones—and a chance to set a good example for the younger generation. Another woman in that focus group said, "I'm working on the exercising, me and my daughter and my grandbabies. I love it."

"Well, I go to the gym like three times a week," says Ruth, 70. "Sometimes I take a Tai Chi class; sometimes I lift some weights by myself; and sometimes—let me just be honest—I sit in the whirlpool. I may not look my age, but some days I feel it in my bones."

Since retiring, Ruth has made her self-care a priority. She consults part-time for extra money. She also volunteers for several weeks each year at a holistic health spa. "I might spend part of the day crying and cutting up onions, but I also get to go to workshops where I learn about my health." The new friends she makes at the spa keep in touch throughout the year and help encourage her to maintain her healthy lifestyle.

Sexual and Reproductive Health

Women are capable of being sexually active well into their senior years, but other factors can make sexual relationships difficult. Many of us are socialized to think we should not be having sex anymore, so even if we are in relationships, we may not be surprised when our partners seem uninterested.

Across the life stages, Black women face an even greater shortage of available partners than do our peers of other backgrounds. If we are not in a relationship and want to be, since the life expectancy of Black men is lower than that of Black women, we often end up alone. When we do enter sexual relationships, we may be surprised to discover that our partners have a hard time keeping pace: many older men have issues with their prostates, experience erectile dysfunction, or have other health problems that impede their ability to have sex. "If an older woman has a partner who's her peer, her partner may be struggling sexually," Dr. Wyatt says. "There's a lot of negotiating and frustration, because women are still able to enjoy sex but their partners may not be."

Chronic disease and other conditions can interfere with sexual performance and pleasure for women as well as men. "I was mad at my doctor about that, to tell the truth, because I wondered why and he never spoke of it," says one focus group participant of her experience with bladder cancer when she was 51. "My condition affected my sexual ability, so quite naturally it affected my relationships. But I was scared to say anything because I didn't want him to think I was a sex maniac or something like that. So I just went on with the program. As I got older I realized: Gee, I should have said something."

Senior sex doesn't necessarily mean safer sex—quite the opposite: when older Black women do have sex, we often do not have the skills to protect ourselves from modern perils. "A woman in her 60s has been socialized some 40 years ago or more for what the rest of the population calls dating, but she might call courting. She's totally unprepared for the 21st century," says Dr. Wyatt, herself in her mid-60s. "These are the women who were socialized to douche. They equate venereal disease—which is the word that they grew up with—with unclean, unsavory people, and they don't associate with those people, as far as they know. They have a lot to unlearn to take care of their own bodies."

The STD epidemic extends right through the elder years, as does the danger of HIV/ AIDS. Yet in spite of elders' unique vulnerabilities, HIV-prevention information doesn't take us into consideration or target us with meaningful messages. "They need information that incorporates where they are in their lives, not just telling them how to use condoms," says Dr. Wyatt, who also serves as the associate director of UCLA's AIDS Institute. "Most HIV prevention info doesn't acknowledge the religious, cultural, or age-dependent situations that women are in. We have to acknowledge the fact that if a woman is sexually inactive, she may become sexually active with someone she meets and not be prepared."

To protect ourselves, we need to talk about sex with our partners. But many older Black women don't talk about sex. If we are widowed or divorced, we probably didn't talk about it with our husbands, and our modesty or religious views may add to the restraint. Compounding matters, the characteristics that older Black women find desirable in a man are out of synch with the realities of many people's lives. "Older women don't ask the right questions," says Dr. Wyatt. "They are not going to be suspicious, especially if he's nicely dressed and well spoken, or if he goes to church. They're looking at those kinds of criteria instead of the ones women need to live in a world where sex can kill you."

Tobacco and Substance Use

Smoking cigarettes has been identified as the number one cause of preventable death and disability. While we take pride in knowing that we are not big smokers, the consequences of tobacco use are particularly devastating and perplexing to us. Lung cancer, heart disease and other smoking-related diseases are at the top of the deadly list for older Black women. How can that be?

Those of us who don't start smoking when we're younger tend not to start once we are adults. However, those who begin to smoke in middle age find that the hassles and stressors of being a mother, worker, and caregiver are getting in the way of being cigarette free. Since quitting smoking leads to weight gain, many Black women who are already overweight are often unwilling to trade one health risk for another.

Less than 10 percent of elderly Black women are current smokers—less than White women in any age group—although larger percentages are former smokers. With Black women less likely to smoke, why are Black women more likely to die from lung cancer than white women? Smoking is the biggest risk factor for lung cancer, and research suggests that Blacks who smoke are more likely to develop lung cancer than other smokers.[10]

Many smokers and former smokers get emphysema or chronic obstructive pulmonary disease (COPD). These are terrible ways to live your life, as they all make their sufferers feel as though they can't catch their breath, a sensation that some people liken to the sense that they are drowning.

Like smoking, anyone at any age can have a drinking problem. Aunt Gracie may have always had a drink socially, but now that she is alone after her husband's death—she needs a few drinks or more to get her through the day and night. Drinking can be a common problem among the elderly but just as common are families ignoring their older relative's or neighbor's drinking. Alcohol slows down brain activity and even more so for older women. Because alcohol affects alertness, judgment, coordination, and reaction time--drinking increases the risk of falls and accidents.

Older black adults have had a rate of past month alcohol use that was considerably lower than the national average of older adults 20.3 vs. 38.3 percent. (Figure 2). Their rates of binge alcohol use and illicit drug use, however, did not differ significantly from the national averages.

As people age, the body's ability to absorb and dispose of alcohol and other drugs changes. Like smoking, heavy alcohol consumption is associated with chronic health problems, such as liver cirrhosis.[11]

Since alcohol, is itself a drug, older Black women need to be aware of its harmful effects if mixed with prescription or over-the-counter medicines. This is a special problem for older Black women because they are often heavy users of prescription medicines and over-the-counter drugs.

Throughout their lives, older Black women have been exposed to elevated levels of individual and socioeconomic stressors, such as violence, undue burden of diseases and low wages. Being alone and unsure of what the next day will bring could very likely contribute to the slight increase in substance use, which makes them especially vulnerable.

Past Month Substance Use Among Black Adults Aged 65 or Older Compared with the National Average: 2004–2008

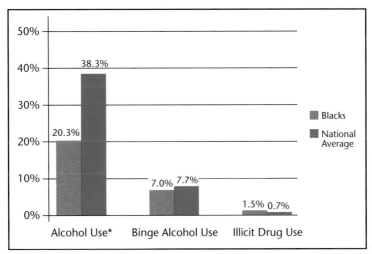

The difference between blacks and the national average is statistically significant at p < .05.

Source: 2004 to 2008 SAMHSA National Surveys on Drug Use and Health (NSDUHs).

The Emotional Tightrope

When we think of diseases of aging, such as heart disease or diabetes, we often consider their physical effect—getting tired when walking up the stairs or losing our vision, for instance. But chronic health conditions affect Black women emotionally as well. Of course, there's the natural fear that we experience when our bodies are out of control or behaving in ways that we don't understand. And then there are the adjustments and impediments that having a chronic condition often impose on our lives.

In fact, Black women with chronic conditions give the least positive assessment of their emotional well-being. Nearly 40 percent of Black women with arthritis report that their emotional health is fair or poor.[12] Whether or not we are suffering specifically in body, the very fact of aging can be hard for some of us to confront. "I think about the years that are gone and the things I could have done, and I mean it's just too late," laments Lilly, 68, a mother of three and grandmother of 11. "A lot of things it's just too late to do." Many Black women who suffer from chronic conditions feel this way, and it's a natural and understandable response—but it doesn't have to be a life sentence.

In this stage of life, we may become depressed or anxious over our diminished horizons or capacities, grieve the potential we didn't live up to, or feel betrayed by people who don't support us as much as we supported them. Eventually the pain may become so severe that we finally put our "strong Black woman" armor down so that we can get the support we need.

Barbara prided herself on not having to ask for anything from anyone. After she suffered a stroke and needed help more than ever, her children weren't available. "I finally broke down one day and just started crying," she admitted. "I said to my doctor, 'Look, I just don't know what to do.' And I think that's when our relationship changed. I said, 'There's so much that's going on, and I'm poppin' pills, and I'm trying to walk, and I can't get up in the morning. What is going on?'"

At that point, the doctor whom she hadn't trusted and whose direction she'd resisted just held her hand and promised to be there to help her.

"That was one thing I had to do for myself," Barbara recalls. "To finally break down and just say look, I need your help."

It is often understood that older Black women have been guided by a unique spiritual understanding for centuries. In fact, had it not been for older Black women's keen understanding and ability to connect with Spirit, it is doubtful that years of survival would have even been possible, given our history of oppression.

As our bodies age and our independence is reduced, we may become frustrated due to our growing need for the assistance of others: transportation to and from our places of worship become difficult; our ability to read our holy text becomes challenging as our eyesight weakens; and our physical strength may limit our mobility to express a praise dance, for example. While this may be discouraging, it is important to realize that our spiritual selves are infinitely awakened no matter our physical location. We can commune with Spirit through the stillness in our own homes or through receiving and sending love to people in our communities. Connecting with new people in our circles, allowing our family members to come visit us and help us with household chores, scrapbooking old photos, or even picking up a new hobby are all examples of how we can create a new peace of mind. It becomes more important as we age to realize that living in the spirit is truly about binding ourselves in the universe through intimacy and valuing our one-on-one human connections.

Why Prevention Is Better Than Cure: Recommended Later Life Screenings

About 95 percent of Black elders report that they have a usual source of health insurance, though only 35 percent of Black elders had both Medicare and supplementary private health insurance, as compared to 54 percent of all elderly who had both forms of coverage. There's evidence, though, that trust is an obstacle when it comes to seeking and receiving care. In community forums and focus groups, many Black elders relate stories of surgeries "gone wrong," being misdiagnosed or treated for conditions they don't have, and prescribed medication they believe they don't need. Commonly they chalk these experiences up to some "money-making scheme" perpetrated by doctors and the health-care industry.

Blacks generally have difficulty trusting health-care providers and the system in general. Many express displeasure over the disrespect and insensitivity displayed by medical specialists treating chronic disease or pain. "My name was called and I went in to see the doctor," said one woman. "'Oh, Ms. Lewis, how are we?' We? I told him how I felt and he wrote out the prescription for Vioxx. I really felt resentful because, well, how in the heck does he know what's wrong with me? He never even touched me. He was sitting as far away from me as that table is from here. I think that's the thing that causes people not to go to the doctor—they have the feeling that the doctor really doesn't care."

Others get intimidated by white coats and typically White faces, the fast pace, their prescriptions' adverse effects, and many providers' lack of effort to translate medical-speak into plain English, or tune in to what their patients are saying. "I can't seem to be able to get them to understand what's happening to me," says one focus group participant, and many others echo her words in different ways. "Sometimes I think, 'I'm just going to shut down and say forget it.'"

"It wasn't until I told them I hear phones ringing and people walking up steps, and I'm in the house by myself, and I feel like I'm losing my mind, that he said, 'Well, that's a side effect of the medicine,'" said Barbara. "All right, so then give me another one, okay? That one just had me itching and scratching. So my fear is what is going to happen when I tell you these things? Are you really and seriously going to help me in getting a little bit better? For the past 27 years, Black women in the Imperative and others have voiced concerns like these.

By contrast, some women believe their primary care or "regular" doctor explains tests well, really cares about how they are feeling, and treats them with respect. Whether our experiences have been positive or negative, Black women are beginning to speak out and speak up for our health; we know that prevention is better than cure.

RECOMMENDED HEALTH SCREENINGS AND VACCINATIONS
MATURE ADULT WOMEN 65 AND OLDER

SCREENING TEST	WHEN TO GET THE TEST
GENERAL HEALTH	
Full checkup, including weight and height	Discuss with your health-care provider.
Thyroid (TSH) test	Discuss with your health-care provider.
HIV test	Discuss with your health-care provider.
HEART HEALTH	
Blood pressure test	At least every two years
Cholesterol test	Discuss with your health-car provider.
BONE HEALTH	
Bone density screen	Get a bone mineral density test at least once. Talk to your health-care provider about repeat testing.
DIABETES	
Blood glucose or A1c test	Every three years.
BREAST HEALTH	
Mammogram (x-ray of breast or digital mammography)	Every 1–2 years discuss with your health-care provider.
Clinical breast exam	Yearly
Breast self-examination	Perform breast self-examinations at the same time each month.
REPRODUCTIVE HEALTH	
Pap test	Discuss with your health-care provider. Women 70 years of age or older who have had three or more normal Pap tests in a row and no abnormal Pap test results in the last 10 years may choose to stop having cervical cancer testing.
Pelvic exam	Yearly

Chlamydia test	Get this test if you have new or multiple partners.
Sexually transmitted infection (STI) tests	Both partners should get tested for STIs, including HIV, before initiating sexual intercourse.
MENTAL HEALTH SCREENING	Discuss with your health-care provider.
COLORECTAL HEALTH (USE OF THESE THREE METHODS)	
Fecal occult blood test	Yearly. Older than age 75, discuss with your health-care provider.
Flexible sigmoidoscopy (with fecal occult blood test)	Every five years. Older than age 75, discuss with your health-care provider.
Colonoscopy	Every 10 years. Older than age 75, discuss with your health-care provider.
EYE AND EAR HEALTH	
Comprehensive eye exam	Every 1–2 years
Hearing test	Every three years
SKIN HEALTH	
Mole exam	Monthly mole self-exam. Annual exam by a health-care provider as part of a routine full checkup.
ORAL HEALTH	
Dental exam	Routinely; discuss with your dentist.
IMMUNIZATIONS	
Influenza vaccine	Discuss with your health-care provider.
Pneumococcal vaccine	One time only
Tetanus-diphtheria-pertussis booster vaccine	Every 10 years
Herpes zoster vaccine (to prevent shingles)	Starting at age 60, one time only. Ask your health-care provider if it is okay for you to get it.

PART TWO

BEATING
the
ODDS

Chapter 5

Top Ten Health Risks
for Black Women

Cancer

Depression

Diabetes

Heart Disease

HIV/AIDS

Kidney Disease

Obesity

STDs

Stroke

Violence

*Staggering under the weight of racial and gender discrimination,
and all too often poverty, Black women consistently suffer
the highest rates of chronic illnesses and conditions.*

*Beating the Odds highlights 10 of the most troubling health conditions
that lead to higher mortality rates as well as higher rates
of stress, disability, shame and despair.*

The section is organized alphabetically to serve as a handy reference to the most pressing health risks, from cancer to violence. We provide you with these top ten health risks so that you can be informed about the best way to approach making personal health decisions to take control and getting answers to questions about what health risks and factors you should be most concerned about. You will find also personal stories of women who serve as a testimony that empowerment and change are possible. Some of the names have been changed to honor privacy and others fully agreed to chronicle their stories.

CANCER

No three words can shake us to our core like these: "You have cancer." Those words evoke emotions from fear to rage and everything in between. Once we hear them, our lives are changed forever, and we begin thinking about those things in life that we love and stand to lose. For many of us, our focus shifts not to ourselves and our next steps for treatment, but instead to our loved ones: *Who will take care of my children? How will my family manage without me?*

Our family histories are filled with relatives and friends who had the "Big C," and we can all recall hearing how "Miz Johnson had that operation and the next thing you know she has cancer." We've all heard the myths about how cancer forms or is spread when "air hits it" through surgery or some injury. And while many people equate the word "cancer" with a horrible disease or certain death, most may have a good bit of difficulty actually defining the word. Simply put, cancer is a term used to describe a group of diseases in which abnormal cells in the body begin to divide and develop out of control, forming masses called tumors, which can eventually invade other tissues and organs in the body and interfere with their functions. Cancer is not just one disease; in fact, there are over 100 different kinds of cancer. Most cancers take the name of the location in the body (organ or cells) where the cancer starts. For example, cancer that starts in the colon is called colon cancer.

Types Of Cancer[1]

Cancer types can be grouped into broader categories. The main categories of cancer include:

- **Carcinoma:** cancer that begins in the skin or in tissues that line or cover internal organs

- **Sarcoma:** cancer that begins in bone, cartilage, fat, muscle, blood vessels, or other connective or supportive tissue

- **Leukemia:** cancer that starts in blood-forming tissue such as the bone marrow and causes large numbers of abnormal blood cells to be produced and enter the blood

- **Lymphoma and myeloma:** cancers that begin in the cells of the immune system

- **Central nervous system cancers:** cancers that begin in the tissues of the brain and spinal cord

Although cancer deaths have declined for both Whites and Blacks living in the United States, Blacks continue to suffer the greatest burden in each of the most common types of cancer. For all cancers combined, the death rate is 25 percent higher for Blacks than for Whites. Although cancer is the leading cause of death for Black women ages 35 to 74, very little is known and discussed about cancer in the Black community. The reasons for this inequality are complex and likely include our lower overall standard of living, including income level and education. These economic and social barriers reduce our access to quality cancer treatment, prevention, and early detection: studies have documented inequities in the care Black women receive compared to White women. Our inherited or genetic differences make only a small contribution to the unequal burden of cancer in our community. In the past ten years, this cancer racial disparity has begun to shrink; however, our death rate from all cancers continues to be about 33 percent higher in Black men and 16 percent higher in Black women than in our White counterparts—just one of the reasons why our overall life expectancy is more than five years shorter.

How Do I Know If I Have Cancer?

The symptoms of cancer may vary depending on the type of disease. For breast cancer, changes in the appearance of the breast or the way it feels may indicate the possible presence of a tumor. Unusual pain, bleeding, or vaginal discharge, as well as changes in bowel habits or the appearance of stools, may be signs of other cancers and reason to investigate.

Just as there are different symptoms for various types of cancer, there are different ways of diagnosing it. For some types of cancer, screening methods such as mammograms or Pap smears can help to detect its presence early. For breast cancer, regular clinical and self-exams can be used to detect growths. For other types of cancers, it may be necessary to insert a small scope or camera into the body to check for disease. Biopsies—a procedure in which samples of tissue are examined for the presence of disease—are also used to test for and diagnose cancer.

BREAST CANCER

Since becoming a nurse in my mid-twenties, I was always proactive about my breast health. I made sure I did my monthly breast self-exam; I never missed my annual visits with my primary-care physician and gynecologist. I even embraced healthy living. But on April 15, 2008, the unthinkable happened: I was diagnosed with triple negative breast cancer at the age of 35.

After hearing the news, I was paralyzed with fear, anger, and resentment. I was 35, a mother of three, and here I was just diagnosed with breast cancer. I didn't even know I was at risk at such a young age.

It was only by chance that I was diagnosed when I was. I had gone to my doctor with a severe case of hives that left me short of breath and my skin covered in swollen, painful red wheals. Both my primary-care physician and my gynecologist put me through a series of tests to determine the cause of the sudden breakout, but the tests showed nothing. My gynecologist reviewed my results with me and concluded that my hives probably were a reaction to stress or an insect bite. Just as I was about to leave, he said, "Erika, wait one moment. I want to give you a referral for a mammogram." He explained that since Black women were more likely to have breast cancer diagnosed late—and to die as a result—he thought it was a good idea for his Black patients to get their first mammograms at 35, rather than at 40 as recommended for the general population.

When I receive these types of referrals, I usually throw them in the back of my car, forget about them, and remember just weeks before my next doctor's appointment that I should finally schedule the exam so my doctor won't be annoyed with me. But this time I got back to work and called for an appointment right away.

Luckily, the radiology department at the medical center where I worked could take me the next afternoon. So the next day, I went for my first mammogram. "You're so young, you probably don't have anything to worry about," the radiologist told me. Two weeks later, I got a letter in the mail saying that more tests were needed, and one week later I had a second digital mammogram. A week after that, I was referred to a breast specialist at St. Joseph Medical Center in Towson, Maryland, who requested an ultrasound for me.

At this point, I was in denial because everyone just kept saying, "Don't worry; it's probably nothing. We just want to be certain." The radiologist who performed the ultrasound just kept going over the same spot over and over and over again. I was getting annoyed and asked her to stop. Then she said, "I need to get the doctor."

Hearing those sobering words confirmed it for me—something was wrong, and it was time to be concerned. As I waited for the doctor to come in, I found myself crying uncontrollably. I was scared and all alone. I didn't think to ask anyone to come with me to the appointment, because who would have thought I would have breast cancer?

Within seconds of seeing the images on the monitor, the specialist knew that I had stage I breast cancer and that a biopsy needed to be scheduled right away. The biopsy showed it was an aggressive form of cancer called triple negative, and right away I thought I was going to die. My first thought was, "Who will take care of my children?"

But my diagnosis wasn't a death sentence. I got treatment, and I have been cancer-free for two and a half years. I meet with my medical team—a breast health specialist, a medical oncologist and a radiation oncologist—every three months and get a mammogram every six months. I'm being vigilant about monitoring my breast health so that I can make it to the five-year mark; that's considered "out of the woods" for triple-negative survivors. It would have been a different story if my doctor didn't recommend a baseline mammogram at 35; my cancer might have gone undetected for much longer.

As it is, I'm optimistic—and determined. I'm an advocate for my health now. I don't let any doctor tell me that it's going to be okay. If something doesn't feel right, I demand an examination and testing. Even if everything feels right, I don't miss my annual physicals, and I gather as much information as I can about what can affect my health as a Black woman.

—Erika Jones

Breast Cancer and Black Women

Breast cancer is perhaps the most feared disease that women face, and the most personal. It touches an astonishing one in eight women during their lives, and many of us know someone—a mother, sister, church member, or friend—who has had it. Sadly, we may also know someone who has died from it. Breast cancer is the second leading cause of death among American women, killing about 40,000 women each year.

Breast cancer affects 118 of every 100,000 Black women.[2] Like all women, we need to guard against this far too common, life-altering, and potentially life-threatening disease—and for a number of reasons we need to be even more alert.

The disease tends to affect Black women earlier in life, when many of us assume we are not at risk. Black women under age 40 have a greater incidence of breast cancer than White women in the same age group. Also, while our overall incidence of breast cancer is 10 percent lower than it is for White women, across all age categories and all stages of the disease we are more likely to die of it. The five-year survival rate for Black women is only 77 percent compared to 90 percent for White women. While the breast cancer survival rate has improved overall, the survival rate for Black women has stayed about the same for the past two decades.

Just as troubling, we are about three times more likely than other women to develop triple-negative breast cancer. In triple-negative breast cancers, the three hormonal factors known to fuel most breast cancers are not present, so these cancers don't usually respond to hormonal treatments or targeted therapies; they are harder to treat, more aggressive, and more likely to recur than other cancers. Thirty percent of Black women with breast cancer develop these aggressive tumors, compared with just 11–13 percent of other women. Still, thousands of women survive breast cancer every year, often catching it in its early stages. Through educating ourselves about this type of cancer, Black women can help lead the fight against our higher risk.

Researchers are beginning to look into a number of factors that may explain why breast cancer tends to appear in Black women earlier than in other women, and in deadlier forms. Some of these factors include higher rates of obesity, stress, and genetic predisposition to the disease. Others include our access to health-care and the quality of the care we actually get from our providers:

- We are more likely to be uninsured than White women and therefore less likely to have a primary health-care provider. Uninsured women, in turn, are less likely to be screened for breast cancer, less likely to catch it early, and therefore more likely to die from it.

- We are less likely to have access to digital mammograms and other advanced technologies, such as tomosynthesis, which creates a three-dimensional picture of the breast using X-rays.

- We are less likely than White women to be told about abnormal mammogram results or to have the results of our tests adequately explained.

- We are less likely to live in areas with good breast cancer treatment facilities. Among women with advanced breast cancer, White women are five times more likely than Black women to receive advanced therapies and more than three times more likely to receive chemotherapy.

- We are more likely to experience delays in follow-up and treatment once we are diagnosed with breast cancer or other breast abnormalities.

- Most Black women are less likely to participate in breast cancer clinical trials. A history of mistrust of the health-care system, limited access to care, and bias on the part of health-care providers may contribute to Black women's low participation in clinical trials.

No one knows why some women develop breast cancer and others do not. Still, research[3] has found that those who have the following risk factors may have an increased chance of developing the disease:

- **Age.** Our risk of developing breast cancer increases as we get older. Black women are more likely than other women to develop it early.

- **Personal history of breast cancer.** Women who have been diagnosed with breast cancer are three to four times more likely to develop a new cancer in the other breast or a different part of the same breast.

- **Family history of breast cancer.** A person may also have a higher risk for breast cancer if she has a close relative who has it. About 20–30 percent of women with breast cancer have a family history of the disease.

- **Dense breasts.** Women who have a high percentage of dense breast tissue (as seen on a mammogram) have a higher risk of breast cancer than women of similar age who have little or no dense tissue in their breasts. Unfortunately, dense breast tissue can also make it harder for doctors to spot problems on mammograms and may require additional screening with more advanced technologies, such as ultrasound or magnetic resonance imaging.

- **Genes.** Some people have mutations in genes—specifically, BRCA1 and BRCA2—that make them more prone to developing breast cancer. These genes normally produce proteins that protect you from cancer. If you inherit a defective gene, you have less protection.

- **Menstrual cycle.** Women who started their periods early (before age 12) or went through menopause late (after age 55) may be at increased risk for breast cancer.

- **Alcohol use.** Drinking more than 1–2 glasses of alcohol a day may increase your risk of breast cancer.

- **Childbearing.** Women who have never had children, or who had their first child after age 30, may have increased risk.

- **DES.** Women who took diethylstilbestrol (DES)—a drug given to women from the 1940s through the 1960s to prevent miscarriage—may have an increased risk of breast cancer after age 40.

- **Hormone replacement therapy (HRT).** A woman is at higher risk for breast cancer if she has received hormone replacement therapy for several years. (Many women take HRT to reduce the symptoms of menopause.)

- **Obesity.** Obesity has been linked to breast cancer, although this link is controversial. The theory is that obese women produce more estrogen, which can fuel the development of breast cancer. From this perspective, obesity poses an even greater breast-cancer risk for women after menopause, when their estrogen production would normally drop significantly—if not for the excess estrogen produced by their fat cells.

- **Radiation.** Women who received radiation therapy as children or young adults may have a significantly higher risk for developing breast cancer. The younger a woman started such radiation, the higher her risk—especially if the radiation was given when her breasts were developing.

How Do I Know if I Have Breast Cancer?[4]

Breast cancer does not usually cause any noticeable physical symptoms in its early stages. In many cases, the first outward sign of breast cancer comes in a later stage, showing itself as a slight change in the breast. Any of the following unusual changes in the breast can be a symptom of breast cancer:

- A lump in or near your breast or under your arm.

- Thick or firm tissue in or near your breast or under your arm.

- A change in the size, shape, or color of your breast.

- Nipple discharge (fluid that is not breast milk).

- Nipple changes, such as an inverted nipple, one that turns inward into the breast.

- Changes to your breast skin, areola, or nipple, such as itching, redness, scaling, dimpling, or puckering.

The process of diagnosing breast cancer may start when you notice (or your doctor notices) a change in your breast, or when a routine mammogram reveals an abnormality that needs checking out, as in Erika's case. If your doctor suspects you have breast cancer, he or she may order a biopsy. The tissue sample will be sent to a lab and tested for cancerous cells.

If the test results are positive, the next step will be to determine what kind of cancer it is and what stage it has reached. Breast cancer, like many cancers, is classified in four stages, from stage I, which is early and localized in the organ or tissue where it originated, to stage IV, cancer that has spread to other organs in the body. There are many types of breast cancer, each with different treatment options.

Reducing Your Risk of Breast Cancer[5]

While there is no sure way to prevent breast cancer, living a healthy lifestyle may lower your chances of getting it, even if you have risk factors that can't be controlled, such as age and a family history of the disease. Eat a healthy diet, exercise regularly, keep your weight down, drink alcohol in moderation or not at all, and take hormones as little as possible.

Early detection is vital to successfully treating—and surviving—breast cancer. As we've seen, Black women need to be especially vigilant, since we are more likely to develop the disease early in our lives and yet less likely to have it detected early in its progress. Stay in control of your breast health with these essential screenings:

- **Mammogram.** A low-dose X-ray exam of the breasts to look for changes that are not normal. Women age 40 and older should have screening mammograms every year. Depending on factors such as family history and your general health, your health-care provider may recommend a mammogram before age 40 (as Erika's doctor did). Free and low-cost programs can help lower-income women get breast cancer screening (see Resources). Remember, that although mammography is the gold standard for screening, younger women and women with dense breasts should seek more advanced imaging for better views and early detection of cancer cells.

- **Clinical breast exam (CBE).** During an examination, your health-care provider looks at and feels the breasts and under the arms for lumps or anything else that seems unusual. Women in their twenties and thirties who have dense breasts or other risk factors should have a CBE as part of a regular health exam. After age 40, all women should receive a breast exam by a health-care provider every year.

- **Breast Self-Exam.** No one knows what your breasts should look and feel like better than you. Do a breast self-exam every month, preferably after your period. Here are three simple steps to follow:[6]

  - **Step 1:** Begin by looking at your breasts in the mirror with your shoulders straight and your arms at your sides. Check your breasts for any changes in size, shape, color, or position and any skin puckering or dimpling. Inspect your nipples and look for any sores, peeling, or change in the direction they point.

  - **Step 2:** With soapy hands, place one hand on your hip and use the other to feel your underarm for any lumps or thickening. Repeat on the other side.

  - **Step 3:** Raise one arm behind your head and use the flat part of the fingers of your other hand to press gently into the breast. Follow an up and down pattern, covering the entire breast. Repeat on the other side.

  Be sure to feel all the tissue, from the front to the back of your breasts: for the skin and tissue just beneath, use light pressure; use medium pressure for tissue in the middle of your breasts; use firm pressure for the deep tissue in the back. When you've reached the deep tissue, you should be able to feel down to your rib cage. Most women have lumpy breasts, so don't be alarmed—the key is to determine what is normal for you so that you will know when your breasts don't feel normal.

  If you detect any changes, visit your health-care provider right away.

Taking Control of Breast Cancer

In dealing with breast cancer, it's crucial to be proactive in seeking and demanding the best care. This includes pushing for a quick diagnosis; asking for and getting referrals to the best physicians when you or a loved one, receives a positive diagnosis; inquiring about and doing your own research on the most effective treatments and clinical trials, if they are relevant (see Resources); and ultimately getting the best treatment possible to fight breast cancer. Your treatment may include surgery, radiation therapy, and/or chemotherapy; depending on the stage of your cancer, your doctor may recommend two or more types of treatment to be used at the same time or one after the other. Do your homework and learn as much as you can about your options so you can be a true partner in your cancer treatment.

Just as important, during every step in the process you should be treated with respect and compassion. It is important to have a trusted relative or friend present to offer you some support. Having your hand held or even a shoulder to cry on can be critical when going through such a life-changing medical diagnosis, and your health-care provider should respect your need for outside encouragement and emotional support. In fact, your health-care provider should take all your concerns seriously and answer all your questions. When you walk out of your doctor's office, you should feel as if he or she has your best interest at heart and is doing everything possible to help you get healthy.

Erika Jones Akers, whose story you read earlier, offers this advice to all women: "Get to know your breasts—feel them, look at them, and touch them. Be an advocate for your health—seek information, be persistent with your health-care providers and, ask questions." And she charges women who have been diagnosed with breast cancer to empower themselves with information.

Erika is a survivor. Thousands of women survive breast cancer every year—and by educating ourselves about it, Black women can help lead the fight against it.

Resources:

For free mammography sites in your area, go to http://www.cdc.gov/cancer/NBCCEDP/. For clinical trials, go to http://www.clinicaltrials.gov.

African American Breast Cancer Alliance
PO Box 8981
Minneapolis, MN 55408
(612) 825-3675
www.aabcainc.org

Avon Foundation for Women
1345 Avenue of the Americas
New York, NY 10105-0196
(866) 505-AVON
www.avonfoundation.org

Black Women's Health Imperative, Moving Beyond Pink to End Breast Cancer Disparities Campaign
1726 M Street, NW, Suite 300
Washington, DC 20036
(202) 548-4000
www.moving beyondpink.org

Sisters Network, Inc.
National Headquarters
2922 Rosedale Street
Houston, TX 77004
(713) 781-0255
(866) 781-1808
www.sistersnetworkinc.org

Tigerlily Foundation
11654 Plaza America Drive #725
Reston, VA 20190
(888) 580-6253
www.tigerlilyfoundation.org

Susan G. Komen for the Cure
5005 LBJ Freeway, Suite 250
Dallas, TX 75244
(877) 465-6636
www.komen.org

CERVICAL CANCER

I am a mother and a poet, and in 1999, I was diagnosed with stage II cervical cancer. The news was devastating. My treatment included 28 days of intense radiation and a procedure in which doctors placed a cancer-fighting implant inside my cervix. This procedure was done twice, and each time, I had to lie on my back for three days without moving. These treatments left me severely anemic, and my digestive tract still has not recovered. Yet, I am still alive, and I'm working to help other women who have cervical cancer and those who are at-risk for this disease.

When I was diagnosed, I was working at Tennessee's state health department, and that's where I met Dr. Wendell Inman, director of the Breast and Cervical Cancer Early Detection Program. She turned out to be a true inspiration. I originally approached her about helping me release my poetry, but after hearing about my struggle, she asked me to personally share my story and invited me to appear at a cancer seminar. Dr. Inman continued to encourage me after this first appearance. She eventually suggested I start a cervical cancer organization, and I thought she was kidding! I had no business experience and little desire to run an organization. After seriously thinking about it and praying about it, I founded the Cancer Coalition of Tennessee in September 2001.

While still keeping my job at the health department, I began to appear at as many events as possible. Being part Cherokee, African American, and Portuguese helps me relate to a variety of women. Most often, I handled these events by myself, but my daughter and friends helped me as well. In the beginning, I invested my own money to start this organization, and the "office" was my apartment. I am especially proud of our growth. In 2002, we created posters and bus advertisements that appeared on 100 buses in Nashville, Memphis, and Chattanooga, and we now have an office space. I plan to continue to help other women overcome this disease.

—Navita

Black Women and Cervical Cancer

Cervical cancer is caused by abnormal cells that grow, divide, and spread in the cervix, the lower, narrow part of the uterus, or womb, that opens into the vagina.[7] It tends to occur during midlife, with half of women diagnosed between the ages of 35 and 50. Although the rate of new cases of cervical cancer, as well as death from cervical cancer, has declined approximately 50 percent in the United States over the past three decades, the disease remains a serious health threat, especially to Black women. While it occurs most often in Hispanic women, Black women tend to have lower five-year survival rates and to die from the disease more often than any other race. In fact, Black women have the second-highest death rate from cervical cancer in the United States despite the fact that it is preventable through vaccination, Pap smears, and HPV screening (to detect cellular changes before cells become cancerous).

How Do I Know if I Have Cervical Cancer?[8]

Early cervical cancer generally shows no signs or symptoms. This is why regular screening is so important. A woman may develop symptoms only when the cancer has become invasive and spread to nearby tissue. When this happens, the most common symptoms are abnormal vaginal bleeding; unusual discharge from the vagina—separate from a normal menstrual period; bleeding following intercourse, douching, or after a pelvic exam; and pain during intercourse. Symptoms of advanced cervical cancer may include loss of appetite, weight loss, fatigue, pelvic pain, back pain, leg pain, a single swollen leg, heavy bleeding from the vagina, leaking of urine or feces from the vagina, and bone fractures.

The first-line screening for cervical cancer is the Pap smear, administered by your gynecologist, in which a small sample of cells from your cervix is removed and examined under a microscope. If your Pap results are abnormal—or if your doctor suspects cervical cancer because of your symptoms—he or she will order a colposcopy. This is an examination of the cervix with a colposcope, a lighted instrument that remains outside of the vagina and magnifies the cervix so it can be examined. Another way your doctor may opt to take a tissue sample is through a cone biopsy, in which a cone-shaped tissue sample is removed under general anesthesia. The tissue your doctor collects from any type of biopsy will be sent to a lab and tested for cancerous cells. Results generally come back in less than two weeks.

If your Pap smear results show cellular changes, your doctor may remove the affected tissue. There are several procedures for doing this, depending on the extent of the changes; some take only a few minutes and can be done in your doctor's office. If the test results come back positive for cervical cancer, the next step will be to determine what stage the cancer is in. There are four cervical cancer stages, with stage I being early cervical cancer and stage IV being cervical cancer that has progressed and spread to other organs in the body.

Reducing Your Risk of Cervical Cancer

Cervical cancer is almost always caused by a high-risk strain of the human papillomavirus (HPV), an STD that about 80 percent of sexually active people in the United States have. Each year there are more than 6.2 million new HPV infections in both men and women, 10 percent of whom will go on to develop persistent dysplasia or cervical cancer. HPV can trigger alterations in the cells of the cervix, which can lead to the development of cervical intraepithelial neoplasia, which can lead to cancer.

However, most women infected with HPV will not get cervical cancer. You are more likely to develop cervical cancer if you have HPV and smoke, have HIV or reduced immunity, or don't get regular Pap smears. Pap smears look for changes in the cervical cells that could become cancerous if not treated. Other risk factors for cervical cancer include having many sexual partners, a chlamydia infection, exposure to the hormonal drug diethylstilbestrol (DES), and a family history of the disease.

Taking Control of Cervical Cancer

If it is detected early, cervical cancer is one of the most successfully treatable cancers. Treatments usually include radiation and chemotherapy before a hysterectomy is considered. The choice of treatment depends on the type and stage of the cancer. Your doctor will talk to you about your treatment choices and the side effects associated with each treatment.[9] He or she will also take into account your age, overall health, quality of life, and desire to have children.

Being screened for cervical cancer is your first and most important line of defense against the disease. In general:

- All women should begin cervical cancer screening within three years after they start having sex, and no later than age 21 whether or not they are sexually active. Screening should be done every year with a regular Pap smear.

- Beginning at age 30, women who have had three normal Pap smear results in a row may get screened every two to three years. Women older than 30 may also get screened every three years with a Pap smear plus an HPV test.

- Women 70 years of age or older who have had three or more normal Pap smears in a row and no abnormal Pap smear results in the last ten years may choose to stop cervical cancer testing.

- Women who have had a total hysterectomy may also choose to stop having cervical cancer testing, unless the surgery was done as a treatment for cervical cancer or a precancerous condition. However, women who have had a hysterectomy without removal of the cervix should continue cervical cancer screening according to the guidelines above.

Young women today have another defensive weapon at their disposal: the HPV vaccine. There are two vaccines available, designed to be given in three doses over six months; both protect against the types of HPV that cause most cervical cancers, and one also protects against most genital warts, which also result from HPV. Ideally, girls should get the vaccine before they are sexually active. The Centers for Disease Control and Prevention recommends the vaccine for 11- to 12-year-old girls, though it can be given to girls as young as age 9. The vaccine is also suggested for females ages 13 through 26 years of age who did not get any or all of the three recommended doses when they were younger.

Resources:

Gynecologic Cancer Foundation
230 West Monroe, Suite 2528
Chicago, IL 60606
(312) 578-1439
www.wcn.org

National Cervical Cancer Coalition (NCCC)
6520 Platt Avenue #693
West Hills, CA 91307
(800) 685-5531
www.nccc-online.org

National Cervical Cancer Public Education Campaign
230 West Monroe, Suite 2528
Chicago, IL 60606
(312) 578-1439
www.cervicalcancercampaign.org

Tamika and Friends
PO Box 2942
Upper Marlboro, MD 20773
(866) 595-2448
www.tamikaandfriends.org

COLORECTAL CANCER

The first thing I noticed was a pain in my hip. Since I am a firm believer in alternative medicine, I went to an acupuncturist. In fact, I went back three times because the pain never got better. The last time I went, the acupuncturist told me that I should go see a doctor before getting any more treatments, so I did. They discovered that I had colorectal cancer when I was 45.

I have been a big girl all my life. Not really overweight, but solid and tall. I've been six feet tall since I was a teenager. I look healthy. I always felt I was big and strong so I could take anything that came my way. I could tough it out. I think women are used to ignoring pain; we go through menstrual cramps and other aches and pains and we are supposed to keep going and take care of everyone else. It was really hard for me to ask people for help, but I had to. I realized that it didn't make me weak to ask for help.

There is a lot of cancer in my family. If you have a family history of any kind of cancer, you should be screened earlier rather than later. Don't get me wrong—the screening test for colorectal cancer is not fun, but the prep is worse than the test itself. In fact, the test is nothing. I found out that there are other ways to prep for the test, but you have to ask about them.

I still get screened even though I am cancer free now. I feel really good, really healthy. I am more willing to ask for what I need now and take time for myself. I learned a lot about myself. The biggest thing I learned is how to be strong on the inside as well as looking strong on the outside."

—Barbara

Colorectal Cancer and Black Women

Colorectal cancer is cancer that develops in the colon and/or the rectum. (The colon is the part of the digestive system where waste is stored; the rectum is the end of the colon that connects to the anus.) Most colorectal cancers develop first as colorectal polyps, which are growths inside the colon or rectum that may later become cancerous. Colorectal cancer is the third most common cancer in American women and men and the second leading cause of death from cancer in the United States

Black women are at great risk for colorectal cancer, yet we don't perceive ourselves as being at risk. Because of this widespread misconception, 70 percent of Black women over the age of 45 have not received the lifesaving screening for colorectal cancer that's recommended for everyone starting at that age. If they have polyps—or tumors—they don't know it, and their cancer may not be discovered until it has progressed into a late, less treatable, stage.

How Do I Know if I Have Colorectal Cancer? [10]

There are numerous symptoms for colorectal cancer, which often make it difficult to diagnose. They include fatigue, weakness, shortness of breath, change in bowel habits, narrow stools, diarrhea or constipation, red or dark blood in stool, weight loss, abdominal pain, cramps, and bloating. Other conditions such as irritable bowel syndrome, ulcerative colitis, Crohn's disease, diverticulosis, and peptic ulcer disease can have symptoms that mimic colorectal cancer.

If your doctor suspects you have colon cancer, he or she may order either a lower GI series, also called a barium enema X-ray, or a colonoscopy to confirm the diagnosis and to localize the tumor. If these tests reveal cancerous growths, your doctor may order a biopsy to confirm the diagnosis. If colon cancer is confirmed, there are further examinations to determine whether the cancer has spread to other organs. Since colorectal cancer tends to spread to the lungs and the liver, these tests usually include chest X-rays, ultrasonography, or a CT scan of the lungs, liver, and abdomen.

Unfortunately, colorectal cancer can be present for several years before symptoms develop. This is why screening for the disease is critical. Black women should begin getting screened for this type of cancer once they reach age 45. There are several screening options, including fecal occult blood testing, which can be done annually, and a colonoscopy that can be done every ten years.

Reducing Your Risk of Colorectal Cancer [11]

Doctors are unsure what causes the disease; however, there are certain known risk factors, including high fat intake, a family history of colorectal cancer and polyps, the presence of polyps in the large intestine, and chronic ulcerative colitis. Colorectal cancer is also more likely to occur in older people. More than 90 percent of people with this disease are diagnosed after age 50. The average age at diagnosis is 72.

Because the cause of colorectal cancer is unknown, there is no guaranteed preventive measure. However, you can lower your risk for it by eating a variety of fruits, vegetables, and whole grains; drinking alcohol in moderation, if at all; quitting smoking; and exercising regularly. Maintaining a healthy weight is also critical. Studies have shown that people who carry excess fat around their waist are more prone to developing colorectal cancer, and there is also evidence that they are more likely to die from it if diagnosed.

Taking Control of Colorectal Cancer

There are four main types of treatment for colorectal cancer: surgery, radiation, chemotherapy, and targeted therapies such as monoclonal antibodies.[12] Depending on the stage of your cancer, two or more types of treatment may be used at the same time, or used one after the other. Surgery is usually the primary treatment for rectal cancers that have not spread to distant sites, and common procedures include a colonoscopy, laparoscopy, and open surgery. Talking with your health-care provider will help to determine the best treatment program for you.

Being diagnosed with colorectal cancer, like any cancer, can be traumatic, and fighting it can be demanding. It is important to have a strong network of family and friends around you from the time you learn you are diagnosed to when you're recovering. You may also consider joining a support group to benefit from the company and counsel of others who are in your position—and to inspire them with your presence, too.

Resources:

Colorectal Cancer Coalition
1414 Prince Street, Suite 204
Alexandria, VA 22314
Office: (703) 548-1225
Answer Line: (877) 427-2111
www.fightcolorectalcancer.org

The Colon Cancer Alliance
1025 Vermont Avenue, NW, Suite 1066
Washington, DC 20005
(877) 422-2030
www.ccalliance.org

American College of Gastroenterology
PO Box 342260
Bethesda, MD 20827-2260
(301) 263-9000
www.acg.gi.org

American Society of Colon and Rectal Surgeons
85 West Algonquin Rd., Suite 550
Arlington Heights, IL 60005
(847) 290-9184
www.fascrs.org

LUNG CANCER

I remember saying, I'm only 35—this can't be happening to me. Yet it was. Lung cancer, in my mind, was always a disease other folks got, someone older, someone I didn't know. As I approach the five-year anniversary of being a cancer survivor, I know how blessed I am to have my big, loud, and loving family, whose members took turns holding my hand, hearing my doubts, regrets, and stories, and giving me the love and support I needed during those rough months of sadness and despair.

From the very first day that my doctor diagnosed the soreness in my right shoulder blade and the fatigue—the kind of fatigue you have when you are pregnant, the kind that just drains half the life out of you—as lung cancer, I realized that I had not lived my life as I could have. That I had a lot of living left to do.

My journey began six months after that first chest CT. I was sitting in the lounge of the hospital, feeling stressed about my upcoming surgery the following morning, and for the first time in my life I actually wished I was a smoker. Maybe that could justify what was happening to me, maybe that could answer the question of why me. Those hours and days were the most stressful of my life—not knowing and not believing.

After the surgery and months of recovery I started chemotherapy. I was exhausted physically and emotionally. I truly felt like I would die. During this time that I was feeling sorry for myself, my sister became my guardian angel. Determined, stubborn, and supportive, she knew that I needed something or someone to help me have hope, to let me know that others do okay and survive lung cancer. I began reading, seeking out organizations, talking about my cancer and my rough time recovering, and I decided to join an organization that was raising awareness of lung cancer. Two years after my surgery, I made a promise to myself and my sister that I would be walking in cancer awareness events every year. Since I lost my lung, I have gone on to live a pretty rich life and do some pretty remarkable things, such as finishing a 20-mile walk, and, I hope, inspiring others to feel this dreaded disease can be beaten.

—Mary

Lung Cancer and Black Women[13]

Over 71,000 women die from lung cancer every year, and although this type of cancer takes the lives of more women each year than breast, ovaria, and uterine cancers combined, it doesn't get the amount of attention it deserves. Behind breast cancer, lung cancer is the second most diagnosed cancer in women.

Lung cancer is the uncontrolled growth of abnormal cells in one or both lungs. These abnormal cells do not carry out the functions of normal cells and do not develop into healthy lung tissue; instead, they can form tumors and impede the function of the lung. Lung cancer is very deadly. The five-year survival rate is only 16 percent, compared to an 89 percent five-year survival rate for breast cancer.

Many people know that smoking is the main cause of this disease, but the story doesn't end there. Only about 18 percent of Black women smoke—fewer than White women—yet we are just about equally likely to be diagnosed with lung cancer and more likely to die from it.

How Do I Know if I Have Lung Cancer?

Early lung cancer may not cause any symptoms. Many times, lung cancer is found when an X-ray is done for another reason. When symptoms do appear, they depend on the specific type of cancer you have, but may include:

- A cough that doesn't go away

- Coughing up blood

- Shortness of breath

- Wheezing

- Chest pain

- Loss of appetite

- Losing weight without trying

- Fatigue

It's important to know that these symptoms usually don't indicate lung cancer; they may be due to a wide variety of other causes. However, you should still consult your doctor to find out what they mean for your health.

If your health-care provider suspects you have lung cancer, she or he will perform a physical exam and ask questions about your medical history. You will be asked if you smoke, and if so, how long you have smoked. When listening to the chest with a stethoscope, a health-care provider can sometimes hear fluid around the lungs, which could, but does not always, suggest cancer. She or he may order tests, such as:

- Chest X-ray

- Sputum cytology test to look for cancer cells

- Blood work

- CT scan of the chest

- MRI of the chest

- Positron emission tomography (PET) scan

Reducing Your Risk of Lung Cancer

Smoking is directly responsible for 80 percent of lung cancer deaths in women in the United States each year, making it one of our most preventable diseases. In fact, women who smoke are 13 times more likely to die from lung cancer than women who have never smoked.[14]

Cigarettes may be small and light, but their list of harmful ingredients isn't. Each cigarette contains about 600 ingredients. When burned, they create more than 4,000 chemicals. Many are poisonous and at least 50 are known to cause cancer. And it doesn't have to be your mouth puffing a cigarette to put you at risk for lung cancer. Secondhand smoke is also potentially deadly. Approximately 3,400 people in the United States die from lung cancer annually due to exposure to secondhand smoke, and 65 percent of these are women.

It's true that some people who never smoked a day in their life still get lung cancer. About 1 in 5 women and 1 in 12 men diagnosed with the disease have never smoked. Beyond smoking, other risk factors include:[15]

- **Radon.** Radon, a radioactive gas that you cannot see, smell, or taste, forms in soil and rocks. People who work in mines may be exposed to radon, and in some parts of the country radon is found in houses. If you live in an area with high levels of radon coming from the bedrock (see www.epa.gov/radon), consider having your house tested for radon exposure. If radon levels are too high, a device can be installed to reduce them.

- **Asbestos and other substances.** People who work in certain jobs (such as those in the construction and chemical industries) have an increased risk of lung cancer due to their exposure to asbestos, arsenic, chromium, nickel, soot, tar, and other substances. The risk is highest for those with years of exposure.

- **High levels of air pollution.** Air pollution may slightly increase the risk of lung cancer.

- **Family history of lung cancer.** People with a parent or sibling who has had lung cancer may be at slightly increased risk for the disease.

- **Personal history of lung cancer.** People who have had lung cancer are at increased risk of developing a second lung tumor.

- **Age over 65.** Most people are older than 65 years when diagnosed with lung cancer. However, part of the reason is that lung cancer can take years to develop.

Remember that it is never too late to stop smoking. Your risk of lung cancer drops dramatically the first year after you quit. Also, remember that cigarettes are very addictive and it may take much more than willpower alone to help you quit. Being open to a variety of methods and trying again and again—no matter whether, or how often, you relapse—is key. Finally, keep in mind that other people are likely depending on you to quit as well. Even if you are the type of smoker who goes outside the house to take a quick puff, you could still be putting your family at risk, including your children. The odds of developing asthma are twice as high among children whose mothers smoke more than ten cigarettes a day. If you are pregnant, you have yet another reason to quit: smoking during pregnancy accounts for 20–30 percent of low-birthweight babies, up to 14 percent of preterm deliveries, and about 10 percent of all infant deaths.

Taking Control of Lung Cancer

If you are diagnosed with lung cancer, your health-care provider may refer you to a specialist with experience treating lung cancer. If not, you should ask for a referral. You may have a team of specialists participating in your care. Specialists who treat lung cancer include thoracic (chest) surgeons, thoracic surgical oncologists, medical oncologists, and radiation oncologists. Your health-care team may also include a pulmonologist (a lung specialist), a respiratory therapist, an oncology nurse, and a registered dietitian. Don't be afraid to ask questions of—and about—anyone who's entrusted with your care. Getting the best possible people to treat you can mean the difference between life and death.

Resources:

Visit www.lungusa.org for tools like Freedom From Smoking Online.

Lung Cancer Alliance
888 16th Street, NW, Suite 150
Washington, DC 20006
(202) 463-2080
www.lungcanceralliance.org

American Lung Association
1301 Pennsylvania Avenue, NW, Suite 800
Washington, DC 20004
(800) 586-4872
www.lungusa.org

National Cancer Institute Smoking Quitline
(877) 784-8669
www.smokefree.gov

The American Lung Association's helpline at 1-800-LUNG-USA.

OVARIAN CANCER

Christmas of 2009 started off great. I had actually started my holiday shopping early and was just about finished—two weeks ahead of schedule. Christmas was going to be a big deal this year because my oldest son had been away at school and this would be his first time home in months. My husband and I were busy as usual with work, keeping up with the kids, and living life. So I was trying not to pay attention to the constant fatigue, bloating, and weight loss I was feeling. I just chalked it all up to being busy. I knew I didn't feel quite right, but convinced myself that I would be fine and would get everything checked out after the holidays.

A few days after Christmas I started having some pretty bad abdominal pain, but because it went away after a day or two I thought it was just stomach flu. But when the pain came back around New Year's I knew something was wrong. I went to the hospital and spent the day there getting a load of tests done—blood work, CT, and ultrasounds. They found I had a large amount of abdominal fluid, but couldn't tell me what was causing it. I was admitted and told I would be having a procedure the next morning to help remove some of the fluid.

Well, the next morning my whole world changed. The surgeon who had ordered the CT and ultrasounds took a second look at them himself and called in a gynecological oncologist. My doctor then came and told me that a gynecological oncologist would be examining me. When I heard "oncologist" I was terrified, but he confirmed that there was a grapefruit sized mass on my right ovary. The whole time he was talking, I kept thinking, "I don't want to hear this!"

All I could think about was how this was going to ruin what was left of my son's time at home and the rest of our holiday. My doctor performed a total hysterectomy, and two days after the surgery I got the good news that the cancer had not spread to my lymph nodes.

After I had been home for about a month, I started chemo and was warned that half the women who have this treatment can't complete the full six cycles. Well, that doctor and that treatment didn't know me and everything I was fighting for, and I finished all six cycles! I was on maintenance for another year after the chemo and I can now say that I am almost a two-year survivor.

—Victoria Mann

Ovarian Cancer and Black Women

Ovarian cancer is a type of cancer that begins in the ovaries. All women are at risk for it, but older women are more likely to get the disease than younger women. About 90 percent of women who get ovarian cancer are older than 40 years of age, with the greatest number aged 55 years or older.

In 2006, the most recent year for which statistics are available, nearly 20,000 women in the United States were diagnosed with ovarian cancer, making it the second most common gynecological cancer, after uterine (endometrial) cancer. Ovarian cancer accounts for only about 3 percent of all cancers in women; however, it causes more deaths than any other gynecological cancer in the United States

Of those 20,000, White women had the highest incidence of ovarian cancer. Black women's rate was among the lowest—but Black women had the second highest rate of death from ovarian cancer after White women.[16]

How Do I Know if I Have Ovarian Cancer?[17]

Signs and symptoms of ovarian cancer may include abdominal pressure, fullness, swelling, or bloating; pelvic discomfort or pain; persistent indigestion, gas, or nausea; changes in bowel habits, such as constipation; changes in bladder habits, including a frequent need to urinate; loss of appetite or quickly feeling full; increased abdominal girth or clothes fitting tighter around your waist; a persistent lack of energy; and low back pain. These symptoms mimic those of many other more common conditions, including digestive and bladder problems, which is one reason why ovarian cancer often goes undiagnosed until it is advanced.

Reducing Your Risk of Ovarian Cancer

It is not clear what causes ovarian cancer. We do know that, while all women are at risk for it, some women may be more likely to get the disease than others. These include women with inherited gene mutations, a family history of ovarian cancer, or a previous cancer diagnosis, as well as women who have never been pregnant.

The majority of ovarian cancers—like far too many diseases—are diagnosed late, after the cancer has spread. So even though the symptoms of early ovarian cancer are elusive, it's important not to put off going to the doctor when you know something is not quite right with your body and to encourage other women to do the same.

Taking Control of Ovarian Cancer

If your doctor suspects you have ovarian cancer, she or he will likely start with a pelvic examination, then order various other tests and procedures as needed, such as an ultrasound to create pictures of your ovaries or surgery to remove samples of tissue for testing. You will probably also be given a CA 125 blood test. CA 125 is a protein found on the surface of ovarian cancer cells, as well as on some healthy tissue.

If your doctor says that you have ovarian cancer, you may be referred to a gynecological oncologist—a doctor who has been trained to treat cancers like this. This doctor will work with you to explore your option and create a treatment plan.

Fighting ovarian cancer—and any type of disease—can put an enormous strain on anyone. In addition to seeking the support of family and friends, finding a support group for those who have ovarian cancer and talking with ovarian cancer survivors can strengthen your spirit.

Resources:

National Ovarian Cancer Coalition
2501 Oak Lawn Avenue, Suite 435
Dallas, TX 75219
(214) 273-4200
www.ovarian.org

Ovarian Cancer National Alliance
910 17th Street, NW, Suite 1190
Washington, DC 20006
(866) 399-6262
www.ovariancancer.org

FORCE: Facing Our Risk of Cancer Empowered
16057 Tampa Palms Boulevard West, PMB #373
Tampa, FL 33647
(866) 288-7475
www.facingourrisk.org

Gynecologic Cancer Foundation
230 West Monroe, Suite 2528
Chicago, IL 60606
(312) 578-1439
www.wcn.org

UTERINE CANCER

I am an eight-year survivor of uterine cancer, diagnosed at age 45. I had gone through early menopause and noticed some spotting. I called my obstetrician-gynecologist and made an appointment for a checkup. At that time, he did a biopsy. They found cancerous cells, which he said were an aggressive form. I was referred immediately to a gynecological oncologist, who told me the best treatment would be a complete hysterectomy. During surgery, they discovered the cancer had spread from the uterus to some of the pelvic lymph nodes, so I would need more treatment—a course of 30 radiation treatments, five days a week for six weeks.

I was symptom-free for four and a half years until I developed a cough. Scans revealed spots on my lungs and stomach. My doctor recommended I undergo chemotherapy—once a month for five months. I have remained symptom free since.

Throughout all of this I have been mostly pain free, able to have fun with my kids and my husband, and I have great family and friends. It may sound strange, but this journey has been a positive and eye-opening experience for me. Yet I have to admit that I've been scared. What has helped me most in dealing with the fear is the support group I found and some great relationships I've developed with other women just like me. I try to maintain a positive attitude and live each day as fully as I can.

—Deloris

Uterine Cancer and Black Women

Uterine cancer is the most common gynecological cancer in the United States, with an estimated 40,100 new cases and 7,470 deaths occurring in 2008.[18] There are many types of uterine cancer; the most common type is endometrial cancer, which starts in the endometrium, the lining of the uterus. Most cases of endometrial cancer occur between the ages of 60 and 70 years, but a few cases may occur before age 40.

The survival rate for all stages of uterine cancer is approximately 84 percent, but if diagnosed at its earliest stage, survival increases to 90–95 percent. The incidence of uterine cancer is lower among Black women than among White women, but our overall rate of deaths from cancer is higher, so prevention, early detection, and treatment are vital for us.

How Do I Know if I Have Uterine Cancer?

Uterine cancer symptoms include bleeding between normal periods before menopause, vaginal bleeding or spotting after menopause, extremely long, heavy, or frequent episodes of vaginal bleeding after age 40, lower abdominal pain or pelvic cramping, and a thin white or clear vaginal discharge after menopause.

There are three ways of diagnosing uterine cancer: an endometrial biopsy, a dilatation and curettage (D&C), and imaging tests. Endometrial biopsy involves inserting a narrow tube into the uterus through the vagina and removing a small amount of tissue from the uterine wall. This tissue is tested in a lab for cancerous or precancerous cells. The procedure takes just a few minutes and is usually done in the doctor's office. A D&C involves widening the cervix and inserting an instrument to scrape or suction the uterine wall and collect tissue; it takes about an hour and is usually done in a hospital because it requires anesthesia. Imaging tests are used in patients who have certain medical conditions, such as severe high blood pressure, obesity, diabetes, or other types of cancer, since these patients may not be able to tolerate anesthesia safely.

Reducing Your Risk of Uterine Cancer

Although the exact cause of uterine cancer is unknown, increased levels of estrogen appear to play a role. Estrogen helps stimulate the buildup of the lining of the uterus. Studies have shown that high levels of estrogen in animals result in excessive endometrial growth and cancer.

There are many known risk factors for uterine cancer. They include diabetes; estrogen replacement therapy without the use of progesterone; history of endometrial polyps or other benign growths of the uterine lining; infertility; infrequent periods; taking the drug Tamoxifen to treat breast cancer; never being pregnant; obesity; polycystic ovarian syndrome; starting menstruation at an early age; and starting menopause after age 50.

You cannot prevent uterine cancer, but you can lower your risk by engaging in regular physical activity, eating a diet low in saturated fats and high in fruits and vegetables, and breastfeeding your children. Taking contraceptives that combine estrogen and progestin has also been shown to decrease the risk of endometrial cancer.

Taking Control of Uterine Cancer

If you are diagnosed with uterine cancer, you and your doctor will decide on the best course of treatment based on the type of cancer and the degree to which it has progressed. Options include surgery, radiation therapy, and chemotherapy. For women with early stage I disease, a hysterectomy may be recommended, usually involving removal of the fallopian tubes and ovaries in addition to the uterus.[19]

Resources:

Society of Gynecologic Oncologists
230 West Monroe Street, Suite 710
Chicago, IL 60606
(312) 235-4060
www.sgo.org

Gynecologic Cancer Foundation
230 West Monroe, Suite 2528
Chicago, IL 60606
(312) 578-1439
www.thegcf.org

Taking Control of Cancer

While doctors often cannot explain why one person develops cancer and another does not; we do know that there are certain risk factors that can increase the chances of developing it. Among the most common are tobacco use, alcohol use, a family history of cancer, and simply growing older. We have already discussed how being overweight or obese, eating a poor diet, and not getting enough physical activity can put Black women at risk for other conditions, such as diabetes and heart disease. These characteristics of our lifestyle are risk factors for cancer, too, and knowing this may help motivate us to make the changes we need.

Although researchers are still working to find cures for different types of cancer, there are steps that we can take to reduce our chance of developing the disease and improve our chances of treating it successfully if we do. For instance, various screening practices, such as mammograms and Pap smears, can help to detect the presence of cancers early in their development. For some cancers (for example, cervical cancer), vaccines may be an effective way to decrease risk. While no research findings and no doctor can tell someone how to completely eliminate his or her risk, our individual health-care and self-care practices—such as regular medical checkups—may reduce our risk and improve our prognosis. Here are a few things you can do:

Decrease Tobacco Use. One of the most important ways to lower the risk of cancer is to avoid the use of tobacco products. Smoking can increase a person's chance of developing several types of cancer, including cancers of the lung, mouth, throat, esophagus, bladder, kidney, larynx, pancreas, cervix, and stomach. Even for those who do not smoke or use tobacco products, exposure to cigarette smoke—secondhand smoke—may put them at increased risk for cancer.

Maintain a Healthy Weight. Results from several studies suggest that people who are overweight or obese may be at a greater risk for developing a number of cancers. You'll read more about what "overweight" and "obese" mean—and the many ways Black women are affected by excess weight—in chapter 6. For now, keep in mind that increasing your physical activity and eating more healthful meals are two essential steps to achieving and maintaining a healthy weight.

Limit Alcohol Use. Regular consumption of alcoholic beverages can increase risk for several types of cancer, including cancers of the throat, mouth, and larynx. The findings from many research studies also suggest that alcohol use can increase the chance of developing liver, breast, and colorectal cancers.

DEPRESSION

———————◆———————

Looking in the mirror, I was the first depressed Black woman I ever saw. No one else in my family admitted that they were in pain, and so it made me feel isolated and crazy. Today, I have committed myself to sharing my journey through depression—a journey that led to attempted suicide, and ultimately to self-care.

Now, at 33 years old, I realize that I have always had a melancholy disposition. Even looking back on my childhood pictures, I remember being the odd girl in my family, the only one who had what I call an "oceanic blue" countenance. For me, the chaos of being a Black girl transitioning to womanhood resulted in an inner chaos that sometimes seemed too much to bear.

To me, oceanic blue perfectly describes the difference between me and my sister. Even though we grew up under the same roof, everything about my sister was always sunny, and she was always able to find the positive in her circumstances. But that just wasn't me. Oceanic blue is a kind of blue that would make me feel sad on any given day. Some moods were lower than others, but at the core, I was always blue—the hue of the deepest part of the ocean, with countless shades of low and sad moods, a state that I eventually learned was depression.

As a child, I had no language to express what was happening—because no one ever told me— and I have moved through waves of depression my entire life. No one ever explained or reacted to the chaos that went on in my life, so I felt very alone or crazy. I was always taught to "just suck it up and keep it moving." I always compared myself to the Black women around me, who taught me to take whatever life threw at me without having an emotional reaction. We Black women are trained to mimic our mothers, who have become masters of disguise—this is how we've been conditioned to survive. Watching the Black women in my family march around, knowing that they were dealing with disappointment, and heartache, and barely making ends meet, I never saw anyone cry. These strong Black women were always walking with their heads held high. I was always told never to let anyone see you vulnerable, to bite your lip when you were about to cry, to do whatever you could to mask how you felt inside.

Domestic violence, poverty, abandonment, and incarceration were all traumas that my family faced, yet I was the first one to be depressed? It was hard because no one around me ever said that they were hurting, too. It would have made me feel much less crazy if the women in my family weren't so occupied with putting on those masks of being fine when they were really suffering from some type of pain. Even my family's reaction to me seeking professional therapy was dismissive and confusing. They would chastise me by saying, "That's White women's shit. What do you have to talk to someone else for?" They made me feel like I was somehow an inauthentic Black woman.

Most Black women don't even realize how we are burying an emotion that's actually coming from a true place of hurt. My grandmother, for example, when she got emotional, always got angry. I now realize that her anger was simply the way she protected herself, so that her sadness or tears wouldn't be perceived as weakness.

As a child, I saw a counselor, but it was never really helpful. While my counselor was nice, I felt that I needed to censor myself because I didn't trust that I could reveal my personal truths to an older White man. Since I was well trained, I never wanted to air my family's dirty laundry. This bottling-up of emotions was something that I carried around for years. Not smiling, not feeling upbeat, and yet not having anything necessarily bothering or weighing on me made this constant state of oceanic blue—or depression—even more difficult to handle. I was never able to tell my mother, or even understand for myself, what was really wrong; it never occurred to either of us that I was just sad for no reason.

Thinking back, I can chart my depression with more awareness. I recognize that a sad mood could be brought on by a change in weather or some moment of disappointment when my spirits would plummet and I'd feel physical pains in the pit of my stomach. Many Black women are quick to dismiss their depression this way—they're just tired, or having a migraine—but I have learned that those low moods are really our minds and hearts trying to cope with our true feelings.

I have a tendency to remember the things that hurt me the most, and my thoughts become a negative tape player message on repeat, telling me that there was no point in living, even though I knew that was irrational—because depression is not rational. This cycle of negative thinking led me to contemplate my death, and eventually I attempted suicide several times. Fortunately for me and the other Black women I have been able to inspire through my raw journey with depression, my attempts were never successful.

I can now say with pride that instead of thinking about dying, I am planning to live. It has taken years for me to get to this point, because the depression was always there, like my second skin, for nearly three decades. But I am now learning that in taking it one day at a time, I am able to manage being content and prioritize self-care. I was able to write a lot through my pain, and that became my ultimate coping mechanism. The pain fades, though it never goes away, but every day I grow more and more aware and comfortable with myself. While I used to fantasize about my own death, as a young child and even into my college years, I have found my real strength by wanting to live.

Today, I am proud to say that I am not a strong Black woman. I think the notion of the strong Black woman is a myth—one that can eventually kill us. Because we are multiply oppressed, we cannot afford to wear our vulnerabilities on our sleeves. Our sadness, denied an outlet, often shows up as anger. We come across as being perpetually upset and unapproachable. Black women sometimes just need someone to take care of us and listen to our challenges. We never acknowledge that Black women's lives and our stories are traumatic because we're too busy talking about how resilient we are and how we overcome. Breaking the conspiracy of silence has revealed my true strength to me.

The change came through maturity and becoming more secure with my depression. I used to cry in secret, but now I cry out of necessity. My tears became a cleansing—a soul cleansing—absolving me from all the past memories that lingered in guilt. I began crying out everything that I had been carrying around. The tears carry the weight of my pain—you have to let it out to heal.

—Robin

Depression and Black Women

Many Black women remember when Ntozake Shange brought the realities of Black women's lives to the stage in *For Colored Girls Who Have Considered Suicide When The Rainbow Is Enuf.* That powerful play laid bare the challenges that Black women are expected to suffer silently. Issues of rape, violence, love and love loss, abandonment, abortion, poverty, and shame are just some of the complexities expressed by the ladies of the rainbow. The play presents a host of painful truths embedded in our lives on and off stage. *For Colored Girls* explores the material defeats and the psychological abuses that Black women endure.

Yet Black women aren't given the space or time to really heal from any of our traumas; we aren't even supposed to acknowledge them. Our responsibilities are exponential and the discrimination we experience is chronic. There is a name for this constant stress buildup and emotional pain that Black women feel. And no, it's not called the angry Black woman syndrome. It's called clinical depression.

"Why are you depressed? If our people could make it through slavery, we can make it through anything." "You should take your troubles to Jesus, not some stranger/psychiatrist." Statements like these all too often reflect the real beliefs that are held in our community. The National Survey of American Life[20] studied the racial, ethnic, and cultural influences that impact mental health disorders and concluded that Black people's long histories of shame, secrets, and mistrust dating back to slavery teach us to avoid our emotions in order to survive. That technique has been passed down by our grandmothers and mothers, churning a cycle of suppression.

The study captured some of the common reasons why Black women kept their depression and other mental health battles a secret instead of seeking treatment. Most interesting was that the explanations were always focused on other people and never on the women themselves, reinforcing the concept of the strong Black woman who takes care of everyone but herself.

These were the common reasons Black women gave for not admitting their emotional pain or seeking treatment:

- It might hurt my family.

- It might ruin my career.

- People might think I'm crazy.

- I can't afford to appear weak.

- I'm ashamed.

We've all heard time and time again that Black women are supposed to be strong— strong for our children, strong for our families, strong for our communities, strong for our friends, strong for the whole world, and, if that wasn't enough, strong for ourselves, too. But what about our own mental health? If we are caring for everyone else's needs, how do we manage our own? By and large, we don't, and our coping strategies to survive (emotionally and mentally) are made up as we go along, because very few of us have ever seen a healthy way of confronting and processing emotional chaos.

Instead, a lot of Black women have learned to deal with depression through displaced anger. It's so common among us that we've even been misdiagnosed as having the angry Black woman syndrome we mentioned above—a loose term for Black women who are perceived as being evil or perpetually on edge. But this is a dangerous stereotype that oversimplifies the pain and emotional distress a lot of us have felt we've needed to internalize. Psychologist and author, Dr. Brenda Wade reminds us that "Your Body will talk to you." It will tell you that you feel mad, not sad. She counsels that " . . . when you see an angry Black woman, you're seeing a depressed woman."

FROM STRESSED TO DEPRESSED

When sisters tell me that they're evil, I often suggest that they read Brenda Lane Richardson and Dr. Brenda Wade's book, *What Mama Couldn't Tell Us About Love: Healing The Emotional Legacy of Slavery, Celebrating Our Light.* In the chapter called "You're Not Evil, But You Might Be Depressed," they do a wonderful job of showing us the connections between depression and seeming mean-spirited, impatient, or overly critical behavior:

Many of us mask our depression with the attitude of [got it all under control]. The deep feelings of grief continue [without stopping] because they don't fit into our schedule. So we get mad because we tell ourselves we can't feel sad. When people see that many of us are hyper irritable, which is a symptom of depression, they mistakenly call us evil. In fact, many of us are depressed and exhausted.

How sad but true. Many of us act out our pain, yet don't believe we're entitled to feel it, much less address it! Wouldn't it be better to know why we feel irritable and negative, why we may be hurting the feelings of those around us, than to continue to live with a feeling of low-grade misery? I think the answer is yes, but of course that's easier said than done. For generations, Black women's pain threshold has simply been too high. We have been taught to minimize our problems, take on more than we can handle, always put ourselves last, and never slow down, because maybe if we're running we won't fall. Although this strength has often been the backbone of the Black family, it has also meant that we are unable to recognize when we've reached our emotional breaking point—when we're just stressed that hell out!

Lately, I can tell that I'm feeling stressed when I start feeling irritated over little things, in other words, acting "evil." I don't intend to be rude, but sometimes when I'm overworked and can't handle another phone call or e-mail, I just snap! I'll cut people off on the phone, raise my voice, stop listening when someone is speaking, or let my impatience show. Nowadays I'm *trying* to get to a place where I can stop before the stress reaches that point. By the time I'm that stressed, there are already dozens of fires I'm trying to put out and it feels like I'm about to go up in flames myself. Instead of acting evil, I need to learn to set boundaries and ask for help before I feel completely and totally overwhelmed.

Karin Grant Hopkins, a longtime colleague, told me this story about being "evil":

> I remember my first awareness that something was wrong with me. I was in my early teens. Back then my family labeled me "evil" because I would retreat into my own world. As I grew older, I bought into it—I would warn friends and lovers so they would not be surprised when I became "evil." In truth, at those times, I was emotionally unavailable, and ignorant of the underlying medical condition; but to everyone around me, I was just a bitch. Insanely, this was a status booster. Unlike my bubbly cousins, I was tough and in control. If only they had known how fragile and out of control I really was.

Through the years I felt like war was raging inside me, compounding the pain. The "bitch" image had been around so long that even I believed it. So when soft, sad Karin would take over, all hell would break loose in my psyche. For many reasons, I could never verbalize this in detail to anyone. My friends were accustomed to leaning on me during hard times. I think I felt I owed it to them to always be their rock of strength. My family saw me as a symbol of success. I just couldn't burst their bubble. They loved to brag about my accomplishments, first as a television news anchor and later as a public relations executive. My depression would have stolen their pride.

Being evil and seeming bulletproof are the female versions of swagger and machismo in men: It's a painfully common cover-up for depression. What we call "evil" is really the inability to set boundaries for ourselves, to say, "Hey, this is more than I can handle right now. I need some help, or some downtime, and preferably both!"

—Terrie Williams, author of *Black Pain: It Just Looks Like We're Not Hurting*

Williams emphasizes that it's the masking and internalizing of pain that causes us to be so easily irritable, quick tempered, and snappy. Forever taught to minimize our problems, we dismiss the fact that we're exhausted and depressed.[21] So when our emotional pain, responsibilities, and pressures to be the best and meet everyone else's expectations do spiral out of control, we blow up! That breakdown is what people see—just another hostile or rude Black woman—when in reality it's a depressed Black woman who needs some help and self-care in her life.

What Does Depression Look Like?[22]

Depression is not simply a bad day or an isolated moment of sadness. Everyone has bad days, but when those days start adding up until *every* day becomes an emotional and psychological battle—or when you feel periods of emptiness and unwarranted anger, anxiety or fatigue you can't explain—you could be experiencing clinical depression. Sometimes there's an obvious trigger: grief over a loss, post traumatic stress, or the birth of a child that sends a woman into post partum depression. Often, as in Robin's case, there's no way to pinpoint a cause.

Depression is one of the most common mental disorders, yet it's often under diagnosed and under treated, especially among Black women. Our rate of depression is roughly 50 percent higher than that of White women,[23] yet only 7 percent of us get treated for it, compared to 20 percent of White women . In our community, depression is often normalized as a mere "rough patch" in a Black woman's life; in fact, studies show that almost two-thirds of Black women think that depression is a personal weakness, so they ignore the signs and put off or decline treatment. So not only are we bottling up our depression (increasing our risk for a sudden mental breakdown or attempted self-harm), we are also less likely to get the care we need to meet the challenges of depression that becomes chronic.[24]

How Do I Know If I'm Depressed?

Depression manifests in a variety of ways, but typically begins with low moods, a sudden loss of interest or pleasure in things that were once enjoyable, feelings of guilt or low self-value, interrupted and irregular sleep patterns, an inability to focus, constant fatigue, and over eating or not eating at all. Because of the cultural stigma around depression, most people don't know that depression is among the leading causes of disability-adjusted life years[25] (DALYS), which means the total number of years of potential and productive life lost due to premature death and disability. In other words, depression can easily cut your life short if not treated with some form of intervention, such as counseling, medication, or psychotherapy.

These are the hallmarks of depression:

- Persistent sad, anxious, or "empty" feelings

- Feelings of hopelessness and/or pessimism

- Irritability, restlessness, anxiety, mood swings

- Feelings of guilt, worthlessness, and/or helplessness

- Loss of interest in activities or hobbies once pleasurable, including sex

- Fatigue and decreased energy

- Difficulty concentrating, remembering details, and making decisions

- Insomnia, waking up during the night, or excessive sleeping

- Overeating, or appetite loss

- Thoughts of suicide, suicide attempts

- Persistent aches or pains, headaches, cramps, or digestive problems that do not ease even with treatment

- Inability to enjoy pleasurable activities or have fun

In *Black Pain*, Terrie Williams also identifies symptoms of depression that are overlooked in the lives of Black superwomen. Such super sisters might be surprised to find themselves hidden in this well-camouflaged depression checklist.

- You are always too busy and you don't take care of yourself.

- You are running from something.

- You keep things that bother you locked up inside, you hold grudges for far too long, you are afraid to speak out about disappointment, hurts, and fears.

- You can't ask for what you need.

- You lie about everything—even simple things.

The symptoms of depression can put us at risk for other health problems, including obesity, anorexia, bulimia, self-inflicted harm, bipolar disorder, and substance abuse.[26] New research is starting to show connections between depression and fibromyalgia, as well as depression and anxiety. One common coping mechanism to deal with the emotional pain of depression—self-medication through the abuse of alcohol and drugs—can create even bigger problems that are even harder to treat. Most often associated with depression, however, are the irreversible consequences of self-inflicted harm (such as cutting) and the ultimate "permanent solution to a temporary problem"—suicide.

We know that Black women are disproportionately affected by poverty, racism, and sexism. Carrying such societal burdens on top of the ups and downs of everyday life makes Black women more vulnerable to depression, yet less able to deal with it in a healthy and responsive way. "Living is hard. Living with oppression is harder. I think we all sometimes or at some point, like Fantasia, just want the noise to stop," writes one blogger, recalling her own hidden bouts with depression. She was finally able to admit her cycling depression, she says, when Fantasia Barrino's public story of attempted suicide circulated[27] in the news.

There's a popular notion that Black people don't commit suicide, but this is a tragic misconception. The reality is that Black Americans try to kill themselves with almost the same frequency as the general population (4.1 percent compared to 4.6 percent). The Centers for Disease Control and Prevention reported in 2004 that, between 1999 and 2004, suicide was the third leading cause of death among Black people between the ages of 15 and 24 . Not much is known about how those numbers reflect Black women specifically, because of the relentless stigma associated with Black women and emotional pain. What we do know is that while White women experience depression more often, Black women experience more severe and persistent depression that eventually manifests in other health issues, sometimes with fatal consequences. Depression is silently killing Black women, and at an alarming rate.

Taking Control of Depression

Some of the signs of depression—occasional fatigue, stress, sadness, anger—are part of the human condition, there's no getting around it. However, if you experience more than half of these symptoms consistently for two weeks or more—or if you just know that the hue of your life is too close too, too—i.e., too blue or too angry—you should ask for help. Start with your primary-care doctor, your pastor, a trusted friend—just don't keep it bottled up where it can do you harm.

Your family doctor, psychologist, or psychiatrist may recommend a variety of treatment options to address your situation. Treatment options—range from anti-depressant medications to individual or group counseling or psychotherapy with a licensed mental health professional. Any medications should always be prescribed and monitored by a licensed health professional.

If you begin to experience a funk that doesn't seem to be gaining momentum, consider trying some of the following mood shifters. They can often put the brakes on the blues before it accelerates into a full-fledged downward spiral.

- Fight isolation. Spend time with other people. Remember you don't have to go it alone.

- Get at least 7-8 hours of sleep every night.

- Take 10-minute mind vacations to focus on the things that bring you joy and happiness.

- Eat well.

- Take a load off of your "to do" list. Book your inner superwoman on an extended vacation.

- Talk to someone that you trust (a minister or a close friend) and seek support, guidance, and perspective.

- Avoid alcohol and sedatives.

Here's what you owe it to yourself to remember: feeling that bad just isn't good enough. Being inexplicably mad or moody all the time, overeating, not sleeping, always being tired, crying every day—these are not things we should take lightly or try to overlook in the name of being "strong." We must consider our life experiences and ask ourselves if we are really living or if we are engaged in an artful masquerade.

In *For Colored Girls*, Sister Shange illustrated how Black women always end up last on their own agenda; expected to be strong for others, we are conditioned to neglect our own self-care, and this is one of our greatest challenges in dealing with depression. Yet as the play ends, the ladies of the rainbow come together to demonstrate the power of communal support and womanhood, and healing comes within reach when the Lady in Red declares, "I found God in myself, and I loved her fiercely."

Depression is a universal challenge that does not discriminate; however, Black women are not only at increased risk, but we are also less likely to be able to create the space to deal with depression in a healthy way. To overcome it, we must realize that we are whole beings and deserve to be healthy: mind, body, and soul. We must realize and demand to do more than just survive but to actually enjoy our lives. We must claim our space to cry, or to take "me time" and say "no." More than ever, we must love ourselves fiercely enough to put our health first.

Resources:

Association of Black Psychologists
7119 Allentown Road, Suite 203
Ft. Washington, MD 20744
(202) 722-0808
(202) 722-5941
www.abpsi.org

National Alliance on Mental Illness
3803 North Fairfax Drive, Suite 100
Arlington, VA 22203
(800) 950-6264
www.nami.org

National Organization for People of Color Against Suicide
(202) 549-6039
www.nopcas.org

Black Mental Health Alliance for Education and Consultation
733 West 40th Street, Suite 10
Baltimore, MD 21211
(410) 338-264
www.blackmentalhealth.com

DIABETES

■

It may sound odd, but I was initially relieved when my doctor told me I had type 1 diabetes. I had arrived at her office expecting a far worse diagnosis—a tumor in or near my eye, to be exact. My vision had become poor quite suddenly, which was very alarming considering that just a month before I scored 20/20 during a routine eye exam. During the past month, I had ignored symptoms that pointed to something being wrong: feeling thirstier than usual, running to the bathroom more often, and having my first ever yeast infection. However, the problem with my eyesight was a red flag that was impossible to ignore or expect to go away on its own.

I'm glad I finally listened to my body. And ironically, I'm glad I didn't listen to my doctors. I went to the same two doctors I had seen a month earlier for a regular physical and vision test. When I arrived complaining of poor eyesight, my main physician was a little more than skeptical because the ophthalmologist she'd sent me to had just declared my vision was fine. When I mentioned that my vision problems could be a sign of diabetes and told her about my other symptoms, she flat out said I couldn't have the condition. Being young, healthy, active, and thin made my chances of having it almost nil, she said. Yet I knew she was just making an educated guess that I didn't have diabetes. When it came to my health, I didn't want any guessing to be involved; I wanted to know.

After I pressed further, my doctor said I could get the vision test and she would test me for diabetes depending on the outcome. I agreed to this, but then was floored again when I was told that because of the military insurance I had, the earliest I could see the ophthalmologist would be in ten months. Were my doctors off their meds? That was simply not going to work. It took me talking to my doctor's supervisor, my ophthalmologist's supervisor, and the patient ombudsman at the hospital for them to agree to give me an eye test that day. To my doctors' astonishment, my vision test came back 100/20—I was legally blind. After that, I was given a blood test, and at the end of the day I had my diagnosis: type 1 diabetes.

Though I was thankful I had a manageable condition, I certainly wasn't happy about it. And despite being diagnosed with gestational diabetes four years earlier when I was pregnant with my daughter, it wasn't something I was expecting. As is common with gestational diabetes, it had gone away after I gave birth to her, and while my obstetrician had mentioned that I now had an increased chance of having another type of diabetes later in life, it was not a point that was stressed. I didn't beat myself up, though. While I had my vices like everyone else, I took pretty good care of myself. Also, as I found out, type 1 diabetes is an autoimmune disease that I probably could not have prevented no matter how well I ate or how much I exercised.

I returned home that day knowing that, regardless of the cause of the condition, I had it now and had to take even better care of myself for the sake of my life and that of my beautiful four-year-old daughter, who was depending on me. That meant having to say "ouch" several times a day from pricking my finger to test my blood sugar, as well as injecting myself with insulin two to three times each day. Most diabetics will tell you this is quite a nuisance; however, it's having to meticulously and consistently monitor my diet that is the hardest part for me.

Prior to being diagnosed, I was more casual about my eating schedule. Like most people, I based my food choices on what I had a taste for. Managing my diabetes has required changing my entire relationship with food, and this "relationship" requires giving 100 percent. I have to be very deliberate now about my timing and selection of foods, which means food is always on my mind. As soon as I have finished a meal, I have to think about the next one, and skipping meals is a no-no. I also have had to cut out junk food and say good-bye to most sugars. This is difficult for a person with a "God-given sweet tooth." Still, while I have not managed my diabetes perfectly, I have done very well. I am 48 now, and in the 14 years since I was diagnosed, I haven't had any complications from the disease—and there are many.

This is something I am proud of. I am also proud that I was never ashamed of having the disorder and didn't make it seem like something unbearable. Had I acted this way, my daughter would have been at a great disadvantage when she was diagnosed with type 1 diabetes six years after me.

It was her diagnosis that made me grateful assertiveness was in my genes along with diabetes. Getting her a quick diagnosis proved even harder than it had for me. My daughter was ten at the time, and a month after she had returned from a month-long visit with her grandparents; she quietly showed me what looked like signs of a yeast infection. As I watched her more closely that day, I realized she was thirstier than usual and was making frequent trips to the bathroom. Uh-oh, I thought, and grabbed her hand and headed to the after-hours urgent care clinic. When we arrived, I told the doctor about her three big bright-red flags that pointed to type 1 diabetes. Then I felt like I was having a bad case of déjà vu when I was informed that my daughter couldn't have the condition—she was too young, thin, active, etc. It was suggested that allergies were to blame for her frequent urination and thirstiness, and she was given allergy tablets. If this wasn't foolish enough, the doctor implied that her yeast infection was caused by her experimenting sexually, and the gynecologist didn't want to examine a 10-year-old. By this time, it was late at night and I decided to head home and regroup.

The next morning, I literally had to make ten phone calls and tap dance all over the doctors' heads before they agreed to test her for diabetes—which seemed to be done to appease me. She was tested later that afternoon, and while waiting for the results, we went to grab lunch. When we got back, there was an ambulance waiting for her. My daughter's blood sugar was 985; it should have been between 90 and 180. She did have type 1 diabetes, and her life was in danger.

Thankfully, she received the care she needed over the next several days in the acute care unit at the hospital. They were able to get her blood sugar down and teach her about injections and food choices. Having diabetes myself, I was much better prepared to help her manage the condition in the days, months, and years that followed. In the process, however, I learned that much had changed since I was diagnosed. There were new and easier ways to live with diabetes, and we both benefited from the knowledge I gained.

I have been living with diabetes for 14 years now, and my daughter for 9 years. We both understand that while diabetes is a part of our lives, it doesn't define us. And while we do have to have injections and monitor what we eat and when we eat it, we can still be healthy and shape the direction of our lives. This is what I tell other people who find out I have diabetes, which isn't hard because I share the fact freely. I also let people with or without the condition know that taking charge of one's own health is vital. Too many of us believe our doctors are all knowing, but they are human just like us. They make mistakes and they can be wrong. It's up to us to know our bodies and make informed decisions about our care and about which treatment and approach best fit our needs and lifestyle. Our lives and the lives of our children depend on it.

*—**Tammy Jo Tucker** is a native of Portland, Oregon, who now makes her home in the Washington, D.C., metropolitan area. She considers herself not a superwoman, but a single parent striving to find the balance between her multiple roles—professional, mother, advocate, and empowered Black woman.*

People still talk about the long-term effects of Hurricane Katrina—one of the worst disasters Americans have ever experienced. From handling the loss of loved ones, employment, property, and a place to call home, to simply dealing with the stress that living through such hardship brings, countless New Orleanians are still putting the pieces of their lives back together. I am one of them. However, there is something else I believe Hurricane Katrina left me: the gift of diabetes.

Nine months after the hurricane hit, I was working harder than I had been already through my position as an associate professor of nursing at Southern University in Baton Rouge. Though I had lost my beautiful house and the library that was my pride and joy in New Orleans, I was determined not to let the hurricane set me back more than it already had. I was blessed in that I had kept an efficiency apartment in Baton Rouge in case I didn't feel like commuting home after a long day of work, and I was very thankful I had the foresight. Now I was living there and taking care of my 87-year-old father, and mapping out a plan to rebuild my life.

Though I didn't show it—and perhaps didn't know it—I was still more stressed than I had been at any point in my 54 years on the planet. As a health professional, I knew that long bouts of stress weren't good for the body, but I soon found out exactly how much havoc they would cause.

At some point, I realized that something funny was going on with my body. Regardless of what building I was in and how long I had been in it, I could tell anyone who asked exactly where the bathroom was. I had also unknowingly become a bottled water expert. I could tell you the minute differences between Evian, Dasani, and Fiji, and chances were I had just drunk some water or was about to. It seemed like my thirst was never quenched.

I knew the symptoms of diabetes and didn't waste time heading to the doctor when I put two and two together. My primary care physician, Cornelius Mayfield, an African American man whom I respect greatly, was able to give me a quick diagnosis and excellent treatment. Though I was somewhat expecting the diagnosis, I was still confused. It is true that I was overweight; however, I was still active, felt great despite the stress, and had never been told I was in danger of having the condition. Still, I try to look forward. In this case, I had the illness, I knew it was manageable, and ensuring my health did not suffer because of it became my goal. Before I left my doctor's office, he gave me samples of diabetes medication and discussed what my first step would be to manage the condition: diabetes education class.

The class in Baton Rouge was instrumental in helping me navigate my new world as a person with diabetes. It was eye opening in a very different aspect as well. One day, the diabetes educator asked the 18 people in the class how many of us had survived Hurricane Katrina. It blew my mind when 90 percent of us raised our hands. As a health professional and researcher, I knew *immediately that it was the disasters that had likely pushed many of us over the edge to diabetes—especially those who were pre-diabetic. I have since studied and talked extensively about the post-disaster health effects of Hurricane Katrina.*

The months that followed my diagnosis were extremely trying, especially when it came to food. Not only were my taste buds used to having their way, I lived in the most flavorful city in the United States, where our rich foods are one of the many things we're known for. Being in the South, Louisianans tend to like their sugar, too. This shows in the sweet tea I loved to drink that didn't seem right unless it had at least three to four tablespoons of sugar in it. But I knew I had to significantly reduce—key word being "reduce"—the unhealthy foods and ingredients I was used to, and I did. I soon began grilling foods instead of frying them—you'd be surprised at how good grilled oysters can taste. Doing this helped me eventually lose the addiction to fried foods. So, when I recently went to a jazz fest that featured more fried foods than it did singers, I wasn't that tempted. I went to a Gambian booth and ordered chicken on a stick and spinach and plantains on a saucer. The meal was tasty and healthy, too. I also learned to satisfy my craving for sugar, as well as salt, in better ways. For example, if I want a little bit of both, I simply put a few sprinkles of salt on a watermelon. Delicious!

Planning my meals was perhaps the hardest practice to adopt. Managing diabetes requires eating small meals four to six times a day—even when you don't really want to. But now, both planning and portion control come naturally to me. At restaurants, when everyone else is ordering entrees big enough for two people, I order an appetizer and this serves as my meal. When once I would order a shrimp po'-boy sandwich and eat the whole thing like everyone else, now I just savor half a sandwich. I am also much more active now. I walk and enjoy yoga, and you can even find me in both regular and aquatic Zumba classes showing off my rhythm. Of course, routinely monitoring my blood sugar levels and taking medication is also part of my treatment plan. I inject myself once a day with a drug that stimulates my pancreas to produce insulin.

I have learned much about diabetes since my diagnosis, including that it's essential for people to think differently about having the condition. To show and celebrate this, in 2009, I established and directed 100 African Americans Living Well with Diabetes in Louisiana as part of the Black Women's Health Imperative's Spirit of Health Initiative. As I and others prove every day, diabetes is manageable and not a death sentence.

*—**Dr. Cheryl Taylor** is an associate professor of nursing science at Southern University, a researcher, health policy advocate, and respected community leader. Her many accomplishments include serving as the commissioner of the Katrina National Justice Commission and being inducted into the Louisiana State Nurses Association's Nightingale Hall of Fame in 2011.*

Nearly everyone knows someone who has diabetes. About 7.8 percent of the United States population—23.6 million people—have it. Yet no group has a higher rate of incidence of diabetes than Black women. It affects about twice as many Blacks as Whites and will strike a staggering one in four Black women and half of our young girls during our lifetimes. While it's often referred to as "sugar" in the black community, this disorder is nothing but bitter. It is the fourth leading cause of death for black women. It is also linked to obesity, high blood pressure, high cholesterol, and kidney disease, so that it increases your risk for stroke, heart attack, kidney failure, and other devastating medical emergencies.

Though diabetes is manageable, it can also be debilitating and life threatening, causing serious complications and consequences if left untreated. Black women of all ages need to know exactly what it is, how to prevent it and lower our risk, and how to manage the disease if we have it.

Unfortunately, for many, our lifestyles have resulted in us being the hardest hit by the disease, particularly by the more familiar type 2. Many of the risk factors that can lead to developing type 2 diabetes are far too common among Black women: obesity, high blood pressure and high cholesterol, and lack of physical activity. On average:

- 80 percent of Black women are overweight or obese

- 45 percent of Black women suffer from high blood pressure

- 46 percent of Black women have high cholesterol

- 55 percent of Black women are inactive

However, we have the power to reduce or eliminate these risk factors and live healthier lives. Diabetes is not and does not have to be our destiny.

> *It is projected that an estimated 50 percent of Black females born in the year 2000 and beyond will develop type 2 diabetes in their lifetime.*

How Does Diabetes Work?

Diabetes is a disorder of the metabolism—the process by which the body uses digested food for growth and energy. Most of the food people eat is broken down into glucose, the form of sugar in the blood and the main source of fuel for the body. After digestion, glucose passes into the bloodstream, where cells use it for growth and energy. For glucose to get into cells, insulin must be present.

Insulin is a hormone produced by the pancreas, a large gland behind the stomach. When people eat, the pancreas automatically produces the right amount of insulin to move glucose from blood into the cells. In people with diabetes, however, the pancreas either produces little or no insulin or the cells do not respond appropriately to the insulin that is produced. Glucose builds up in the blood, overflows into the urine, and passes out of the body in the urine. As a result, the body loses its main source of fuel, even though the blood contains large amounts of glucose.

There are three main types of diabetes: type 1 diabetes, type 2 diabetes, and gestational diabetes:[29]

- **Type 1 diabetes** is an autoimmune disease, one in which the immune system turns against a part of the body. In diabetes, the immune system attacks and destroys the insulin-producing cells in the pancreas so that the pancreas produces little or no insulin. A person who has type 1 diabetes must take insulin daily to live. At present, scientists do not know exactly what causes the body's immune system to attack the pancreatic cells, but they believe that autoimmune, genetic, and environmental factors, possibly viruses, are involved. Type 1 diabetes accounts for about 5–10 percent of diagnosed diabetes in the United States. It develops most often in children and young adults, but can appear at any age; it occurs equally among males and females, but is more common in White people.

- **Type 2 diabetes** is much more common than type 1, and this is the type we've mostly been talking about in this book as we describe the health of Black women. About 90–95 percent of people with diabetes have type 2. With type 2, the pancreas is usually producing enough insulin, but for unknown reasons the body cannot use the insulin effectively, a condition called insulin resistance. After several years of this, insulin production decreases. Then the result is exactly what happens in type 1 diabetes—glucose builds up in the blood and the body cannot make efficient use of its main source of fuel. Unlike type 1 diabetes, which often appears without a cause, type 2 is most often associated with older age, a family history of diabetes, a previous history of gestational diabetes, physical inactivity, and ethnicity. Yet the clearest association is with obesity.

About 80 percent of people with type 2 diabetes are overweight. Type 2 diabetes is increasingly being diagnosed in children and adolescents, especially among African Americans. It is projected that an estimated 50 percent of Black females born in the year 2000 and beyond will develop type 2 diabetes in their lifetime.

- **Gestational diabetes** is a condition that about 3 – 8 percent of American women develop late in pregnancy. Gestational diabetes is caused by the hormones of pregnancy or a shortage of insulin. Although this form of diabetes usually disappears after the birth of a baby, women who have had gestational diabetes have a 40 to 60 percent chance of developing type 2 diabetes within five to ten years.

The most common diabetes symptoms include:

Eating and drinking changes. Early symptoms of diabetes often include unusual changes in diet. You may find yourself extremely thirsty, no matter how much you drink. The same can be said for hunger; you may have the urge to eat everything in sight. Some diabetics claim to have a severe sugar craving, especially when they are first diagnosed, but this is not true for everyone.

Weight changes. Even though you're eating excessively, you may find that you are losing a lot of weight. This is usually one of the clearest signs that something is wrong. In almost all serious diseases, unexplained weight loss is a symptom.

Changes in bodily functions. Another common symptom in the early stages of diabetes is an excessive need to urinate. If you notice you have the frequent or persistent need to urinate, it could mean that there is something wrong. Many diabetics have reported the need to relieve themselves many times more than the average person, sometimes as frequently as every hour of the day.

Changes in mental function. If you find yourself becoming tired easily or suffering from ongoing fatigue, then you need to determine the source of the fatigue. You can assume something is wrong if you have not changed your daily habits but you can't handle them as well as you used to. Another symptom is irritability; mood swings and emotional ups and downs are common in the early stages of diabetes.

Frequent yeast or skin infections. Yeast feeds on sugar, and when your blood sugar is high, there is more food available for yeast to feed on. If you suffer from frequent yeast infections, this could be a symptom of diabetes.

Eye problems. One of the most common early symptoms of diabetes is blurry vision. In fact, eye problems are so common with diabetes that most diabetics—diagnosed or not—experience them in the course of their illness.

What are the complications of diabetes and how can they be avoided? [30]

Untreated diabetes can lead to many serious complications, including blindness, amputation, stroke, heart disease, and kidney failure. These complications fall most heavily upon Black women. For example, we are 300 percent more likely than Whites to go blind due to uncontrolled blood sugar and high blood pressure on the tissues and small blood vessels of the eyes. Each year, 82,000 people lose a foot or leg to diabetes, and Black women and men are 1.5 to 2.5 times more likely to suffer from lower limb amputation. We also suffer from terminal kidney disease at rates as high as 5.6 times that of Whites, and diabetes is the leading cause of kidney failure.

Most of these losses are unnecessary because preventing them is simple. Research has found that simply controlling your blood pressure and blood sugar can reduce heart disease and stroke in diabetics up to 50 percent and can lower diabetes-related kidney failure by 33 percent. Regular eye exams and timely treatment could prevent up to 90 percent of diabetes-related blindness and foot-care programs can prevent up to 85 percent of diabetes-related amputations.

How Can I Reduce My Risk of Diabetes?

The keys to avoiding diabetes—or staying healthy as a diabetic—are a healthy diet and regular exercise:

- A well-balanced and vegetable-rich diet that is low in fat and sugar and that balances fats and carbohydrates while also providing vitamins, minerals, and fiber can prevent diabetes and keep those who are already diabetic healthy. Black women with or without diabetes would do well to have their entire families eat this way. This means that cookies, chips, sodas, fried foods, red meat, and other foods high in calories, sugar, cholesterol, salt, and saturated fat should be treated like delicacies—your family should rarely eat them. They don't belong anywhere in your kitchen, car, purse, or backpack.

- Exercise is also a guard against diabetes, as well as key to maintaining a normal weight and lower blood sugar, blood cholesterol, and blood pressure. And it's fun and easy. Try for at least 30 minutes a day of your favorite physical activity—such as walking, dancing, playing tennis, or jogging. If you need to, divide the period into shorter bursts of ten minutes each (no shorter than that). Losing just 5–7 percent of your body weight can reduce your risk for diabetes if you are overweight.

Pre-diabetics need to pay special attention to their risk. They have blood glucose levels that are higher than normal but not high enough for a diagnosis of diabetes. They are likely to develop type 2 diabetes within ten years, unless they take steps to prevent or delay diabetes, which can certainly be done. Pre-diabetes testing is recommended for anyone who has a family history of type 2 diabetes, as well as for those who are obese or have metabolic syndrome. Women with a personal history of gestational diabetes should also be tested.

Yet most of these losses are unnecessary, because preventing them is simple. Research has found that simply controlling your blood pressure and blood sugar can reduce heart disease and stroke in diabetics up to 50 percent and can lower diabetes-related kidney failure by 33 percent. Regular eye exams and timely treatment could prevent up to 90 percent of diabetes-related blindness, and foot-care programs can prevent up to 85 percent of diabetes-related amputations.

What Treatment Will I Receive for Diabetes?[31]

If your health-care provider suspects you have type 1 or type 2 diabetes, you will probably be given a fasting blood glucose test. The test is most reliable when done in the morning. However, a diagnosis of diabetes can be made based on any result of 126 milligrams per deciliter (mg/dL) or higher after an eight-hour fast, confirmed by retesting on a different day.

Once you're diagnosed, what then? It has never been easy to control diabetes, though the exact way people handle diabetes varies and can depend on which type they have. It's important to be among people who support and encourage you.

Your first step should be to see a health-care provider who will help you learn to manage your diabetes. Most people with diabetes get care from primary care physicians—internists, family practice health-care providers, or pediatricians. The team can also include other health-care providers, such as cardiologists and other specialists. The team for a pregnant woman with type 1, type 2, or gestational diabetes should include an obstetrician who specializes in caring for women with diabetes.

Many physicians recommend that their patients take a diabetes education class or join a support group. Not only is the class an excellent way to learn how to manage the condition, but it lets you see that you're not alone in your effort to live well with diabetes. People from all walks of life will be in the class with you.

For people with type 2 diabetes, healthy eating, physical activity, and blood glucose testing are basic management tools. In addition, many people with type 2 diabetes require one or more diabetes medicines—pills, insulin, and other injectable medicine—to control their blood glucose levels.

People should also know that diabetes is not just a physical illness; it affects the mind and soul as well as the body. This is why, as is the case with other illnesses, we have to take a holistic approach to caring for ourselves. Beyond just doing what it takes so our glucose levels don't get out of control, this means getting enough rest and finding ways to alleviate the stress in our lives. And we should be doing this whether we have a medical condition or not.

This is particularly important for Black women to understand. We suffer from so many life-threatening conditions not because we care less about our health than others, but because there are so many other issues we must address. Still, if we aren't well, it hinders our ability to help serve as guardians of our communities. Just as important, it makes it more difficult for us to be the health champions we can be in preventing and fighting diabetes and other conditions. The health of each and every one of us matters. As Tammy Jo and Cheryl are showing all of us, diabetes does not have to define you. It's essential for you to define it.

Resources:

American Diabetes Association
National Service Center
1701 North Beauregard Street
Alexandria, VA 22311
(800) 342–2383
www.diabetes.org

Juvenile Diabetes Research Foundation International
26 Broadway, 14th Floor
New York, NY 10004
(800) 533–2873
www.jdrf.org

National Diabetes Education Program
1 Diabetes Way
Bethesda, MD 20814
(888) 693–6337
(866) 569–1162
www.ndep.nih.gov

HEART DISEASE
(CORONARY ARTERY DISEASE)

———————————◾———————————

It was the end of a typically stressful day when my life changed in a heartbeat. I had a heart attack. At 36 years old, I had a heart attack.

The confused, panicked moments are revealed in the 911 call placed by my live-truck operator that day, Bruce Bookhultz: "My reporter is having a really hard time breathing."

At 5:45 P.M. September 8, 2010, I felt the symptoms of a heart attack. "First I felt pressure inside my chest that seemed very distant. Then I felt my left arm go numb. Then the pain went from zero to ten."

My mother, Maryanne, still remembers the phone call she got: "It wasn't real. It was . . . This couldn't be happening. They had to be making a mistake. This should not be happening. It should be the other way around."

I was rushed to the emergency room at Washington Hospital Center, where I got the news I feared most: I came face-to-face with my mortality.

The doctor—I will never forget—looked me in the face and said, "Your EKG shows that you're having a heart attack." That's when reality set in.

"I don't want to die—I don't want to die," I said through tears. It was the last thing I would ever expect the doctor to say to me. And I didn't want to die there. I didn't want to die without my family. I just didn't expect at 36 years of age that this was going to be it for me.

What led me to this day was a childhood in Fairfax County, where I was raised by my mother, a single parent and a county science teacher. I graduated from Fairfax's Robinson High School and then the University of Virginia, guiding my lifelong dream to become a reporter in the highly competitive world of broadcast journalism. I got lucky enough to be able to do it in my hometown.

Back at the hospital, I was quickly taken to the cardiac catheterization lab, where Dr. William Suddath performed my lifesaving procedure. My right coronary artery, which is the largest vessel, was totally blocked. At that point, a team of doctors had to switch out the catheter and place a wire into my vessels. Through aspiration they were able to remove as much of the clot as possible.

Doctors eventually learned that the heart attack was brought on by a tear in an artery, an extremely rare condition. In fact, the pain I had felt just seconds after my live report was the actual tear.

The heart attack happened at the hospital where they were able to save my life. As I recovered, I had to admit that my mother has been my rock. I know I'm very lucky. I have a mother who has been there for me, always. But she has been tough because I have been emotionally very weak at times. I don't think I'll ever be able to thank my mother enough for what she's done for me.

Nearly two months after my nearly fatal event, I started to rebuild my life by being more active and adjusting my lifestyle. It's gorgeous out and five weeks ago I couldn't walk two blocks, so to be out here at Eastern Market on a Sunday and to have the energy to do that feels great. Opening up to talk about my brush with death and my comeback was not an easy thing for me to do, but there are a lot of reasons why I'm sharing my story.

This is one of the most important stories I may ever tell. I never imagined that, at the young age of 36, I would be facing cardiac rehabilitation after having a nearly fatal heart attack. With every twinge or pain that I feel in my chest, I wonder if it's happening again. Three times a week three months after my heart attack, I began working on my comeback at Washington Hospital Center. It's really what gave me the confidence to exercise because they put me on a heart monitor and watched everything that I was doing. Under close supervision I exercised as a part of my cardiac rehabilitation. I built my confidence back; I built my strength back; I built my heart muscle back. But it was more me rebuilding my confidence.

Although these events are rare and typically happen to women in childbirth, it happened to me. Doctors say a combination of lifestyle, stress, and perhaps even genetics played a role in the tear and my subsequent heart attack. Exercise is just one part of the equation. I am now on an extensive medication regimen and am eating healthier, and I have stopped smoking.

My doctors are happy that I decided to change by taking better care of myself through my new commitment to exercise, improving my diet, and staying on top of my medications. I have made vast progress since that day. I am dedicated to getting better because I almost lost everything.

—Jennifer Dolan

Heart Disease and Black Women

One woman dies every minute from heart disease, a little-known fact often overshadowed by other conditions that make bigger headlines. Heart disease is sometimes called a "silent killer" because in women it often has barely noticeable symptoms—or no symptoms at all. The most commonly recognized symptom is persistent chest pain, pressure, or other discomfort, called angina. This pain results when the heart is getting too little blood or oxygen. It can be felt under the breastbone and tends to accompany exercise or extreme emotional stress. Women, however, are more likely than men to experience a different type of chest pain, which is sharp and temporary, and to mistake it for something else, such as indigestion, or ignore it altogether.[32]

For a condition that used to be known as a "man's disease," heart disease is claiming more than its fair share of women in the United States. The truth is that heart disease is the number-one killer of women in this country, with one in four women dying of the disease. And for Black women, the risks of developing and dying from heart disease are tremendous. Our rates of heart disease overall are twice as high as those for White women; we suffer coronary artery disease (CAD), the most common type of heart disease, at much higher rates than White women do and are much more likely to die of it—35 percent more likely, in fact.

Women with diabetes have more than double the risk of heart attack than nondiabetic[33] women, and we know that Black women suffer disproportionately from diabetes. We are more likely to be overweight or obese, more likely to be physically inactive, and more likely to have high blood pressure and high cholesterol levels–all risk factors for heart disease. We are also more likely to encounter challenges in obtaining care and less likely to be aware of our elevated risks. Small wonder that Black women die from heart disease not only more often than White women, but more often than all other Americans.

What Does Heart Disease Look Like?

Heart disease is a term used to describe a number of problems affecting the heart and the blood vessels of the heart. Coronary artery disease (CAD) is the most common type of heart disease and the leading cause of heart attacks. CAD occurs when the coronary arteries, which surround and supply blood to the heart muscle, lose their elasticity and become hardened and narrowed because of plaque buildup inside them, a process called atherosclerosis.

When your coronary arteries become narrowed, they can't supply enough oxygenated blood to your heart, especially when it's beating hard—for example, when you're physically active, for example. In the beginning the restricted blood flow may not cause any symptoms. But as the plaque continues to accumulate, you may start experiencing chest pain and shortness of breath when you engage in light physical activity or, say, walk up the stairs. If your coronary artery becomes completely blocked, you may have a heart attack, whose classic signs and symptoms include crushing pressure in your chest and pain that spreads to your shoulder or arm, sometimes with shortness of breath and sweating.

But women often don't experience these classic symptoms. Although chest pain is the symptom most commonly associated with a heart attack, for women chest pain may not be the most prominent or troubling symptom, or they may not experience chest pain at all. Instead, they're more likely to experience less-common warning signs, including:

- Atypical chest pain (pain that is sharp and temporary)

- Stomach, back, or arm pain

- Nausea or dizziness (without chest pain)

- Shortness of breath and difficulty breathing (without chest pain)

- Unexplained anxiety, weakness, or fatigue

- Palpitations, cold sweat, or paleness

These nonspecific symptoms have many other possible causes, making diagnosis difficult, whereas crushing chest pressure with physical exertion or emotional stress makes doctors think about a heart-related cause immediately. Even when doctors suspect that a woman's symptoms may be due to coronary heart disease, making a definitive diagnosis can be more challenging than it is with male patients, since traditional diagnostic tests such as the standard stress test (walking on a treadmill while your heart function is monitored) tend not to be as accurate.

According to the American Heart Association,[34] there are a number of possibilities for the differences in heart care between men and women. For one thing, most of the original cardiovascular research studies were conducted on men. The design of newer studies should yield results that are more informative about women, too. In the meantime, to get appropriate treatment, you need to take the initiative with your doctor, communicate clearly, and be aggressive in seeking attention for symptoms and concerns related to your heart.

How Can I Lower My Risk of Heart Disease?[35]

The development of cardiovascular disease begins at an early age, and so can the cultivation of a healthy heart. Fortunately, many of the risk factors for heart disease can be controlled by making small improvements that lead to large benefits. For example, losing only 10 to 20 pounds can help lower your heart disease risk. Other steps to reducing heart disease risk include:

- Engaging in at least 30 minutes of a moderate-intensity activity such as brisk walking or another activity that you enjoy, such as dancing, at least five days a week. If you need to, divide the period into shorter time frames of at least 10 minutes each.

- Eating well-balanced meals that are low in fat and cholesterol and include several daily servings of fruits and vegetables.

- Knowing your numbers–have your blood pressure and cholesterol levels checked regularly to ensure that they are in a healthy range.

- Keeping your blood pressure, blood sugar, and cholesterol under control.

- Limiting your alcohol intake to no more than one drink (one 12-ounce beer, one 5-ounce glass of wine, or one 1.5-ounce shot of hard liquor) a day.

- Not smoking.

Learn the risk factors and the symptoms of heart disease; if you have them, see your doctor. Also, find healthy ways to cope with stress—perhaps by talking to your friends, exercising, or writing in a journal.

What Treatment Will I Receive for Heart Disease?[36]

Your doctor will diagnose heart disease based on your medical and family histories, your risk factors, the results of a physical exam, and diagnostic tests such as an electrocardiogram (EKG or ECG), echocardiogram, stress test, and coronary catheterization. An EKG records the electrical signals traveling through the heart and can often uncover evidence of a previous heart attack or one in progress. An echocardiogram uses sound waves to produce images of your heart. During an echocardiogram, your doctor can determine whether all parts of the heart are working. Parts that move weakly may have been damaged during a heart attack or be receiving too little oxygen—indications of heart disease or various other conditions.

If the signs and symptoms that you experience occur most often during exercise, your doctor may ask you to take a stress test—for instance, by walking on a treadmill or riding a stationary bike during an EKG. As we've mentioned, this type of stress test is not the most revealing for female patients; other types of stress tests exist as well.

If your doctor diagnoses you with heart disease, you'll decide with him or her what treatment is right for you. Treatment options for heart disease include cholesterol-modifying medications to decrease the material that deposits in the arteries; aspirin to reduce the tendency of your blood to clot, diminishing the risk that your coronary arteries will become obstructed; beta blockers to slow your heart rate and lower your blood pressure, decreasing your heart's demand for oxygen; and nitroglycerin tablets, sprays, and patches to control chest pain by opening up your coronary arteries and reducing your heart's demand for blood.

Sometimes more aggressive treatment is needed, such as an angioplasty and stent placement or coronary artery bypass surgery. In an angioplasty and stent placement, your doctor inserts a long, thin tube into the narrowed part of your artery. A wire with a deflated balloon is passed through the catheter to the narrowed area. The balloon is then inflated, compressing the deposits against your artery walls. A stent is often left in the artery to help keep it open. Some stents slowly release medication to help keep the artery open.

In coronary artery bypass surgery, a surgeon creates a graft to bypass blocked coronary arteries using a vessel from another part of your body. This allows blood to flow around the blocked or narrowed coronary artery. Because this requires open-heart surgery, it's most often reserved for cases of multiple narrowed coronary arteries.

Resources:

American Heart Association
7272 Greenville Avenue
Dallas, TX 75231
(800) AHA-USA-1
www.heart.org

National Coalition for Women with Heart Disease
818 18th Street, NW, Suite 1000
Washington, DC 20006
(202) 728-7199
(877) 771-0030
www.womenheart.org

National Heart Lung and Blood Institute Health Information Center
PO Box 30105
Bethesda, MD 20824
(301) 592-8573
www.nhlbi.nih.gov/

HIV/AIDS

———————————————— ■ ————————————————

I became infected with HIV when I was 19 years old and attending college in Nashville. I wasn't the type to carry condoms; I thought it was the man's job. I would never have gotten an HIV test back then; I just thought it didn't apply to me. It took having unprotected sex only once to end up with the virus. My boyfriend had clearly told me that he didn't have a condom, but I chose to have sex anyway.

Still, I was shocked when the doctor told me I had HIV. I had believed my greatest risk from having unprotected sex was pregnancy; yet I had contracted something that I thought I was immune from. All because I didn't know that the "H" in HIV stands for "human," not "homosexual" or "hooker" or "heroin addict" — you know, anyone but me.

At the time I felt like I'd been given a death sentence. Many of the people I'd loved and cared about were scared to touch me, hug me, or kiss me. And once my boyfriend realized that other people knew about my status, he didn't want anything to do with me. I became the laughingstock of my college. Once after I ate in the cafeteria, they actually threw my tray away. There were times when I was forced to eat on paper plates and with paper cups and wash my clothes separately.

I think my boyfriend knew he had HIV, although I later witnessed the fact that he was in denial about it. But I'm over the whole "everybody's-to-blame-but-me" syndrome—too much information is available. Black women worry so much about a person's status or their sexual orientation, when protecting yourself from HIV is not about the other person, it's about the self. Quite simply, I should have loved myself enough to protect myself. I couldn't blame him; it wasn't like I was forced. I simply made a bad decision: having unprotected sex. If I had insisted on using a condom,

I would never be in this situation. I mean, what if he hadn't known that he was infected—and a lot of people don't know—I would still have HIV, right? So you have to protect yourself, and when you protect yourself, you're also protecting them.

Right after I was diagnosed, life was really hard. I wanted my friends and my family to treat me the way they used to, but they didn't. Then after a few months I started realizing that, in a way, HIV was a good thing: it was pushing a lot of negative people out of my life. I figured that since I have HIV I could either take it and run with it or I could keep it to myself and allow other unsuspecting people to get infected and die. So about six months after I was diagnosed, I started telling my story publicly. That gave me a mission—I have a purpose in life. And I know for a fact that I am doing God's work. I use the "no B.S., no sugarcoat" method to help people understand that they have to take responsibility for themselves.

The question I get asked most often is whether I have sex. I always tell the person that my message is safer sex, not abstinence. That gets their attention. Because let's be realistic; I am 25. But most people think that if they have sex with somebody who is HIV-positive that they are going to become HIV-positive also. They are shocked to learn that it doesn't have to happen that way. Generally, I don't have a problem in the dating world. Sometimes I date men who are HIV-positive and sometimes men who are HIV-negative. HIV doesn't define me. If someone really wants to be with you, they don't care about all that because it's not the priority. I always let guys know that I have HIV in the beginning before it gets very far so no feelings are involved. I definitely experience rejection, but I'm not the only person who experiences that, and for every guy who says no, there is usually a guy who says yes. They always have a million questions, so I invite them to come to my doctor with me and let her answer them. Then if we have sex, we simply use a condom and use it correctly.

The worst thing about HIV is taking seven pills a day—I've always been anti-pill, and pills make me nauseous and give me diarrhea. One day, I'd like to have a baby. There's a 98 percent chance that a mother who knows she is HIV-positive can deliver an HIV-negative baby. I guess when the time comes, I'll know whether I'll do it naturally or by artificial insemination.

People always say that knowledge is power, but I think what's powerful is when you use that knowledge. So even though being an AIDS activist is not something I wanted to spend my life doing, I put my own feelings and emotions aside. The most rewarding part of my work is helping somebody make a wise decision, whether they get tested or start using condoms. It's nothing that I would have chosen for myself, but having HIV has taught me to grow up and take responsibility for my life. It scares me to think of where I'd be without HIV. I know that I would be worse off for sure!

—*Marvelyn Brown* is an AIDS activist and author of The Naked Truth: Young, Beautiful and (HIV) Positive

HIV/AIDS and Black Women

In a 2007 Harris Interactive survey commissioned by the Black Women's Health Imperative, one-fourth of the women surveyed stated that HIV/AIDS was the biggest threat to Black women's health—by far the most common answer. But only 11 percent thought that HIV/AIDS was a problem for *them*. A full two-thirds of Black women were "not very concerned" about their personal risk of contracting the virus. This is not just the definition of denial; it's a recipe for disaster.[37]

JUST THE FACTS
BLACK WOMEN AND HIV/AIDS

Black women account for

Percent of population:	12
Total of new AIDS cases:	64%
Total of new HIV diagnoses:	61%

1 in 32: Black women will contract HIV/AIDS in their lifetime

HIV/AIDS as cause of death (rank):

Ages 15–19:	8th
Ages 20–24:	5th
Ages 35–44:	3rd
Ages 45–54:	4th

How women become infected:

Heterosexual sex:	78%
Intravenous drug use:	20%
Unknown:	2%

Source: "Fact Sheet: Black Americans and HIV/AIDS," September 2009, Kaiser Family Foundation; and "Views and Experiences with HIV Testing Among African Americans in the U.S.," Kaiser Public Opinion, June 2009; Racial/Ethnic Health Disparities Among Children with Diagnoses of Perinatal HIV Infection—34 States, 2004–20007. http://www.cdc.gov/mmwr/preview/mmwrhtml/mm5904a2.htm

Black women are far more likely to become infected with HIV than any other American women.[38] We have almost 15 times the AIDS rate of White women and over 4 times the rate of Latinas. No matter how we try to slice or dice our risk—whether by age, income, neighborhood, educational level, or marital status—the reality is that any one of us can be infected.

Yet while many of us are in denial about our own risk, we are very worried about our children's well-being—and we're right to be concerned. Almost 70 percent of new AIDS cases among teens occur among Black youth. In 2010, HIV/AIDS was the third leading cause of death among Black women ages 35 to 44.[39]

The good news is that HIV is 100 percent preventable if we abstain from having sex or taking drugs, and highly preventable if we're sexually active with the right precautions. Even if you get infected, it is no longer a death sentence. If you are diagnosed early, medications can help you manage the disease and even live a normal lifespan. But you can't protect yourself from getting the virus, or get diagnosed early so that you can receive lifesaving treatment, if you won't admit that you may be at risk.

Even during the earliest days of the AIDS epidemic, Blacks were becoming infected in disproportionate numbers. Back then, many experts warned us that the "5 H's"—hookers, Haitians, homosexuals, heroin addicts, and hemophiliacs—were the ones in danger. Still others told us that AIDS was a "White gay man's disease" or, later, that a Black woman's greatest risk factor was having sex with a man on the "down low." These stereotypes are flat-out wrong. *Anyone* who comes in contact with infected blood, semen, vaginal secretions, or breast milk can contract HIV (saliva does not spread the disease).

For many of us that false sense of security lingers. We believe that since we're not "that kind of" woman—whatever that may mean to us—we are somehow safe. But our own behavior isn't all that counts—and research shows that, compared to Whites, Blacks with few sex partners are more likely to have sex with people who themselves have many partners. Many Black women who are HIV-positive became infected through unprotected sex with someone they loved and trusted.

YOU'RE AT HIGHER RISK FOR BECOMING INFECTED WITH HIV IF YOU: [40]

- Engage in unprotected anal, vaginal, or oral sex with anyone who is infected;
- Share needles or syringes while injecting drugs or steroids;
- Have a sexually transmitted infection, such as syphilis, genital herpes, chlamydia, gonorrhea, bacterial vaginosis, or trichomoniasis, and have unprotected sex;
- Have been diagnosed with hepatitis or tuberculosis;
- Are exposed to the virus as a fetus or infant before or during birth or through breastfeeding from a mother infected with HIV;
- Received a blood transfusion or clotting factor in the United States anytime from 1978 to 1985;
- Engage in unprotected sex with someone who has any of these risk factors.

Today, a Black woman's risk of getting HIV has less to do with her sexual habits than with her sexual network—the pool of people with whom she may have sex. In the pool of Black people, HIV rates are high. This makes it more likely that a Black woman[41] will get HIV than will a woman of another race who engages in the same behavior.

HERE ARE OTHER KEY REASONS WHY BLACK WOMEN ARE AT SUCH HIGH RISK:

- Biologically, women are simply at greater risk than men. A woman has a larger area of tissue (vaginal and cervical) exposed to her partner's body fluids during sex, so the virus has more opportunity to enter her bloodstream—especially if, as often happens, her vagina has microscopic abrasions from sexual activity or STDs.

- Black men are becoming infected in high numbers. Today, there are approximately 1.1 million people living with HIV/AIDS in the United States, including approximately 545,000 who are Black. Analysis of national household survey data found that in 2008, 2 percent of Blacks in the United States were HIV-positive, higher than any other group. However, the rates among Black men are actually much higher: approximately 3 percent of Black men in the United States are HIV-positive, and 1 in every 16 Black men will be diagnosed with HIV in their lifetime. So as long as we're having sex with Black men—and most of us are—our chances of infection are higher.[42]

- Black women have higher rates of STDs. One recent study showed that of 206 sexually active Black girls ages 14–19, almost 50 percent of them had an STD. Young Black women have significantly higher rates of chlamydia, gonorrhea, and syphilis than any other racial or ethnic group . Women who already have an STD are more vulnerable to HIV, because STDs can create those microscopic abrasions in our vaginas and in our genital region that make it easier for the virus to enter.[43]

- Our sexual network is relatively small. In 2009, there were an estimated 42 million Blacks in the United States compared to about 270 million Americans of other backgrounds. Black women tend to have sex with Black men—we're more likely to have sex within our race than women of any other group—so Black people pass STDs back and forth.

- Many Black people with HIV don't know they have it. If you don't know you have it, you're less likely to take precautions that keep you from spreading it. While Black Americans get HIV tested more often than other groups—43 percent, including 60 percent of 18–29-year-olds—even this high is too low, given the prevalence of the disease in our community.

- We wait too long to get tested. As a result, we are more likely to develop AIDS within one year of receiving an HIV diagnosis. When we get tested late, we often don't get treatment until our lives are in jeopardy, and the fact that so many of us lack health insurance just worsens the problem. In the meantime, we unknowingly spread the virus to others.[44]

How Do I Know if I Have HIV?

Some people who get HIV experience very pronounced symptoms, whereas others may experience no symptoms at all. Those who do generally have symptoms similar to the common cold or flu: fever, fatigue, and, often, a rash. Other common symptoms can include headache, swollen lymph nodes, and sore throat. These symptoms can occur within days or weeks of the initial exposure to the virus. Many infections that are not HIV can cause similar symptoms, including mononucleosis, viral hepatitis, and other sexually transmitted infections. Stress and anxiety can also produce similar symptoms in some people, even though they do not have HIV.

Because of this, symptoms are not a reliable way to diagnose HIV infection. Testing for HIV antibodies is the only way to know whether you have been infected; however, the HIV antibody test works only after the infected person's immune system develops antibodies to HIV. During the "window" between the initial infection and the point when antibodies are detectable (which can be from two weeks to six months, but is usually around three months), standard HIV antibody testing may be negative, even though a person is infected—it is too early for the antibody test to be positive. However, HIV can be diagnosed during this window period with a test that looks for the HIV virus itself and not the body's response to it.

Taking Control Of HIV/AIDS

We can't always change the societal forces that place us in harm's way. Nevertheless, there are things we can do to protect ourselves, our loved ones and our communities. Consider incorporating some of these strategies into your life:

- Abstain from sexual activity. This is the only 100 percent way to prevent HIV infection.

- Protect yourself and your partners by knowing both your own HIV status and your partner's.

- Discuss the issue of testing and safer sex with your sexual partner.

- Practice safer sex (using protective barriers such as latex condoms or the female condom for vaginal, anal, and oral sex) every time you have sex.

- Take safer sex into your own hands by using a female condom—something like a male condom, made of nitrile or polyurethane plastic with flexible rings at both ends. The smaller ring at the closed end is inserted into the vagina, where the pubic bone holds it in place, and the larger ring remains outside, partially covering the vulva. Inside, the condom material lines the vagina, protecting it from male bodily fluids (and some STDs). This way, a woman whose partner doesn't have or doesn't want to use protection can say, "Okay, I'll use mine."

- Avoid injecting drugs and do not share needles of any kind.

If you believe or know that you're already infected, don't get down on yourself or feel that your life if over. You *will* need to focus on your well-being. The good news is, there's lots you can do:

- Get tested right away. If you are raped, assaulted, or have unprotected sex with someone whose HIV status you do not know, call a health-care provider immediately to discuss your next steps. Talk to your doctor about whether you should take HIV medication prophylactically, as a precautionary measure.

- If you learn that you are HIV-positive, seek treatment immediately. Not everyone has to take medication, but you do need to know your CD4, or T-cell, count (a measure of your immune system's strength), as well as your viral load (how much HIV your system is fighting). If you need medication, there are very effective treatments available.

- If the doctor prescribes meds, take them exactly as she or he directs. HIV can mutate over time. Missing doses of HIV medication can make the virus immune to the medicine.

- Eat healthy foods, get plenty of sleep, and minimize stress to protect your immune system.

"I WISH WE COULD HAVE BEEN MORE OPEN."

Despite Salt-N-Pepa's now-20-year-old warning that we need to talk about sex more openly, many Black moms still don't educate their daughters effectively about "the birds and the bees." Whether they teach their daughters to describe their genitals with street terms like "coochie" or "snatch," tell them that their menstrual period is a "curse," or say nothing about sex at all out of fear that their daughters will "do it," research suggests that mothers' negative portrayals or insinuations around their daughters' sexuality may make girls less likely to care for their sexual health.

Researchers interviewed 34 mothers (ages 46 to 82) and daughters (ages 20 to 55) from diverse educational and socioeconomic backgrounds in an urban Midwestern

---

city. They found that most of the mothers and daughters wished that they had communicated more openly about sexual health when the daughters were younger. The mothers, in particular, regretted not being more forthcoming. "I think I would be more liberal because of the way society is now, because of the diseases that are so prevalent in the world now," said a 66-year-old mom who participated in the study.

Secrecy between mothers and daughters can lead to dangerous situations, such as young women avoiding breast and gynecological exams. One woman spoke about "testing" her mother's orders during her teenage years because she wanted to know more about her body than what her mom told her and what her mother did say didn't make sense to her. Other young women said they felt uncomfortable and ashamed during gynecological exams, so they didn't use the time to ask questions, just wished it was over. Still others learned about sex and sexuality the worst way: from friends. "I would have been saved from a lot of things, from a lot of decisions that I made, if we had an open relationship," 20-year-old Natasha said. Our daughters need us to be positive examples and to offer our wisdom and guidance as they navigate their lives. Take advantage of "teachable moments," when you can talk about sex and sexuality naturally as it comes up in their world or in the media. And plan to talk with your daughter all throughout her youth. Feeling anxious or unsure of your facts? Read a book like *Sugar and Spice: Sexuality and Adolescent Girls* by Sue Leeds. View a video produced by the Black Women's Health Imperative, *Let Me Know What's Going On: My Body, My Self, My Life*. Or schedule an appointment with a counselor or a health-care provider.

Said 26-year-old Keisha: "If the mother is a role model, girls will follow her behavior. If the mom takes care of herself, the daughters will, too."

Source: From "Mothers to Daughters: A Qualitative Examination of the Reproductive Health Seeking Behaviour of African American Women" by Lari Warren-Jeanpiere. Women's Health and Urban Life 5 (2): 42–61.

Resources:

Balm in Gilead
701 East Franklin Street, Suite 1000
Richmond, VA 23219
(888) 225-6243
(804) 644-2256
www.balmingilead.org

Black AIDS Institute
1833 West 8th Street, Suite 200
Los Angeles, CA 90057
(213) 353-3610
www.blackaids.org

Black Women's Health Imperative
1726 M Street, Suite 300
Washington, DC 20036
(202) 548-4000
www.blackwomenshealth.org

National Association of People with AIDS (NAPWA)
8401 Colesville Road, Suite 505
Silver Spring, MD 20910
(866) 846-9366
(240) 247-0880
www.napwa.org

National Black Leadership Commission on AIDS
(800)992-6531
(212) 614-0023
www.nblca.org

National Minority AIDS Council
1931 13th Street NW
Washington, DC 20009
(202)483-6622
www.nmac.org

SisterLove
709 Bakers Ferry Road, SW
Atlanta, Georgia 30331
(866) 750-7733
(404) 505-7777
http://sisterlove.org

TheBody.com
www.thebody.com

KIDNEY DISEASE

For the longest time I thought the worst health problem anyone in my family had to worry about was high blood pressure. It seemed that too much salt, and perhaps a little too much stress, led to many of my relatives having this condition. Being in the health-care field, I knew that high blood pressure was nothing to play with, so I did my best to keep mine in check. Yet it turned out there was something much more sinister than high blood pressure stalking my family: polycystic kidney disease (PCKD).

Even as I saw my grandmother on my father's side suffer from kidney problems, and then die from kidney failure, I didn't consider this something that I would one day face, nor did anyone else in my family. Part of the reason was that we didn't know the name of her condition, and thus we did not realize we were at risk for it, too. Not only is PCKD life threatening, it is hereditary as well. Very hereditary. If one parent has the disease, there is a 50 percent chance the gene for the disease will pass to a child. This basically meant that everyone on my father's side of the family was at risk for PCKD, including me.

At 32, I began having the first symptoms of PCKD while I was pregnant with my son. I was tired—very tired. When I told my doctor how sluggish I felt, he assumed that it was because of the pregnancy and that I was anemic. This made sense to me, because many women I knew experienced a drop in their iron when they were pregnant and complained of feeling like slug bugs. My husband and I guessed I would just have to suffer through this, too.

A year and a half after I gave birth I still felt very tired—but on and off. I held off going to a doctor until a problem I couldn't deal with hit me: diarrhea. Now, this was not my first time having diarrhea, and I knew by the rate in which this one had me running to the bathroom that something was definitely wrong. I just didn't know how wrong. My husband and I headed to my doctor, and after scanning my abdomen he gave us the devastating news that I had PCKD. On my small little kidneys, he said, were numerous fluid-filled cysts that could and would do a lot of damage. The fact is, in many cases of PCKD, the cysts lead to reduced kidney function and ultimately kidney failure.

Wow, I was floored. Here I was worrying about and trying to prevent high blood pressure, breast cancer, and all these other conditions likely to affect me as a Black woman, and I now had something else I was almost guaranteed to get? It hit me like a ton of bricks. But after getting past the initial shock, I quickly began researching and learning as much as I could about PCKD. It was then that I realized it was what my grandma had died from. As if that wasn't bad enough, it occurred to me that my father and brother probably had it as well. They had both been dealing with high blood pressure nearly all of their adult lives, which was probably being caused by this condition. They wouldn't have known it, however. Like too many Black men, they stubbornly refused to go to the doctor unless they were at death's door.

I sounded the alarm in my family shortly after I was diagnosed, urging everyone on my father's side to get checked. Most did—though it took some a lot longer than others. My sister went immediately, as did some cousins, uncles, and aunts. Others, like my still stubborn brother, took their sweet time. We soon learned that PCKD had hit our family even harder than expected. Our first question had been who had it, but we ended up wondering who didn't have it. Not many, it turned out. Not only did my father have PCKD, as well as my sister and brother; at least seven of my dad's eleven siblings and many of my cousins were touched by the disease, too.

We all found out at different times and handled it in different ways. I decided shortly after being diagnosed that PCKD was not going to steal my life and take away my joy or that of my worried husband, son, and daughter.

I had been working as a coder specialist for a diagnostics lab for a number of years, and had even been a phlebotomist, so I was at ease talking with my doctor. I also knew the importance of following my doctor's orders. Fresh fruits and veggies became staples in my diet—canned would not do. And potato chips and bacon—two of my favorite things—soon became something I ate only as treats. I had to work double duty at controlling my blood pressure now, my doctor explained. This also meant taking my blood pressure every day, along with three pills to control it and boost my iron. And there was still more to do: I had to have blood work done every month to ensure I had all the right chemistry levels in my blood. When something was off, I had to immediately get myself in balance. For example, when my iron was very low I had to have iron injections every week until it returned to normal.

Kidney Disease

Needless to say, all this was not fun. Neither was the fatigue that had returned in full force. I thought I had it pretty bad—but 13 years after my initial diagnosis I learned what "bad" truly was. Despite taking great care of myself, I was diagnosed with end stage renal disease (ESRD) and learned that I would have to go on hemodialysis. Hemodialysis—the process that would be used to clean my blood of toxic waste since my kidneys refused to do so—was no joke. It meant I would pretty much have to quit my job.

I had been a trooper up until that point, but being diagnosed with ESRD and forced to go on dialysis was just too much for me. It all became so real and I had to get my mind, body, and soul ready. So, I asked the doctor to give me more time. He agreed, saying, "You will call me before I call you." Umm, what does that mean? I wondered. A few months later I found out. It was this unbearable pain—far worse than that of natural childbirth—that made me finally leave my job to start dialysis.

It was as bad as I thought. Two "I can't believe you are going to stick those in me" needles had to be inserted into my arms each time I received the treatment, which was every other day for four hours. Still, I had taken time to pray and made a commitment to trust God for what was about to happen in my life. Thankfully, God and my family helped see me through the pain and frustration that came with dialysis. And soon, because I had been adamant with my doctor about returning to work, I got great news—I could get a machine and have hemodialysis at home. This was pleasing, and after quickly learning how to work the machine, in no time I was sticking myself with the needles—something I thought I could never do. But with a little help from some great numbing cream and my family, I became a pro. The only "little" catch was I had to have dialysis six days a week. Still, I could go back to work and, even more important, spend more time with my family. I took my little machine on vacation to Vegas and to Miami! What a blessing!

I was doing pretty well on dialysis, but after two years of being stuck on a machine six days a week I became frustrated. There were many a day and night that I had to hide myself away from everyone and just pray to God for strength. Eventually, my prayers were answered. I was approved for a kidney transplant. I got the call on October 1, 2009—my 49th birthday.

The new kidney I received meant a better quality of life, free of dialysis, and nearly getting back to my normal, outgoing self that was always on the move. Of course, I take about 16 pills every day so my body doesn't reject the kidney, and sometimes I still get very, very tired, but I have no room to complain. Because of my transplant, I have so much more than just a fighting chance of living a long and fulfilling life despite my PCKD.

I do wish I could say the same for others within my family. While I was having my own personal PCKD battle, my father and my brother were, too. Despite my pleading and trying to *scare them into taking care of themselves, they didn't listen. My father died soon after we learned of his illness, at age 49, and my brother years later at age 43. My sister, who got on top of the disease as soon as she found out, lost her resolve when she was told she had to go on hemodialysis. She was on peritoneal dialysis—a simpler procedure that was done not by filtering the blood, but by administering fluid in the abdomen while she slept at night. It didn't require needles; hemodialysis did. "I'm not getting stuck by those needles," she told me quite frankly. It has hurt me since to watch her suffer from several strokes and other PCKD complications. Still, I know firsthand that this disease is not easy. I also recognize that many people don't understand the complications that it will cause if you don't do all you can and talk to your doctors to get the full understanding.*

I hope that others with kidney disease—which is largely preventable—make the choice to fight it no matter what. I can say that it's been a blessing in disguise, because it has made me a stronger and more faithful person. It's also made me love life more and made me willing to do whatever it takes to preserve it.

*—**Karen V. Hill** and husband Gregory have been married for 27 years and have two children, Danielle and Gregory, Jr. Karen loves to laugh and enjoys this beautiful life God has given her.*

Kidney Disease and Black Women

The human body is amazing, and so are the internal organs that keep it functioning. Yet while many people know what the heart, lungs, and even the liver do, our kidneys often don't receive the attention they deserve. Considering the huge role they play in keeping us healthy—from filtering toxins and waste out of the blood to controlling blood pressure and preserving bone health—it's a mistake to overlook them. Just as important, we also shouldn't ignore the kidneys' most serious ailment and one of the leading killers of black women: chronic kidney disease (CKD). This is a potentially life-threatening condition in which the small blood vessels in the kidneys are damaged, causing waste to build up in the blood and making the kidneys unable to do their many jobs. Though our kidneys are tough organs, CKD is usually irreversible and can lead to kidney failure, also called end stage renal disease (ESRD), if not treated.

More than 26 million Americans[45]—one in nine adults—have kidney disease, and millions more are at increased risk for getting it but don't know it. Black women are no exception. In fact, our risk is especially high. CKD is most often caused by diabetes or high blood pressure—the high levels of blood sugar caused by diabetes can overwork the kidneys, and high blood pressure can damage their blood vessels—and these two conditions disproportionally affect Black women. About 45 percent of us have high blood pressure and nearly 12 percent of all Black women ages 20 and older have diabetes—the fifth leading cause of death for Black women after 55. Other risk factors for kidney disease include heart disease—

WHY ARE YOUR KIDNEYS SO IMPORTANT?

- They make urine.
- They remove waste and extra fluid from your blood.
- They remove drugs and other toxins from your blood.
- They regulate the chemicals in your blood.
- They help control your blood pressure.
- They help keep your bones healthy.
- They help you make red blood cells.

also prevalent in the Black community—a family history of kidney failure, and lupus.

Black women and men constitute about 29 percent of all patients treated for kidney failure in the United States, a high number considering we make up only about 14 percent of the U.S. population. Just as distressing, we also develop kidney failure at an earlier age than White Americans; the average age of Blacks at the start of treatment for kidney failure is 56, compared with 66 for Whites. One of the reasons for this distressing fact is that we are less likely to know that we have kidney disease in its early stages, and thus we don't act to prevent or delay kidney failure through adequate treatment.[46]

What Does Kidney Disease Look Like?

Kidney disease can arise in a number of ways, from the major risk factors of diabetes and high blood pressure to inherited disorders such as PCKD (polycystic kidney disease, the family illness that Karen Hill faced) to various forms of inflammation and infection.

Kidney disease tends to start slowly, and its subtle early signs may be hard to detect—or it may produce no symptoms at all in the early stages. Most people do not have severe symptoms until their kidney disease is advanced. However, you may notice that you feel more tired and have less energy, a poor appetite, trouble concentrating, muscle cramps at night, puffiness around your eyes, especially in the morning; dry itchy skin and frequent urination more often, especially at night. Signs of more advanced disease include back pain, fever, chills, and increased urination. If you notice these symptoms, you should get tested and treated right away.

Kidney failure itself may not produce any additional symptoms. The symptoms that do occur are due to the buildup of waste products in the body as the kidneys' function slows down; this may cause weakness, shortness of breath, lethargy, and confusion. In addition, the inability to remove potassium from the bloodstream may lead to abnormal heart rhythms.

If you suspect you have kidney disease, or if you have diabetes, high blood pressure, or heart disease, you should speak with your doctor about getting tested for CKD. There are three simple tests that your doctor may give you: an estimated glomerular filtration rate (eGFR) test, a urine test, and a blood pressure test:[47]

- **eGFR.** This test tells your doctor how well your kidneys clean your blood. Your doctor will test your blood for a kind of waste called creatinine, because healthy kidneys filter creatinine out of your blood. Your doctor will then use your creatinine test result to figure out your eGFR. An eGFR of less than 60 for three months or more may be a sign of kidney disease.

- **Urine test.** This test tells your doctor if there is blood or protein in your urine, a sign of kidney disease. Your doctor may test your urine in the office or ask you to collect your urine at home.

- **Blood pressure test.** This test tells your doctor how hard your heart is working to pump your blood. High blood pressure can cause kidney disease, but kidney disease can also cause high blood pressure.

How Can I Reduce My Risk of Kidney Disease?

The best way to prevent CKD is to take good care of your kidneys and heart. People whose kidneys have failed are three times as likely to have heart disease and high blood pressure. Steps you can take to protect both your kidneys and heart: don't smoke, as smoking is the strongest modifiable risk factor for both kidney and heart disease; control your blood pressure, because high blood pressure causes both kidney and heart disease; and eat a diet low in salt and high in vegetables and low fat dairy products.

What Treatment Will I Receive for Kidney Disease?

Once you've been diagnosed with kidney disease, the goal of treatment is to prevent or slow additional damage to your kidneys. If you have diabetes or high blood pressure, you and your doctor will create a plan to treat and manage these conditions, which could include a range medications and changing your diet.

Steps you can take to control your kidney disease include making exercise a routine part

PREVENT CKD!

- Eat a diet low in fat and salt.
- Exercise most days of the week.
- Have regular check-ups with your doctor.
- Avoid tobacco.
- Limit alcohol.

of your life; avoiding medicines that can affect kidney function, such as over-the-counter pain pills containing ibuprofen, naproxen, and ketoprofen; avoiding dehydration; and getting immediate care for symptoms, such as diarrhea, vomiting, or fever, which can cause you to lose fluids. You should not smoke, drink alcohol, or use illegal drugs.

Your diet also plays a role in preventing further kidney damage. For example, since the kidneys of people with CKD cannot easily remove excess water, salt, or potassium, you may need to limit your intake of foods high in potassium, which include bananas, apricots, and salt substitutes. It may also be important to limit your intake of phosphorus, an often-forgotten chemical that tends to become elevated in kidney failure because poorly functioning kidneys can't remove excess from the blood. Too much phosphorus can leach calcium from the bones and cause osteoporosis and fractures. Foods with high phosphorus content include milk, cheese, nuts, and cola drinks.

Even with the right treatments, CKD often leads to kidney failure. There are only two treatments that allow you to go on living when your kidneys stop functioning: dialysis and kidney transplantation.[48] During dialysis, a special machine is used to filter the blood and remove built up waste. One type of dialysis has to be done in a clinic; for another kind of dialysis, the machine is so small it can be strapped to your body while you go about your daily activities. Many people are reluctant to go on dialysis because of the constraints it puts on one's time—or because of a fear of needles. But not taking advantage of this life-saving treatment can lead to complications like stroke and eventually an early death—outcomes far worse than needles.

In a kidney transplant,[49] you receive a healthy kidney from a donor. Only one donated kidney is needed to replace two failed kidneys, which means that it's possible to receive a kidney from a living donor, often a relative. If a compatible living donor isn't available for a kidney transplant, your name may be placed on a waiting list to receive a kidney from a deceased donor. The wait could be a year or more. Unfortunately, Blacks are less likely than Whites to receive a kidney transplant, and we are less likely to donate our kidneys as well.

Karen hopes that others with kidney disease—which is largely preventable—make the choice to fight it no matter what. It's also made her love life more and made her willing to do whatever it takes to preserve life. Fighting this disease is your choice—take the chance to live and love life, as Karen does.

Resources:

American Association of Kidney Patients
3505 East Frontage Road, Suite 315
Tampa, FL 33607
(800) 749-2257
(813) 636-8100
www.aakp.org

National Kidney Foundation
30 East 33rd Street
New York, NY 10016
(800) 622-9010
www.kidney.org

PKD Foundation
9221 Ward Parkway, Suite 400
Kansas City, MO 64114–3367
(800) 753-2873
(816) 931-2600
www.pkdcure.org

OBESITY

———————————◼———————————

When I was 12, I was told that I was obese.

"Jump on the scale," the school nurse said to me the day of my exam. She muttered something that sounded like, "If you can jump."

"Just as I thought," she said. "You are obese," she said, dragging the word out for what felt like an eternity: "Ooooooooooo—beeeeeeeeeeeeeese."

She went on to say that if I didn't stop eating so much, I would become very sick and might die before I reached the age of 40.

I was only 12 years old, but I was being told that overeating would be the cause of my death. Back then my family was extremely poor, so we hardly ever had enough to eat and we certainly didn't have enough to overeat. Little was known about the impact of genetics on adiposity and even less was understood about the connection between improper nourishment and weight gain. All the nurse knew was that I was fat, and I was unhealthy. The stigma and stereotyping I experienced in my youth were just the beginning of what society would have in store for me.

After graduating from high school, my talent and smarts and several exceptional educators helped me to go to college, but again I faced the discrimination that comes with weight. I joined the show choir, a choral group like the one on the television show Glee, *that does dance moves while singing, and was shocked by the ridicule of audience members who laughed out loud when I approached the microphone. But as I opened my mouth to sing, the powerful gospel tones and phrases took over and I was rewarded with standing ovations. Even so, the director told me I could not come back unless I lost weight, which, he informed me, was distracting people from my talent.*

I was angry and embarrassed, but I did not confront him. That summer, I starved myself and exercised so much that I lost 80 pounds. I looked incredible. Old friends didn't recognize me and everyone wanted my secret.

At the end of the summer, I passed out while playing racquetball and ended up in the hospital. I spent a week there being treated for malnutrition and severe dehydration. I had achieved weight-loss success at the cost of my health, but no one cared about the price I had paid. I looked great, and that was all that mattered.

A few years after finishing my doctoral degree, I became an entertainer and lecturer and soon landed a nationally syndicated television talk show, The Bertice Berry Show (1991–1992). *Now, in case you haven't already heard, television is said to add 10 pounds, but I know from experience that the stress from television executives actually adds about 50.*

One day, while I was hosting the television show, I was instructed by the show's executives to watch the viewer focus-group research video tapes. The initial overall reaction was extremely positive, with viewers stating that they loved the show and felt that I was a well-informed and lively host. Not satisfied with these answers, the interviewer in an authoritative voice asked the participants if they thought I should lose weight since I was on television representing African Americans and women . . . Eventually, the participants, ages 20–45, relented and began to make disparaging remarks. "She has gained a lot of weight since she first came on television," one woman commented. Another said that she felt that I represented the stereotyped image of the loud, big-butt Black woman.

At the time of this event, I weighed between 145 and 155 pounds. Years later, when I ballooned up to 290 pounds, I looked back at pictures and tapes from that period and realized how small I really was. A few years ago, and 35 years after I first heard that I was "obese," I heard the same thing again. This time though, it was coming from a successful cardiologist. "You need to have gastric bypass surgery," he proclaimed. After a quick examination, he said that my health issues were becoming more and more serious and that my weight had been the cause of them all.

"You need to do something fast," he said, "or things will only get worse."

I had no intention of undergoing any form of what I perceived to be unnecessary surgery. At the time, I weighed 250 pounds and I had thought of gastric bypass as a last resort for people who weighed more than 500 pounds. When I told the physician this, he said that the surgery was being done on people who weighed even less than I did and that they were now living healthy lives. I knew that it wasn't as easy as he made it sound.

During this time, my 87-year-old mother suffered from several serious illnesses, including a brain tumor and a series of strokes and heart attacks. I had been caring for her along with my children. I became even more stressed, and my weight got up to 290 pounds. My doctor told me that I was depressed and that my weight had caused other health issues. He said that unless I did something quickly, I'd be joining my mother in heaven.

After caring for my mother and my five adopted children and touring all over the country teaching other people to love themselves and the work they did, I found that I had spent very little time on me. I suffered from several serious illnesses and needed more medical coverage. Again I tried to increase the coverage by switching policies, and again I was declared "uninsurable" because of "obesity." I ran back to my old provider and looked for ways to get healthy.

I soon learned that there was no one program designed just for me. I then looked through research findings and holistic materials for a plan of attack. As I started out, I knew that I had to redefine what a healthy body would look and feel like. I was shocked by how large I had become. I soon came to understand that weight, like everything else about the human body, was linked to genetics and was as unique and varied as our genes. I learned that true wellness, not the number on a scale, was the real prize.

The beginning of any life change must start in the mind. I decided to give myself at least a year to "get well," and I soon noticed that my wellness plan had a life of its own. The pounds seemed to drop off, and my physical exams were improving rapidly.

"When a person seeks their purpose, the Universe conspires to make it happen."

By combining proper nutrition, well-balanced exercise, massage therapy, and proper rest and hydration with visualization, meditation, and sleep therapy, I have enabled my body to heal itself. I have learned to love and embrace the thick thighs that have carried me and be grateful for my large round behind that never let my back down. As I have shown love to my entire body, it has rewarded me with good health. At 50, I look and feel better than I did at 30. I have lost over 150 pounds. The journey has not been easy, but it has been beautiful, wonderful, and powerful.

As I have learned, you too will need to forget what you think you know about weight loss. You will have to open your mind and your heart to a whole new approach to being well in spirit, mind, and body. You must come to see that losing weight is a result of getting well, not the other way around.

Be prepared to change from the inside out, and most of all, get ready to start loving you.

—**Dr. Bertice Berry** *is a sociologist, lecturer, educator, and author of* A Year to Wellness and Other Weightloss Secrets.

Obesity and Black Women

America's growing obesity problem is all over the nightly news. But many Americans don't have to turn on the tube to know about the crisis; they can just look in the mirror. That's how many of us are experiencing our own personal battles with weight gain. Weight is on the rise across age, race, and gender lines in the United States, with nearly two-thirds of adult Americans categorized as being overweight or obese and nearly one-third as obese. Three hundred thousand people die annually of causes related to obesity, and the medical care of obese people costs us $100 billion a year.

For all Americans, obesity is a serious health challenge. For Black women and our families, it's an epidemic. We are more likely to be obese than women of any other racial group, more prone to the diseases that obesity contributes or connects to, and more likely to die from those diseases.

Black women have higher-than-average rates of obesity for many different reasons. As you will read in Chapter 6, we use the same flawed food supply that causes many Americans to struggle to maintain good health. Beyond these common challenges, Black women are fighting a particularly steep uphill battle. Some of us lack the knowledge, resources, or motivation to do what's right for our health. Many of us don't get the exercise we should (55 percent of Black women get little or no exercise), whether because we don't have time, can't afford a gym, or don't want to sweat out our hairdos. Some of us are so drained by meeting our families' basic needs that we don't have time to cook—or maybe we only have fast food and convenience-store canned goods in our neighborhoods.

Then there's the question of how Black women view food—and the even more important question of how we view ourselves. A number of women in Imperative focus groups[50] talked about the dietary habits they were taught growing up. Food as a centerpiece of gatherings and celebrations—it's a part of our lifestyle and our heritage, one that's hard to unlearn. More than that, our daily lives are often filled with stress that takes a heavy emotional and physical toll. We just keep on going and keep on giving, and we use food as a way to relieve our anxiety, frustration, anger, and guilt. Many Black women may not realize they are emotional eaters; one focus group participant said she thought she didn't have a lot of stress in her life, until her doctor asked her to keep a food diary of what she ate and how she felt. She soon realized she was stuffing her emotions by eating—and tipping the scales at 240.

A lot of us are engaged in a similar self-deception: though two out of three Black women are overweight or obese according to standard health guidelines, far fewer of us *think* of ourselves as overweight. Our community accepts being overweight as normal, and this distortion leads us to think we're healthier than we really are.

There's a paradox here: although we buy into the standard by which fat really isn't fat, people who carry excess weight—especially young girls—are subjected to major stigma and ridicule. In this sense, obesity is an increased emotional risk factor because it sets us up to feel like failures, out of control and ashamed. Those feelings hurt, and we often turn to food even more to soothe the pain. Eventually our bodies start to suffer, and we fall ill, and then we take pills to keep us functioning as we spiral down. This happens when we don't love ourselves enough to treat ourselves with care.

What Does Obesity Look Like?

Being obese is more than being just a few pounds on the heavy side. Overweight and obesity are both labels for ranges of weight that are greater than what is generally considered healthy for a given height. The terms also identify ranges of weight that have been shown to increase the likelihood of certain diseases and other health problems.

For adults, overweight and obesity ranges are determined by using weight and height to calculate a number called the body mass index (BMI). BMI is used because, for most people, it correlates with the amount of body fat they have.[51] While many black women may complain that BMI doesn't apply to them because of their extra curves, it is still very useful in determining whether you need to reduce your weight and setting goals for weight loss. You will read more about BMI in Chapter 6.

A wide variety of factors can cause an increase in body weight, starting with the most basic: eating more food than your body can use. Being physically inactive is another clear culprit: you're not using up the energy you're taking in. Dieting or missing meals can, ironically, cause your metabolism to slow down; so can hormonal issues and certain medications. Drinking excess alcohol is another way to pack on the pounds.

There are many causes of obesity as well. Most attention focuses on just one—overeating. But obesity also results from genetic disorders, insulin resistance and metabolic syndrome, depression, and stress, as well as other health factors. The idea that obesity is always caused by overeating feeds the stereotyped ideas about fat people: that we are fat because we are also lazy, unmotivated, and greedy. It's bad enough when ordinary people are misinformed; what's worse is that all too often the physicians who are charged with helping us project the same misconceptions and myths into our treatment and recommended care.

What Does Obesity Do to Us?

Many women who struggle with their weight complain that they can't find cute clothes to fit them, that they have to buy larger sizes and they look frumpy in them. However, obesity is more than a cosmetic problem. It's a medical condition, and it is one of the leading preventable causes of death worldwide. In fact, obesity could become more dangerous to your health than smoking cigarettes. Larry Cohen of the Prevention Institute[52] warns that our focus on blaming the individual, without taking into account the social and economic influence of where we live, work, and play, ignores the unintended consequences. In addition to our obsession with weight loss that shifts us away from good nutrition, there are two other very serious consequences that Black women should pay attention to:

- Internalizing the pervasive stigma and stereotypes of being lazy and lacking self-control—in other words, the fat bias. Living with this stigma takes a toll on our mental health, making us more prone to depression, suicidal thoughts, and suicide attempts.

- Feelings of being judged after receiving a negative health "report card" at the doctor's office. These feelings prevent many Black women from seeking medical care, so that we delay or avoid preventive health-care services when we need them most.

OBESITY RISKS AND RELATED HEALTH CONDITIONS

ARTHRITIS

Osteoarthritis (OA)

- Associated with the development of OA of the hand, the hip, the back, and especially the knee.

- At a BMI greater than 25, the incidence of OA has been shown to steadily increase.

- Modest weight loss of 10 to 15 pounds is likely to relieve symptoms and delay disease progression of knee OA.

Rheumatoid Arthritis (RA)

- Related to RA in both men and women.

BIRTH DEFECTS

- Maternal obesity (BMI > 29) has been associated with an increased incidence of neural tube defects (NTDs) in several studies.

- Folate intake, which decreases the risk of NTDs, was found in one study to have a reduced effect with higher pre-pregnancy weight.

CANCERS

Breast Cancer

- Postmenopausal women with obesity have a higher risk of developing breast cancer. In addition, weight gain after menopause may also increase breast cancer risk.

- Women who gain 45 pounds or more after age 18 are twice as likely to develop breast cancer after menopause as those who remain weight-stable.

- High BMI has been associated with a decreased risk of breast cancer before menopause.

- Premenopausal women diagnosed with breast cancer who are over-weight appear to have a shorter life span than women with lower BMI.

- The risk of breast cancer in men is also increased by obesity.

Cancers of the Esophagus and Gastric Cardia

- Strongly associated with obesity; risk becomes higher with increasing BMI.

- The risk for gastric cardia cancer rises moderately with increasing BMI.

Colorectal Cancer

- High BMI, high calorie intake, and low physical activity are independent risk factors.

- Larger waist size (abdominal obesity) is associated with colorectal cancer.

Endometrial Cancer (EC)

- Women with obesity have three to four times the risk of EC of women with lower BMI.

- Women with obesity and diabetes are reported to have a threefold increase in risk for EC above the risk of obesity alone.

- Body size is a risk factor for EC regardless of where fat is distributed in the body.

Renal Cell Cancer

- Associated with renal cell cancer, especially in women.

- Excess weight was reported in one study to account for 21% of renal cell cancer cases.

CARDIOVASCULAR DISEASE (CVD)

- Increases CVD risk due to its effect on blood lipid levels.
- Weight loss improves blood lipid levels by lowering triglycerides and LDL ("bad") cholesterol and increasing HDL ("good") cholesterol.
- Weight loss of 5% to 10% can reduce total blood cholesterol.
- Effects of obesity on cardiovascular health can begin in childhood, which increases the risk of developing CVD as an adult.
- Increases the risk of illness and death associated with coronary heart disease.
- Major risk factor for heart attack.

CARPAL TUNNEL SYNDROME (CTS)

- Established as a risk factor for CTS.
- Risk for obese patients four times greater than that of non-obese patients.
- Found in one study to be a stronger risk factor for CTS than workplace activity that requires repetitive and forceful hand use.
- 70% of persons in a recent CTS study were overweight or obese.

DAYTIME SLEEPINESS

- Persons with obesity frequently complain of daytime sleepiness and fatigue, two probable causes of accidents.
- Associated with increased daytime sleepiness even in the absence of sleep apnea or other breathing disorders.

DEEP VEIN THROMBOSIS (DVT)

- Increases the risk of DVT, a condition that disrupts the normal process of blood clotting.
- Increased risk of DVT after surgery.

DIABETES (TYPE 2)

- As many as 90% of individuals with type 2 diabetes are reported to be overweight or obese.

- Found to be the largest environmental influence on the prevalence of diabetes in a population.

- Complicates the management of type 2 diabetes by increasing insulin resistance and glucose intolerance, which makes drug treatment for type 2 diabetes less effective.

- A weight loss of as little as 5% can reduce high blood sugar.

END STAGE RENAL DISEASE (ESRD)

- Direct or indirect factor in the initiation or progression of renal disease, as suggested in preliminary data.

GALLBLADDER DISEASE

- Established predictor of gallbladder disease.

- Obesity and rapid weight loss in obese persons are known risk factors for gallstones.

- Gallstones appear in persons with obesity at a rate of 30% versus 10% in the non-obese.

GOUT

- Contributes to the cause of gout—the deposit of uric acid crystals in joints and tissue.

- Associated with increased production of uric acid and decreased elimination from the body.

HEAT DISORDERS

- Found to be a risk factor for heat injury and heat disorders.
- Poor heat tolerance is often associated with obesity.

HYPERTENSION

- Over 75% of hypertension cases are reported to be directly attributed to obesity.
- Weight or BMI in association with age is the strongest indicator of blood pressure in humans.
- Association between obesity and high blood pressure has been observed in virtually all societies, ages, and ethnic groups and in both genders.
- Risk of developing hypertension is five to six times greater in obese adult Americans, age 20 to 45, than in non-obese individuals of the same age.

IMPAIRED IMMUNE RESPONSE

- Found to decrease the body's resistance to harmful organisms.
- A decrease in the activity of scavenger cells, which destroy bacteria and foreign organisms in the body, has been observed in patients with obesity.

IMPAIRED RESPIRATORY FUNCTION

- Associated with impairment in respiratory function.
- Found to increase respiratory resistance, which in turn may cause breathlessness.
- Decreases in lung volume with increasing obesity have been reported.

INFECTIONS FOLLOWING WOUNDS

- Associated with increased incidence of wound infection.
- Burn patients with obesity are reported to develop pneumonia and wound infection with twice the frequency of the non-obese.

INFERTILITY

- Increases the risk for several reproductive disorders, negatively affecting normal menstrual function and fertility.

- Weight loss of about 10% of initial weight is effective in improving menstrual regularity, ovulation, hormonal profiles, and pregnancy rates.

LIVER DISEASE

- Excess weight is reported to be an independent risk factor for the development of alcohol-related liver diseases, including cirrhosis and acute hepatitis.
- Most common factor of progressive liver disease.

LOW BACK PAIN

- Plays a part in aggravating a simple low back problem and contributes to a long-lasting or recurring condition.
- Large waist size is risk factor for low back pain.

OBSTETRIC AND GYNECOLOGIC COMPLICATIONS

- Women with severe obesity have a menstrual disturbance rate three times higher than that of women with normal weight.
- High pre-pregnancy weight is associated with an increased risk during pregnancy of hypertension, gestational diabetes, urinary infection, and toxemia.
- Reportedly associated with the increased incidence of overdue births, induced labor, and longer labors.
- Higher incidence of blood loss during delivery, infection and wound complication after surgery, and Cesarean deliveries.
- Complications after childbirth associated with obesity include an increased risk of endometrial infection and inflammation, urinary tract infection, and urinary incontinence.

PAIN

- Bodily pain is a prevalent problem among persons with obesity.
- Greater disability, due to bodily pain, has been reported by persons with obesity compared to persons with other chronic medical conditions.
- Known to be associated with musculoskeletal or joint-related pain.

- Foot pain located at the heel, known as Sever's disease, is commonly associated with obesity.

PANCREATITIS

- Predictive factor of outcome in acute pancreatitis.
- Patients with acute pancreatitis found to have a higher body-fat percentage and larger waist size than patients with mild pancreatitis.

SLEEP APNEA

- Most significant risk factor for obstructive sleep apnea.
- Incidence of obstructive sleep apnea 12 to 30 times higher among morbidly obese patients compared to the general population.
- Among patients with obstructive sleep apnea, at least 60% to 70% are obese.

STROKE

- Elevated BMI is reported to increase the risk of ischemic stroke independent of other risk factors, including age and systolic blood pressure.
- Abdominal obesity appears to predict the risk of stroke in men.
- Risk factors for ischemic and total stroke in women.

SURGICAL COMPLICATIONS

- Risk factor for complications after a surgery.
- Surgical patients with obesity demonstrate a higher number and incidence of hospital-acquired infections compared to normal-weight patients.

URINARY STRESS INCONTINENCE

- Well-documented risk factor for urinary stress incontinence and involuntary urine loss, as well as urge incontinence and urgency among women.
- Strong risk factor for several urinary symptoms after pregnancy and delivery, continuing as much as 6 to 18 months after childbirth.

Source: Reprinted with permission from the American Obesity Association.

As the Obesity Risks and Related Health Conditions chart suggests, many diseases and conditions, such as type 2 diabetes and heart disease, disproportionately affect black women because of our higher-than-average rates of obesity. And being in poor health is not the only thing to worry about—death is a real consequence too. The degree to which obesity increases risk varies by cause of death, and most of this increased risk is due to the strain that excess weight puts on the heart. Obesity is a risk factor for all the leading chronic conditions and has a direct link to the alarming increase in death rates among young Black women.

Taking Control of Obesity

In order for us to have a fighting chance in this battle against obesity, we must first embrace creating a healthy lifestyle as an achievable goal. It starts with taking stock of our life practices—what we eat, how we eat, how we move, how we handle stress—and making a commitment to plan and problem-solve in order to make some needed changes in our lives. For more guidance on taking control of obesity, see Chapter 6, "Healthy Body."

Resources:

The Obesity Society
8757 Georgia Avenue, Suite 1320
Silver Spring, MD 20910
(301) 563-6526
www.obesity.org

Obesity Action Coalition
4511 North Himes Avenue, Suite 250
Tampa, FL 33614
(800) 717-3117
www.obesityaction.org

Weight Control Information Network (WIN)
1 WIN Way
Bethesda, MD 20892-3665
(877) 946-4627
www.win.niddk.nih.gov

SEXUALLY TRANSMITTED DISEASES

Imagine being a teenage girl and being too scared to tell anyone you think you might be pregnant. That was how I remembered feeling at age 15, when I thought I was pregnant. I didn't know what was happening to my body; I was on birth control and did not know I needed anything else. I went to the clinic for a pregnancy test and instead they told me I had chlamydia.

After my diagnosis, I remember feeling ashamed and not wanting anybody to know that I had an STD. I didn't tell anybody, not my mom or the guy I had sex with. A teacher at my school talked to me and helped me by telling me where I could go for treatment.

I went for treatment, but still felt so ashamed and angry that I ran away from home and began drinking and having risky sex. My shame and anger never left me, so I kept on using sex and drinking as an escape.

When I was around 17 or 18, I had a discharge but didn't know what it meant. I got tested and found out I had gonorrhea. When I first heard the news, I was really scared, thinking I wouldn't ever be able to have kids. I wanted to talk to my boyfriend about it, but when I told him that I had gonorrhea, he beat me up. I was so ashamed and embarrassed; I couldn't tell anybody what was happening.

When I went for treatment, the staff at the clinic was really supportive; they were people that I could talk to. They made me feel very comfortable and helped me feel less ashamed. It was a little while after that that I decided I needed to start being more careful and taking better care of myself.

I started talking to my partners about protection and made sure that I did not have sex unless

---

it was with a condom. I started educating myself about STDs and different ways to be better pro-tected. I started going to the doctor and insisted that unless a man was willing to go to the clinic with me to be tested, I wouldn't have anything to do with him.

This is something I insist on and information I share with my daughters as well. I tell my daughters and any other young women out there that there is more in life that you can do than to lay down with a boy. You have a choice about what your tomorrow will be.

—Lola

Sexually Transmitted Diseases and Black Women

Black women are experiencing an STD epidemic. By some estimates, 48 percent of us between ages 14 and 49 have genital herpes, a common STD. Black women accounted for 64 percent of new AIDS cases among women in 2009, even though we represent only 12 percent of the population. The good news is that most STDs are preventable.[53]

You may be a bit confused about some of the terms we hear today. Years ago, we were warned about the dangers of venereal disease, or VD. Then we learned about sexually trans-mitted diseases, STDs, and how to avoid getting them. More recently, we hear the term sexually transmitted infection, or STI. With all these terms, the question remains . . . what are we talking about?

Medically speaking, many diseases begin with an infection first; after the infection creates symptoms, it is considered a disease. Sexually transmitted infections—or STIs—are caused by viruses and bacteria that are most commonly passed from one person to another through sexual contact. Once a person begins to develop symptoms from an STI, it is considered a sexually transmitted disease, or STD. We may hear the terms STI and STD used inter-changeably, but for the purpose of this book, we're using STD.

Sexually transmitted diseases are infectious diseases spread through intimate contact—typically vaginal intercourse, oral sex, or anal sex. What is less well known is the fact that they can sometimes be transmitted through skin-to-skin contact or a visible or microscopic sore, by sharing drug needles, during childbirth or breastfeeding, and even while using sex toys. Bacterial vaginosis, chlamydia, gonorrhea, hepatitis, herpes, HIV/AIDS, human papil-loma virus (HPV), syphilis, and trichomoniasis are among the most common STDs.

How Do I Know If I Have an STD?

For women, many STDs have signs that are few or extremely mild—or there may be no signs at all. In other cases, their symptoms are hidden by folds of skin, under the pubic hair, or in an obscure location that's hard to see. No wonder many people pass them along without even knowing they have them. When STDs do have symptoms, they vary widely, but the most common are soreness, unusual lumps or sores, itching, pain when urinating, and/or an unusual discharge from the vagina. Among the infections that typically show no symptoms is HPV, which can cause genital warts or even cervical cancer.

All STDs are passed through intimate contact, but not all require that you have intercourse. Genital herpes, for instance, can pass through microscopic breaks in the skin. "My outbreak sometimes goes down my thighs," says one 34-year-old Houston resident. Some people are shocked to discover they have an STD in their throat, an all-too-common outcome from oral sex—and something parents of teens should be aware of, whether their children have had intercourse or not.

Whether you have symptoms or not, you should be tested immediately if you have any reason to believe that you may have been exposed or within a couple of months of having sex with a new partner—particularly if you've had unprotected sex—so that any infection can be caught before it harms your immune system and damages your body or someone else's. Since everyone is at risk—even married people—some doctors advise that patients get tested yearly no matter what. "You know only what you're doing; you don't know what anybody you're having sex with is doing," says Dr. Natalie Achong. "I'd even say that sex is risky in a so-called monogamous relationship."

It's also important to have a yearly Pap test and pelvic exam. However, many women mistakenly believe that just because they're getting a pelvic exam, their doctor is screening them for STDs. They're wrong. When a doctor looks for signs of abnormalities by using a Pap test, this is not a test for HPV or any other STD—there is a separate test for HPV. So if you or your doctor believes you're at risk for one STD, you should get tested for all of them. An STD screening can involve a pelvic and physical exam in which your doctor looks for signs of infection, such as a rash, discharge, or warts. The doctor may also use a swab to collect discharge, cells, or saliva in order to look at them under a microscope; or prick your finger or use a needle to draw blood; or ask you to urinate into a special cup.

Taking Control Of STDs—Common Treatments

The only way to prevent an STD is to abstain from sex until you are 100 percent certain that you are in a monogamous relationship with someone who is also STD free and that the relationship remains monogamous. Establishing this with certainty, though, is virtually impossible. You can insist that your partner be screened for STDs before you engage in sexual intercourse or have oral sex; however, because you cannot ensure another person's faithfulness, it is best to minimize your risk by using a condom each and every time you have sex. Even this approach isn't fail-safe, which makes regular testing so important.

Treatments for STDs differ depending on the type of infection the doctor discovers; they may involve taking oral or topical medication, or getting a shot. For incurable STDs, such as herpes and HIV, treatment helps to relieve or control the symptoms. In the case of HIV, early diagnosis and treatment can help the infected person live a normal lifespan.

If you are diagnosed with an STD, you should use only the medicines prescribed or recommended by your doctor. Some products sold over the Internet falsely claim to treat or prevent STDs, including HIV, but they don't work and they haven't been safety tested. Users may experience unintended effects.

Because there is such a wide range of sexually transmitted diseases—and we may not be familiar with them all—what follows here is a sort of "STD 101" that examines some of the most common STDs.

Chlamydia

About a year ago I got a phone call from my former boyfriend telling me he had tested positive for chlamydia. It was the worst phone call I have gotten in my life. Of course I went right away to get tested and the results were positive. After getting my result, I cried for days. I was upset with my boyfriend, the situation, and myself for not being more responsible for my body and protecting myself. Months have passed and I'm cured now, but I still get very worried and stressed because I have been told that having a child could be very difficult for me now.

—Karmen, age 19

Chlamydia and Black Women [54]

Chlamydia is a common and curable sexually transmitted disease (STD) caused by the bacterium *Chlamydia trachomatis*, which can damage a woman's reproductive organs and lead to infertility in some cases. It can be transmitted during vaginal, anal, or oral sex or spread from an infected mother to her baby during vaginal childbirth. While people of all ethnicities have been affected by this disease, in recent years Black women have had the most diagnosed cases. An estimated 10 percent of us between the ages of 15 and 24 have chlamydia.

It's possible, though, that this figure is misleading. The stigma associated with sexually transmitted infections encourages health-care providers to test young Black women more frequently than White women. Despite the recommendation that all women under age 25 who are sexually active be screened for chlamydia, providers are less likely to screen White women for the disease. This could explain the overwhelming racial disparities in sexual health outcomes and suggest that White and Black women's rates of chlamydia might be more similar than reported.

How Do I Know If I Have Chlamydia?

Symptoms of chlamydia infection include lower abdominal pain, pain or burning with urination, unusual vaginal discharge, and painful sexual intercourse. However, symptoms vary from one woman to another, and many women experience no symptoms at all, especially in the early stages of the disease. Showing no symptoms doesn't mean there is no problem, however: serious permanent damage can be done to the reproductive tissues even if you don't feel a thing.

There are different tests your doctor may give you for chlamydia. Some can be performed with urine; other tests require that a specimen be collected from a site such as the cervix.

Taking Control Of Chlamydia

Chlamydia can be avoided by abstaining from sexual intercourse or by being in a long-term, mutually faithful relationship with a partner who has been tested and is known to be uninfected. Considering the high rate of infection among Black women, it's wise to always use a condom as well, even in such a monogamous relationship. Latex condoms, when used consistently and correctly, can reduce the risk of transmission of this and other STDs.

If you do become infected, chlamydia can be treated and cured with antibiotics. All sex partners of someone who's found to be infected should be evaluated, tested, and treated as well. People with chlamydia should abstain from sex until they and their sex partners have completed treatment; otherwise, they may reinfect one another.

Gonorrhea[55]

> *An old boyfriend told me he was infected with gonorrhea. Although he had been embarrassed to reveal it at first, after reading a health brochure his doctor gave him and learning that gonorrhea was curable but that left untreated it could lead to infertility, he decided to tell me. He was embarrassed to make the call, but he knew that I wanted to have children some day. I was tested and was able to get treatment before any complications occurred.*

> *—Nita, age 27*

Gonorrhea and Black Women

Gonorrhea is so common in the United States that an estimated 700,000 people are infected with it each year. Black women should be especially wary: in 2009, those between the ages of 15 and 19 had the highest gonorrhea rate of any group, second only to Black men.

Gonorrhea, often called "the clap," is a sexually transmitted disease (STD) caused by bacteria that can grow and multiply easily in the warm, moist areas of the reproductive tract—in women, the cervix, uterus, and fallopian tubes. The bacteria can also grow in the mouth, throat, eyes, and anus. It can be transmitted through any variety of sexual contact, which is one of the reasons it is so prevalent.

Once infected, a person runs a high risk of spreading the bacteria to other parts of the body. For instance, a woman with gonorrhea may rub her eye, inadvertently spreading the infection and extending the treatment period. Like chlamydia and some other STDs, the infection can also be spread from mothers to babies during childbirth.

How Do I Know If I Have Gonorrhea?

Initial symptoms and signs in women include a painful or burning sensation when urinating, increased vaginal discharge, vaginal bleeding between periods, anal itching, soreness or bleeding, or painful bowel movements. Infection in the throat may cause a sore throat. However, most women with gonorrhea have no symptoms, and when they do, they are often mild or easily confused with a different infection.

A doctor can obtain a sample for testing from the part of your body likely to be infected. He or she will then send the sample to a laboratory for analysis. A urine sample can be used to diagnose gonorrhea thought to be present in the cervix or urethra.

Taking Control Of Gonorrhea

Gonorrhea can be avoided by abstaining from sexual intercourse or being in a long-term, mutually faithful relationship with a partner who has been tested and is known to be uninfected. Considering the high rate of infection in the Black community, it's wise to always use a condom as well. Latex condoms, when used consistently and correctly, can reduce the risk of transmission of gonorrhea.

Gonorrhea is treated with antibiotics. It is important not to have sexual contact with anyone while you are being treated. If you are treated for gonorrhea and your sex partner is not, you will probably become infected again, so it's important for both sexual partners to get tested even if only one person shows symptoms. If one of you notices symptoms continuing even after receiving treatment, you should return to a doctor to be reevaluated.

Hepatitis

I was one of those women devoted to my career. As a social worker, I spent most of my time working to ensure that my clients had the assistance that they needed. I'd spent a lot of time working in health-care facilities, so I was familiar with many of the problems—both medical and nonmedical—that my clients encountered.

Although I was often tired because of the long hours I spent at the office, I had begun to notice that I was feeling a bit more run down than usual. I tried to get more sleep and eat healthier, but I still continued to experience bouts of fatigue. Finally, after deciding that I might need to go for medical assistance—after all, I did work in a health-care facility—I made an appointment with my physician. After describing my symptoms and going for a series of blood tests, I got the diagnosis from my physician. I had been infected with hepatitis B. My doctor explained that there were several types of hepatitis and these various types of the disease could be categorized as one that would last for just a short period or a disease that could possibly be more long term. Although I was devastated by the news, I did not let my diagnosis get me down. I had spent years advocating on behalf of my patients and now I would have to advocate for myself. I continued to help the patients at my job, but I also began to volunteer as a health educator in the community. I wanted to do what I could to make certain that others in my community did not have to go through the same situation.

—Tanya Rose, age 33

Black Women and Hepatitis [56]

The viruses for hepatitis B and C are most often overlooked and misunderstood, but together they infect three to five times more Americans than HIV does, and most of the people who have it don't know it.

Viral hepatitis is inflammation of the liver caused by a virus. The most common types are hepatitis A, hepatitis B, and hepatitis C. Hepatitis A occurs in an acute, time-limited form, while hepatitis B, which is sexually transmitted, and hepatitis C can develop into lifelong chronic illnesses. An estimated 4.5 million Americans have chronic hepatitis B or hepatitis C. Over time, about 15 to 25 percent of people with chronic hepatitis develop serious liver problems, including liver damage, cirrhosis, liver failure, and liver cancer. Black women and men are just as much at risk as everyone else for viral hepatitis, but we have the highest incidence rate of hepatitis B in the United States, with 2.3 cases per 100,000 population based on 2007 data.

Although anyone can get hepatitis B, the risk factors for each type of viral hepatitis vary. In general, those people most likely to become infected include international travelers, particularly those traveling to developing countries; people who live with or have sex with an infected person; people living in areas where children are not routinely vaccinated against hepatitis A; day-care children and employees, during outbreaks; men who have sex with men; substance users; and infants born to infected mothers.

How Do I Know If I Have Hepatitis?

Symptoms of viral hepatitis can include jaundice, which causes a yellowing of the skin and eyes; fatigue; abdominal pain; loss of appetite; nausea; vomiting; diarrhea; low-grade fever; and headache. To determine whether you have viral hepatitis, and which type, a doctor will review your symptoms, give you a physical exam, and run blood tests that check for liver enzymes and viral antibodies. He or she may also talk with you about opportunities you've had to become infected:

- Hepatitis A is spread primarily through food or water contaminated by feces from an infected person. It can also be spread through contact with infected blood, but this is rare.

- Hepatitis B is spread through contact with infected blood, through sex with an infected person, and from mother to child during childbirth, whether the delivery is vaginal or via cesarean section.

- Hepatitis C is spread primarily through contact with infected blood. Less commonly, it can spread through sexual contact and childbirth.

Taking Control Of Hepatitis

There are currently safe and effective vaccines to prevent hepatitis A and B. Although hepatitis C does not have a vaccine yet, there are ways to reduce the risk of contracting it.

Here's what you can do to prevent or reduce your chances of getting hepatitis:

Preventing Hepatitis A (HAV)

Get vaccinated. The hepatitis A vaccine is available for adults and children older than age 1.

Those at highest risk who should be vaccinated include:

- Users of illegal injected drugs

- Restaurant workers and food handlers

- Young people living in dorms or in close contact with others

- Children living in communities that have high rates of hepatitis

- Children and workers in day-care centers

- People engaging in anal or oral sex

- People with chronic liver disease

- Laboratory workers who handle live hepatitis A virus

- If you eat raw shellfish frequently, ask your physician about being vaccinated

Practice Good Hygiene. Hands should be washed with soap and water following bowel movements and before food preparation.

Be Careful When You Travel. People who travel to developing countries where sanitary conditions are poor should be vaccinated two months prior to departure. Avoid tap water when traveling internationally.

Preventing Hepatitis B (HBV)

There is a vaccine for hepatitis B. For people who have not been vaccinated, reducing exposure to the virus is another way to help prevent infection. Reducing exposure through sexual contact means using latex condoms, which may lower the risk of transmission. No one should share anything that could have an infected person's blood on it (toothbrush, razor, nail clipper, body piercing instruments, etc.).

Handle blood spills correctly. If there is blood spill, even a small one; clean it up with a 10 percent solution of household bleach (believed to kill the virus). Wear protective gloves.

Preventing Hepatitis C (HBV)

There is no vaccine for hepatitis C. The only way to prevent the disease is to reduce the risk of exposure to the virus. Reducing exposure means avoiding behaviors like sharing drug needles or personal items such as toothbrushes, razors, and nail clippers.

Treating Hepatitis

The treatment options for viral hepatitis vary according to the type. Hepatitis A usually resolves on its own over several weeks. Drugs are primarily used to treat hepatitis B and chronic cases of hepatitis C. There are a variety of medications available, and they work by slowing the replication of the virus in the body and boosting the immune system.

Herpes (Genital)

When my best friend told me that she'd been diagnosed with herpes, I was devastated. I didn't know much about the disease, but listening to the tone of her voice as she told me that there was no cure not only scared me, it made me start to rethink my own practices.

A few months later, I found myself thinking back to my conversation with my best friend. When I was about to enter into an intimate relationship with someone whom I had been dating, I found myself insisting that we use condoms. My male friend wasn't interested in hearing anything about condoms. He told me that he was healthy and that he hadn't noticed anything wrong. I didn't back down. I told him that most people don't know if they are infected with many types of sexually transmitted diseases and that it's easy to pass a disease on to someone else—especially if you don't use any protection. Although he tried to get me to change my mind by saying that there are medicines that can cure sexually transmitted diseases if something were to happen, I again thought back to my best friend and the news that she'd received about her own health. My friend refused to use condoms, and because I had to make sure that I took care of myself and my health, I decided to break off the relationship with him. If he wouldn't agree to use condoms for me, then I guess he just wasn't worth it.

—Debra, age 27

Herpes and Black Women[57]

Perhaps no one is at greater risk for herpes than Black women. Given the high level of infection in the Black community and the fact that most people who are spreading it do not know it, it is crucial that we take this disease seriously.

Women get herpes more easily than men, so their rates are higher: roughly 25 percent of women versus 13 percent of men have it. But only 10 to 15 percent of people with herpes know that they have it. Recent estimates from the Centers for Disease Control and Prevention (CDC) state that nearly 48 percent of us between ages 14 and 49 have genital herpes, and Black people in general are more than three times as likely as Whites to have the disease.

Herpes, also known as genital herpes, is a lifelong, incurable infection that can cause itchy and painful blisters around the genitals and rectum. It is one of the most common sexually transmitted diseases in the United States, affecting approximately 1 in 6 Americans. Unfortunately, more than 80 percent of those with genital herpes are unaware of their infection, making it a serious public health risk.

Genital herpes is caused by a virus—either the herpes simplex virus type 1 or the herpes simplex virus type 2. While either virus can cause sores on the lips (cold sores), type 2 more often causes genital sores.

How Do I Know If I Have Herpes?

Symptoms of herpes can vary greatly from person to person. The most obvious sign of the disease are the genital lesions it can cause, which may first appear as small red bumps. Lesions can sometimes be found in a woman's vagina and cervix as well.

Some people have flulike symptoms, such as a fever, headache, and muscle aches. Women may also notice an abnormal discharge and pain when they urinate. Unfortunately, most people never have any symptoms, or they have symptoms so mild they do not recognize them as a sign of herpes. People who do notice their infection generally spot it about 2 to 14 days after they are exposed to the virus. The blisters they develop eventually rupture and turn into shallow, oozing sores that take up to 3 weeks to heal. Luckily, the sores heal without scarring. Genital herpes infections can be more severe in people who have impaired immune systems, such as those with HIV.

After the first outbreak, the herpes virus stays in the nerve cells below the skin and becomes inactive. As time goes on, the outbreaks happen less often, heal faster, and don't hurt as much. While it is frustrating not to know when an outbreak may occur, factors such as stress, illness, and menstruation often trigger a reoccurrence.

Your doctor can confirm that you have the virus by looking for signs of sores or lesions and by taking a tissue sample from an infected area. If no lesions are present but you are worried you've been exposed to the virus, your doctor can give you a blood test to detect herpes antibodies. Beware of false-negative results, though; it takes several weeks for herpes antibodies to show up in the blood.

Taking Control Of Herpes

We can keep ourselves free from the disease by practicing safer sex as well as by not being afraid to ask our partners if they have the disease or any of its signs. To be extra cautious, you can request that your partner take a blood test for the disease and show you the results, just as he or she would an HIV test. Abstaining from sex until you are in a monogamous relationship with someone also free from the disease is the surest way to prevent infection. Even then, it's still wise to use a condom every time you have sex. Don't be fooled into thinking you're safe if no symptoms are showing; herpes can be transmitted anytime, not just during an outbreak.

Although there is no cure for herpes, medicine can relieve the pain and itching of outbreaks and help sores heal faster. While herpes is incurable, it is not a death sentence, nor is it a reason to believe your life will be less fulfilling. It also does not mark the end of your sex life, since millions of people living with herpes enter into loving relationships with partners who have the disease and partners who don't. Still, finding out you have herpes can be quite depressing—especially if you feel there is no one you can confide in. Going to counseling and joining a support group can help you get past the emotional pain.

Human Papilloma Virus (HPV)

I was 23 when I found out that I had HPV. I had been in this relationship for a few months, only my second serious boyfriend. I thought I knew all about him . . . but you can never really know. My partner and I both had warts at about the same time and I was so sure that he had cheated on me. Before I was diagnosed, I found about five or six warts (I didn't know what they were at that moment but knew it couldn't be anything good). I looked up STDs on the web and read many articles and saw a picture of genital warts, and I was pretty sure that's what I had.

Anyway, I went to the local health department and was told, "Yes, it's genital warts, also known as HPV." I was given the name of a doctor who could give me treatment. I scheduled an appointment immediately. I had the warts frozen off, and in the process we talked about what had happened. The doctor told me it did not mean my boyfriend cheated on me. That's when I learned that HPV can be in your system for many years and you never know because it doesn't show any symptoms.

—Vicki, age 23

HPV and Black Women[58]

Approximately 6 million new cases of sexually transmitted HPV occur in the United States each year, with at least 20 million people estimated to be infected right now. Most people with HPV, though, do not know they're infected.

The human papilloma virus (HPV) is the name for a group of over 100 virus types. More than 40 types of HPV are transmitted sexually, infect the genital area, and are called genital HPV. Genital HPV is the most common sexually transmitted disease in the United States: an estimated 80 percent of women will have acquired the virus by age 50, and about 9.2 million sexually active youth 15 to 24 years of age are currently infected. HPV can be spread through vaginal, anal, and oral sex. However, unlike other STDs, it is spread through skin-to-skin contact, not through an exchange of bodily fluids.

Most, but not all, HPV infections go away on their own within 8 to 13 months. However, HPV is by no means harmless. Persistent HPV infections are now recognized as the cause of most cervical cancers, and each year about 12,000 women in the United States get cervical cancer. Black women have higher rates of HPV-associated cervical cancer than White women, and we must be particularly vigilant about protecting ourselves against HPV or monitoring the infection if we already have it.

How Do I Know If I Have HPV?

Most HPV infections occur without any symptoms and go away without any treatment. Because of the body's ability to fight the infection naturally, it is common for women who test positive for genital HPV at one point to have a negative result within 6 to 12 months. However, scientists are still not sure if this means that a person's immune system has destroyed all of the HPV or has only suppressed the infection to such a low level that it isn't detected by tests.

Some types of low-risk HPVs can cause warts to appear on or around the genitals or anus. About 1 percent of sexually active adults in the United States have genital warts at any one time. The warts can be small or large, raised or flat, or shaped like a cauliflower.

Women generally find out they have HPV after a Pap test comes back with an abnormal result. The abnormalities shown on the test can range from mild to severe. If your test comes back showing that it's likely you have a mild form of HPV, which would be unsurprising considering the high rate of infection, then your doctor will probably have you come back within a few weeks to check to see if it has cleared. If your Pap test shows you likely have a high-risk form of HPV, your doctor may give you an HPV test—a DNA test that looks for HPV on a woman's cervix. Your doctor can use the same sample of cells taken for the Pap test or a separate sample taken right after the Pap. If you test positive for high-risk HPV, your doctor will need to monitor the infection to make sure it goes away on its own and does not develop cellular abnormalities that could lead to cervical cancer.

Taking Control Of HPV

The best way to keep from becoming infected with HPV—or getting reinfected—is to abstain from sexual intercourse or to be in a long-term, mutually faithful relationship. You should also use condoms if you are having sex, though condoms don't fully protect against HPV.

Two vaccines are available to protect women against the types of HPV that cause most cervical cancers, and these are highly recommended. One also protects against most genital warts. Ideally, women should get the vaccine before they are sexually active. The Centers for Disease Control and Prevention recommends the vaccine for 11- to 12-year-old girls, though it can be given to girls as young as age 9. The vaccine is also suggested for young women ages 13 through 26 years old who did not get any or all of the three recommended doses when they were younger.

HPV itself cannot be treated, but often the body will clear HPV infection on its own—even the high-risk types that can lead to cervical cancer. If the HPV infection has already caused abnormal cell changes that could lead to cervical cancer, your doctor may still choose to wait to see if they will heal on their own. If not, discuss what treatment options may be available for removing the abnormal cells.

Syphilis[59]

One day I noticed some small sores on the palms of my hands. I thought about setting up an appointment with my doctor, but like most people, my hectic schedule caused me to put off making the appointment. I was a little worried because I realized that the sores were unusual, but since they didn't really hurt, I thought that they would probably just go away on their own. It wasn't until I started to notice a few sores on my feet and a rash on my body that I became a little more concerned. I couldn't figure out what could be causing the sores and rash. After reading over information on a few Internet sites, I was shocked to find out that my symptoms could be related to a syphilis infection! Syphilis?! Because the sores were on my hands, feet, and body it didn't even occur to me that they could be caused by some type of sexually transmitted disease. After I got over my initial shock, I immediately called to set an appointment to see my doctor. Unfortunately, my test results revealed that I was right—I did have syphilis. My doctor told me that I was fortunate in some ways because I'd been diagnosed early. He explained that, left untreated, syphilis could have caused health problems for me for many, many years. Although I was freaked out when I was told my diagnosis, I made a promise that I would take better care of myself. Since then I have made it a point to always use protection and always be careful.

—Iris, age 45

Syphilis And Black Women

The Black community has been the hardest hit of any by this STD. In 2009, the syphilis rate among Blacks was nine times that of Whites, and young Black women between the ages of 20 and 24 had the most cases of this infection.

A pregnant mother infected with the disease can pass it to the baby developing in her womb, and Black babies are particularly at risk. Of the 431 congenital syphilis cases reported in the United States in 2008, nearly 50 percent were in infants born to Black mothers in the South.

Syphilis is a sexually transmitted disease (STD) caused by the bacterium *Treponema pallidum*. It has often been called "the great imitator" because so many of the signs and symptoms are the same as those of other diseases. Without treatment, syphilis moves through the body in stages, damaging many organs over time. Infected persons are highly infectious during the early stages.

How Do I Know If I Have Syphilis?

Signs and symptoms of syphilis in its early stages include a firm, round, small and painless sore on the genitals, anus, or mouth, or a rash on the body, especially on the palms of the hands or the soles of the feet. People with secondary syphilis may also have fever, fatigue, rash, aches and pains, and loss of appetite. However, some people have no symptoms. Other people notice symptoms but mistake them for other skin conditions such as psoriasis.

In the late stages of syphilis, the disease may damage the internal organs, including the eyes, heart, blood vessels, liver, bones, joints, nerves, and brain. Signs and symptoms of the late stage of syphilis include difficulty coordinating muscle movements, paralysis, numbness, gradual blindness, and dementia. This damage may be serious enough to cause death.

A doctor can diagnose syphilis by examining material from a chancre (infectious sore) using a special microscope called a dark-field microscope. If syphilis bacteria are present in the sore, they will show up when observed through the microscope. A blood test is another way to determine whether someone has syphilis. Like HIV, syphilis is a reportable infection. This means that doctors must report any cases of syphilis to public health authorities so that potentially infected sexual partners may be identified and treated.

Taking Control Of Syphilis

The best way to prevent becoming infected with syphilis is to abstain from sexual intercourse or be in a long-term, mutually faithful relationship. You should also use condoms each and every time you have sex.

Syphilis is easy to cure in its early stages, and antibiotics are an effective treatment for the infection. You should avoid sexual intercourse until treatment has been completed. Any and all sexual partners should be treated at the same time, even if they have no symptoms.

Trichomoniasis

I knew something was wrong when I saw the expression on my boyfriend's face. When I asked him what was wrong, he was silent for a few minutes, but then he slowly began to speak. Robert told me that he'd been experiencing some health problems over the past few days but he was afraid to go and see a doctor. When he described his symptoms, I knew that I had better make an appointment with my own doctor. I had also been experiencing some discomfort while urinating and during sex, but I had not mentioned it to Robert. Although we didn't always use condoms, I was not concerned about contracting a sexually transmitted disease because Robert and I were in a serious relationship, and I'd been tested for a number of STDs during my last gynecological visit. After being informed that all of my test results for various STDs were negative, I wasn't concerned because I'd assumed that we were monogamous. However, after I returned to my gynecologist and realized that I had tested positive for trichomoniasis, I immediately began having doubts. Once I confronted Robert about my positive test results for trichomoniasis, and revealed that I'd previously tested negative for a number of sexually transmitted diseases, Robert admitted that he'd been unfaithful. He'd been intimate with other women. The relationship eventually ended. Fortunately for me, Trichomoniasis is curable. Still, I learned a hard lesson. I promised myself that I would always use protection unless I was absolutely certain that I was in a totally monogamous relationship!

—Leslie, age 33

Trichomoniasis and Black Women [60]

Trichomoniasis is the most common curable sexually transmitted disease, more common than both chlamydia and gonorrhea. Anyone can get trichomoniasis. However, in the United States, it is diagnosed more frequently among women than among men. It is also significantly more common among Black women than among women of other races.

Trichomoniasis is a sexually transmitted disease (STD) caused by a microscopic parasite usually found in the vagina and urethral tissues. An estimated 7.4 million new cases of trichomoniasis occur in the United States each year. It is spread through sexual contact with an infected partner, including penis-to-vagina intercourse and vulva-to-vulva contact. The parasite cannot survive in the mouth or rectum.

How Do I Know If I Have Trichomoniasis?

Symptoms of trichomoniasis in women include discomfort with intercourse, itching of the inner thighs, a vaginal discharge that is thin, greenish-yellow and frothy or foamy, vaginal itching, itching or swelling of the vulva, and a foul or strong-smelling vaginal odor.

If your doctor suspects you have Trichomoniasis, he or she will give you a pelvic examination and look for red blotches on the vaginal wall or cervix, or provide an examination called a wet prep to look for infection-causing organisms in vaginal fluids. A Pap smear may also diagnose the condition.

Taking Control Of Trichomoniasis

The best way to prevent becoming infected with trichomoniasis is to abstain from sexual intercourse or be in a long-term, mutually faithful relationship. You should also use condoms each and every time you have sex.

There are antibiotic treatments available to cure the infection. You should also avoid sexual intercourse until treatment has been completed and tell your sex partner that you are infected with the disease so he or she can be tested.

Resources:

American Social Health Association
PO Box 13827
Research Triangle Park, NC 27709
(919) 361-8400
www.ashastd.org

Association of Reproductive Health Professionals
1901 L Street, NW, Suite 300
Washington, DC 20036
(202) 466-3825
www.arhp.org

Hepatitis Foundation International
504 Blick Dr.
Silver Spring, MD 20904
(800) 891-0707
www.hepfi.org

Hepatitis Prevention Programs
444 North Capitol Street, NW, Suite 339
Washington, DC 20001
(202) 434-8090
www.hepprograms.org

Herpes Resource Center
PO Box 13827
Research Triangle Park, NC 27709
(919) 361-8488
www.ashastd.org/herpes/herpes_overview.cfm

National Cancer Institute
NCI Office of Communications and Education
Public Inquiries Office
6116 Executive Boulevard, Suite 300
Bethesda, MD 20892
www.cancer.gov/cancertopics/factsheet/Risk/HPV

National Chlamydia Coalition
Partnership for Prevention
1015 18th Street, NW, Suite 300
Washington, DC 20036
(202) 833-0009
www.ncc.prevent.org/

National Prevention Information Network
CDC NPIN
PO Box 6003
Rockville, MD 20849-6003
(800) 458-5231
www.cdcnpin.org

STROKE

—————————————■—————————————

Yeah right, I thought as I walked out of my doctor's office on a cool, sunny day in March 2002. Of course, I hadn't told him that as he frankly but politely told me I needed to get my high blood pressure, cholesterol, and weight down. And more than anything, he stressed, I had to stop smoking if I wanted to live the long life I was expecting. I simply nodded my head yes and then promised I would get all four under control—the blood pressure and cholesterol with medication, the weight with a better diet, and the smoking with willpower and patches.

But on my way home, I considered how my 57-year-old body felt, which was just fine, thank you! While I certainly didn't feel like a spring chicken, I didn't feel bad either. I wasn't stressed, I thought as sharply and clearly as I ever had, and I had enough energy to bowl, garden, go on frequent vacations, and keep up with my grandkids. I took them to the zoo in the summer and helped them build snowmen in the winter—more than many so-called healthy people half my age could boast. So, even if I did have high blood pressure and cholesterol, it wasn't causing me any problems, I reasoned. And when it came to my weight, the doctor just didn't know what he was talking about. Sure, I might have a few extra pounds on me, but I was thick in all the right places—always had been. While I wasn't against shaving off a few pounds, the 20 to 25 he had suggested just didn't sound right.

The only thing I couldn't argue with was the smoking. I went through about three packs a day and I knew they were bad for me. Now, I hadn't known this 40 years ago, when Lucille Ball and every other actress on television was making smoking seem so sexy and cool. But the labels on every package I picked up now made it clear. The truth is, I had tried to quit a few times before and you might as well have been asking me to give up breathing. I was addicted. Plus, trying to quit had made me feel so irritable, nervous, and depressed that I was willing to deal with the possible consequences of smoking.

So I took the prescribed pills when and if I wanted to, didn't change my eating or exercise habits, and puffed on cigarettes as I pleased. I got away with going against the doctor's orders, and my family's warnings, for another three years. However, when the penalty for ignoring them came, it happened swiftly and left no room for debate.

I was driving to Five Guys Burger & Fries Hamburger with my oldest daughter. We had spent a fun day shopping and hanging out, and we both had a taste for their famous hamburgers. It is simply amazing how one moment your body can feel normal, like it's your own, and the next like you're a stranger inside of it. All of a sudden, my hands wouldn't do what I wanted and my feet wouldn't either—a terrible situation for anyone, but especially for a person driving a car. My daughter noticed there was something wrong and urgently asked me what it was. I tried to respond, but my words came out all slurred and I couldn't help slobbering. We both panicked as the car kept going, but then suddenly it came to a halt in the middle of the street. To this day, I know it could only have been God who stopped that car without any accident because it certainly wasn't me. I couldn't grip the steering wheel or press down on the pedal. After the car stopped, my oldest daughter, who didn't drive, quickly called my youngest daughter to come help. Luckily, she was close by. "You've had a stroke and need to go to the hospital," she said. Though I knew all the symptoms, I just couldn't believe I had really had a stroke. Not me. I shook my head no and said something that sounded like "home." "Home?" she asked. "Are you crazy?"

I was quickly put in the passenger seat of my car and driven to a hospital less than eight blocks away. With my daughters' help, I made it up to the admitting desk, where they informed the receptionist that I had just had a stroke. He looked at me sharply and asked me to say my name. I tried to, but it came out all bungled and a long line of spit dripped from my mouth. That was all he needed to see—within moments we were headed to emergency care.

One of the stroke team's residents turned out to be someone my youngest daughter knew, and she told my daughter that something had to be done fast to increase my chance of regaining speech and movement in my arms and legs. She recommended intravenous tPA, a new drug that, if given within three hours of a stroke, dramatically increases a person's chance of recovery. I didn't want to take any experimental drugs, but I also didn't want to live the rest of my life in this state. When a nurse asked me to blink once for yes and twice for no if I wanted the drug, I made sure my eyes squeezed shut only one time so there wouldn't be any confusion. I was then given the drug, which they might as well rename "miracle." Within one hour of the injection, 95 percent of my function came back. So did my chance of living a healthier life.

Ironically, the advice the doctor had given me three years earlier was the same advice I now had to follow. Take my medication. Eat better. Lose weight. Cut back on the cigarettes and work on quitting them altogether. The only difference was that I was listening now.

The medication was the easy part, and I began taking it every day as required. The food was more difficult. My mother was a Southern woman and I knew how to cook Southern style, which meant I depended a little too much on salt and butter. To remedy this, my oldest daughter, who is a fabulous modern cook, showed me how to make dishes sizzle with spices. I have also given fresh vegetables and fruits a larger place on my plate and learned that baked and grilled foods can taste just as great as their fried counterparts. I now have something fried just once a month; before, I helped myself to fried chicken or pork chops four times a week. I've also started walking more. Combined with my healthier eating habits, this is how I work on my weight.

When it comes to smoking, let's just say I'm hoping slow and steady will win the race. I haven't quit yet, but I have gone from three packs a day to half of one. Smokers know that's no easy feat. I tried using the patches and then began doing something simpler that a counselor suggested. He said, Before you light up, ask yourself, do I want this cigarette, do I need this cigarette, or is it a habit? Then I wait 20 minutes and if I still want to light up, I can. Having to ask myself that question and wait afterward has really helped me. I also spend a lot of time at Starbucks and other places that don't allow you to smoke. Sometimes it's simple strategies like these that make all the difference. My goal is to get down to one cigarette a week, and then none at all.

To my surprise and delight, the story about my stroke and the steps I have taken to prevent another one has been shared with others through Georgetown University's Triumph over Stroke Program. They created a video with me and other stroke survivors and also got a story published with the Associated Press. The program aims to increase the number of African Americans who receive rapid stroke treatment in order to improve the quality of life for stroke survivors in Washington, D.C. This is important to me because receiving the treatment suggested is probably the reason I can talk and walk unencumbered. My next-door neighbor, a Black man, had a stroke not too long after me, but for whatever reason, he didn't receive the drug. He is now in a convalescent home. He isn't the only one who could have had a better outcome. Currently, African Americans have twice the risk of stroke compared to Whites but are less likely to receive the appropriate treatment.

Like this essay, I hope my story helps other people at risk for stroke or other medical problems learn not to ignore the advice they're given. We have to stop rationalizing away the unhealthy habits we have—be it smoking, drinking, overeating, being sedentary, or not taking the medication meant to save our lives. I don't know why my life was spared and others haven't been, but I don't intend to test my luck. If you know there is something you need to change, you shouldn't either.

*—**Edna Wooten** is a widow, mother of four, grandmother of thirteen, and great-grandmother of two. She enjoys spending time with all of the children in her family and traveling within the United States and internationally, especially on cruises.*

Stroke and Black Women

Almost all of us have known or seen a victim of a stroke, witnessed the devastation to body and mind, and wondered how a person once strong could be so weakened in an instant. Yet too few us have considered what we must do to prevent being disabled or dying from this serious health condition. And as Black women, we can't afford not to think about it.

Stroke is the third leading cause of death in the United States, killing 160,000 Americans each year[61]—and the statistics are even worse for Black women. Not only are we twice as likely as White women to have a stroke in the first place, we also have them earlier in life. Just as troubling, while stroke is the leading cause of serious long-term disability among people of all ethnic groups, Black women are even more likely to become disabled and experience difficulties with daily living than people of other hues.

Strokes don't discriminate; they have such an adverse impact on Black women simply because we are more likely to be affected by some of the major risk factors for stroke: high blood pressure, diabetes, and obesity.

Other known risk factors for stroke include sickle cell anemia, the most common genetic disorder among African Americans; a family history of stroke; heart disease; high cholesterol; alcohol use; bleeding disorders; cocaine use; and head injury. Certain medications make blood clots more likely and therefore increase your chances for a stroke. Smoking is a significant risk factor, and though Black women smoke less than many other groups—18 percent of us over age 18—that's still too many. Birth control pills can increase the chances of having blood clots, especially in women who smoke and who are older than 35.

In general, a person's stroke risk increases with age. For each decade after age 55, the risk doubles. Each year, nearly three-fourths of people who suffer a stroke are over 65. However, it's dangerous to dismiss stroke as something only older people have to worry about: Black women and men aged 20 to 44 are 2.4 times more likely to have a stroke than White people in the same age group.

How Do Strokes Happen?

A stroke happens when blood flow to a part of the brain is interrupted because a blood vessel in the brain is blocked or bursts open. If blood flow is stopped for longer than a few seconds, the brain cannot get blood and oxygen. When this happens, brain cells can die, causing permanent damage.

There are two types of strokes, ischemic and hemorrhagic. *Ischemic stroke* occurs when arteries carrying blood to the brain are blocked by blood clots or by the gradual buildup of plaque and other fatty deposits; about 87 percent of all strokes are ischemic. *Hemorrhagic stroke* occurs when a blood vessel in the brain bursts. Hemorrhagic strokes account for just 13 percent of all strokes, yet they are responsible for more than 30 percent of all stroke deaths.

Sometimes people suffer what's called a transient ischemic attack (TIA), or "ministroke." A ministroke happens when blood flow to the brain stops for a short time. The symptoms are similar to, but milder than, those of a full-blown stroke, and they may last only an hour or two. Though you may feel completely normal after a ministroke, it is a serious warning sign that you're at risk for a regular stroke—perhaps very soon—and you should get medical attention right away.

Here's how the risk factors mentioned above set the stage for a stroke:[62]

- **High blood pressure.** Over time, high blood pressure leads to atherosclerosis—a condition in which fatty material collects along the walls of arteries—and hardening of the large arteries. This, in turn, leads to blockage of small blood vessels in the brain and weakening of their walls, which can cause them to balloon and burst: a hemorrhagic stroke. People who have high blood pressure are four to six times more likely to have a stroke, and 45 percent of Black women suffer from the condition—though most don't know it.

- **Diabetes.** Persistently elevated blood glucose levels caused by diabetes contribute to the buildup of plaque in blood vessels. Plaque—a pasty substance made up of cholesterol, calcium, cellular waste, and protein—sticks to the walls of blood vessels and can interfere with blood flow. Diabetes affects more than one in ten Black women ages 20 and up, and one in four Black women ages 55 and up.

- **Obesity.** Excessive fat tissue throughout the body can inhibit blood flow and raise the risk of blockage. It's no surprise that Black women are at high risk on this account—a shocking four out of five of us are overweight or obese.

- **Smoking** Smoking has been linked to the buildup of fatty substances in the carotid artery, the main artery in the neck that supplies blood to the brain. Also, nicotine raises blood pressure, and the carbon monoxide in cigarettes reduces the amount of oxygen your blood can carry to the brain. As if that weren't enough, cigarette smoke makes your blood thicker and more likely to clot.

Strokes are often fatal because people fail to see the warning signs or don't take the signs seriously. Symptoms aren't always as disruptive and obvious as Edna Wooten's sudden inability to control her arms and legs. For example, one common symptom is a headache. Headaches are a normal part of life, so to be on our guard against stroke, we must be aware of unusual headaches, especially ones that come on suddenly and severely; occur when you're lying flat; wake you up from sleep; or get worse when you bend, strain, cough, or change positions.

Other symptoms depend on the severity of the stroke and what part of the brain is affected. They can include:[63]

- Muscle weakness in the face, arm, or leg—usually just on one side

- Numbness or tingling on one side of the body

- Problems with eyesight, including decreased vision, double vision, or total loss of vision

- Change in alertness, ranging from sleepiness to unconsciousness

- Changes in hearing

- Changes in taste

- Clumsiness

- Confusion or loss of memory

- Difficulty swallowing

- Difficulty writing or reading

- Dizziness or abnormal sensation of movement

- Loss of control over the bladder or bowels

- Loss of balance or coordination

- Changes in personality, mood, or emotions

- Changes in sensation, such as the ability to feel pain, pressure, different temperatures, or other stimuli

- Trouble speaking or understanding others who are speaking

- Trouble walking

Here's an example. Imagine you're at a family party and you notice a relative acting strangely. Maybe she was just in the middle of telling a joke, but now her speech is slurred, or maybe she was reenacting a very funny scene but now she's suddenly stopped. It could be that she drank too much spiked fruit punch. It could also be that she's having a stroke and her life is in danger.

The National Stroke Association has come up with a helpful acronym—FAST—to help you detect and urgently respond to a stroke:[64]

- F—FACE:
  Ask the person to smile. Does one side of her face droop?

- A—ARMS:
  Ask the person to raise both arms. Does one arm drift downward?

- S—SPEECH:
  Ask the person to repeat a simple phrase. Is her speech slurred or strange?

- T—TIME:
  If you observe any of these signs, call 9-1-1 immediately. The sooner a stroke victim is treated, the greater her chances of recovering.

How Can I Lower My Risk for Stroke? [65]

While strokes often come on suddenly, the damage to our bodies that sets the stage for a stroke can take years to develop. This is why it's estimated that a full 80 percent of strokes could be prevented. The National Stroke Association offers these strategies as part of its Public Stroke Prevention Guidelines:

- **Know your blood pressure.** If it is elevated, work with your health-care provider to keep it under control. Have your blood pressure checked at least once each year— more often if you have a history of high blood pressure.

- **Find out if you have atrial fibrillation (AF).** Atrial fibrillation can cause blood to collect in the chambers of your heart, where it can form clots and cause a stroke. Your health-care provider can detect AF by carefully checking your pulse. If you have AF, work with your health-care provider to manage it.

- **If you smoke, stop.** If you stop smoking today, your risk for stroke will decrease by 10 percent immediately and by 50 percent within five years.

- **If you drink alcohol, do so in moderation.** Remember that alcohol is a drug—it can interact with other drugs you are taking, and it's harmful if taken in large doses. If you don't drink, don't start.

- **Know your cholesterol profile.** If your numbers are high where they should be low, work with your health-care provider to control them. Though high cholesterol can often be managed with diet and exercise, some people may require medication to bring theirs under control.

- **Control your diabetes.** If you are diabetic, follow your health-care provider's recommendations carefully. Your health-care provider can prescribe a nutrition program, lifestyle changes, and medicine to help control your diabetes.

- **Include exercise in your daily routine.** Dancing, taking a brisk walk, swimming, or other physical activity for as little as 30 minutes a day can improve your health in many ways, including helping you bring or keep your weight under control—and being overweight raises your risk of stroke.

- **Enjoy a lower-sodium, lower-fat diet.** By cutting down on salt and fat in your diet, you may be able to lower your blood pressure and, in turn, lower your risk for stroke.

- **Ask your health-care provider if you have circulation problems.** If so, work with your health-care provider to control them. Fatty deposits can block arteries that carry blood from your heart to your brain, and sickle cell disease, severe anemia, and other diseases of the circulatory system can cause stroke if left untreated.

- **If you have any stroke symptoms, seek immediate medical attention.** Remember FAST!

What Treatment Will I Receive for a Stroke?

The treatment you receive will depend on the severity and cause of the stroke. Strokes caused by blood clots can be treated with clot-busting drugs that must be given within three hours of the start of a stroke to work, and there are tests that must be done first. This is why it is so important for a person having a stroke to get to a hospital fast. A hospital stay is required for most strokes.

- **Treatment in the hospital.** The main goal of treatment in the hospital is to stabilize your condition and minimize the damage done by the stroke. Clot-busting drugs (thrombolytic therapy) may be used if the stroke is caused by a blood clot. These medicines break up blood clots and help restore blood flow to the damaged area. Since strokes often cause difficulty in swallowing—temporary or permanent—you may be given nutrients and fluids through a vein or a feeding tube in the stomach.

- **Long-term treatment.** The goal of ongoing treatment after a stroke, whether in a care facility or at home, is to help you recover as much function as possible and prevent future strokes. It's important to be patient with your body. The body can and often does heal itself, but it takes time. Problems with moving, thinking, and talking often improve in the weeks to months after a stroke, and some people see improvement even years after their strokes.

The effects of stroke may mean that you must change, relearn, or redefine how you live. Rehabilitation is a very important part of recovery for many stroke survivors. Stroke rehabilitation is designed to help you return to independent living. It does not reverse the effects of a stroke; its goals are to build your strength, capability, and confidence so you can continue your daily activities despite the effects of your stroke. Rehabilitation services may include:

- **Physical therapy** to restore movement, balance, and coordination

- **Occupational therapy** to relearn basic skills such as bathing and dressing

- **Speech therapy** to relearn how to talk

- **Swallowing therapy** to restore this function

A stroke isn't a death sentence, and it doesn't necessarily mean life in a wheelchair. As we saw in Edna Wooten's story of surviving and thriving, some stroke victims can recover almost completely if they are treated swiftly. Those who sustain more serious, lasting damage can often still improve their quality of life through these forms of therapy. Though adult brain cells don't regenerate, the brain has been shown to have a remarkable capacity for compensation, even creating new neural pathways to circumvent areas that are damaged. Whether you're working through your own rehabilitation or caring for a loved one who has had a stroke, don't give up—if you press for aggressive rehab, you can make a real difference.

Resources:

American Stroke Association
7272 Greenville Avenue
Dallas, TX 75231
(888) 478-7653
www.strokeassociation.org

National Institute of Neurological Disorders and Stroke
PO Box 5801
Bethesda, MD 20824
(800) 352-9424
www.ninds.nih.gov

National Stroke Association
9707 E. Easter Lane, Suite B
Centennial, CO 80112
(800) 787-6537
www.stroke.org

VIOLENCE

———————◼———————

When I was 16 I became a statistic. I was an accident waiting to happen—when my boy-friend split my lip and blackened my eye in a jealous rage. It wasn't the last time he hit me; it only got worse. His abuse escalated to the point where he even kicked me in my pregnant belly, endan-gering the life of the precious gift inside. On that day, I became the third generation of women in my family to be trapped in the never-ending cycle of violence. Twenty-two years later, my daughter became the fourth generation when her partner tried to kill her and threatened the life of their baby girl, Promise. I decided right then and there, I would not let Promise be the fifth.

Saving Promise, my granddaughter, from becoming a statistic has become my life's mission. Today I am the first person in my family to speak up about domestic violence outside of the walls of our family's home. With an unwavering conviction, in an effort to open up and break the silence, I have begun telling my story of how intergenerational violence has impacted my fam-ily. There is no drama in my story, only the conviction that I will no longer be part of the con-spiracy of silence about an issue that so many Black women face. From the time I was five years old, I have been exposed to domestic violence. All the women in my family have been impacted by abuse: my grandmother was abused by my grandfather; I witnessed my mother's abuse at the hands of my own father; I experienced abuse for years; and my daughter was involved in an abusive relationship.

I still remember the first time it happened to me. I was excited to finally be old enough to date and to have my first boyfriend. Returning with him from a New Year's Eve party and without any clue why, I received my first punch. I fell to the ground; he hit me again; and then of course he told me that it was my fault. Later he apologized and told me that it would never happen again. I believed him.

As an adult I realized that in that first incident, when his fist hit my face, I didn't see my father's fist hitting my mother's as I had seen so many times. I didn't think about the stories that I had been hearing, ever since I was old enough to remember, about my grandfather and the fists that he used against my grandmother and her eight children. Like many other young Black women, I saw only a charming boy who must love me—he cared about how I acted. I didn't know then that love didn't have to hurt and you didn't have to stay in that kind of relationship.

My mother was first beaten at the tender age of 18. My grandmother said to my mother, in her southern dialect, "Go back to your husband." The "that's your husband, go back to him" mentality was what would stick with me throughout my life and sent me the message that love did have to hurt.

Images of violence have always been present in my memory. I recall being aware of the scar from my mother's stab wound, but I was never fully aware of the whole story behind it until I was an adult. I eventually learned that on this one day, my mother tried to resist the abuse from her husband—my father. When he went for her, she grabbed a knife. In the violent scuffle, my father took hold of the knife and stabbed my mom in the leg. More than anything, I wish I could have known about these things sooner and known how they impacted my mom's life. She was silent all those years.

My mother wasn't the type that talked to her children; she talked at us. My mother simply wasn't available for me to confide in, as she too was going through her own abusive relationship. I don't blame my mom, because I always knew that she was doing the best that she could, but I needed her in ways that I have only now come to understand. I needed her to be more affectionate and to tell me that she loved me. I was in my twenties before I ever heard those three words from my mother.

All that time, I didn't connect the dots—I was unable to recognize that I was living in the shadows of my mother's and grandmother's abuse. Violence was so normalized in my family that it was the only story I knew how to tell in my book Color Me Butterfly.[66] In what started off as a career change from corporate professional to writer, I discovered that my book would not only allow me to discover my true passion, but also allow me to see and understand, for the first time, the patterns of abuse. Like so many other Black women, I wasn't able to realize how deeply rooted domestic violence was in my family until I began to write it all down, a journey that eventually allowed me to heal and created a platform for me to help other women heal as well. Yet at the same time that I discovered writing, I discovered that my own daughter was in a violent relationship herself—something that she felt she needed to hide until her abuser threatened her life.

With a renewed relationship with the women in my life, especially my daughter, I became a new grandmother to a baby girl named Promise. Since the silences around the intergenerational violence have finally been broken in my family, we are determined to end the cycle of violence in our family as well as in the community. My message for my granddaughter is "You are a beautiful girl who will grow up to be a beautiful young woman. I want to make sure that you embrace, love, and honor yourself." I want to instill in Promise the imperative to value and appreciate her self-worth—she will need it for her social and emotional journey to being whole.

Now as an advocate dedicated to elevating women's stories, validating their pain, and offering them support, I speak out against domestic violence, domestically and globally. Domestic violence affects women throughout the world. Through my organization, Saving Promise, I am determined and empowered to change the way the world views and responds to domestic violence.

—L. Y. Marlow

Violence and Black Women

We've all heard phrases like "partner abuse," "battering," or "domestic violence" used to describe the painful levels of physical, emotional, sexual, and psychological violence that occur in intimate relationships. We see and hear it through music lyrics or in popular movies or on TV, we see it on the street, and we even see it in our own personal or family relationships. We see it so often that sometimes we almost stop seeing it; we may lose perspective and view a slap or a punch as a normal expression of a lover's frustration—but our nonchalance costs. Too often Black women pay for denial with black eyes, bloodied noses, broken bones, and too often even with our lives.

What Is Domestic Violence? "Domestic violence is a pattern of mental, physical, emotional or sexual abuse where one partner makes the other partner feel scared, weak, isolated, hurt or sad, according to Between Friends, a Chicago-based non-profit agency that provides educational and counseling services for domestic violence victims and advocates."[67]

Domestic violence, partner abuse, and battering refer to the physical, emotional, sexual, and psychological abuse, performed by one person against another. The abuser and victim are involved in or have had an intimate or romantic relationship. It is costly and pervasive, causing victims, as well as witnesses, to suffer incalculable pain and loss and shattering the victims' sense of well-being.

Every 15 seconds, a woman in the United States is beaten by her partner and one in four[68] of us has experienced some form of violence at least once in our lifetime. For Black women, this reality is even more frightening because of the conspiracies of silence that we have been conditioned to maintain. We don't talk about domestic violence in our families, we don't share with our daughters what we went through, and we rarely have the space to confide in someone when we are being abused. As important are the health consequences that are linked to a wide range of chronic illnesses and disabilities: 80 percent more likely to have a stroke, 70 percent more likely to drink heavily and more likely to experience a miscarriage and contract a sexually transmitted disease than women who have not experienced intimate partner violence.

Even the discrimination in our legal system sets Black women up for a sort of double jeopardy because we are aware of our vulnerabilities. We know all too well how racial injustice has devastated our communities when we see that more of our men are behind bars than in school, for example. So when it comes time to report our abusers, we are apprehensive; we don't want to send another Black man to jail. We are perpetually making self-destructive personal sacrifices because our decisions, unlike White women's, are inextricably linked to the needs of our community.

Also, resources that protect Black women are scarce. We rarely have the access that other women have to shelters, service programs, and supportive family members. We are not allowed to bring shame on the family and the community—we do not feel that we can be protected. For this reason, in part, Black women's experiences with intimate partner violence frequently end in death. A 2008 study by the Violence Policy Center[69] reported that Black women are being killed at a rate nearly three times higher than White women. Ten percent of the victims were under the age of 18 and 4 percent were 65 or older. The average age of Black women who were homicide victims was 34 years—and most of these women were killed by someone they knew, a family member, intimate friend, or spouse, rather than a stranger.

Types of Violence

Emotional Abuse

Emotional abuse occurs in some form in all abusive relationships. It is undoubtedly the most common and least recognized type of abuse used by abusive partners to control and cause extreme damage to the woman's self esteem. No one really talks about it because it isn't a crime and leaves no visible bruises. Not only that, most of us don't recognize the attitudes, behaviors and language that wound us deeply and constitute emotional abuse. The name calling, the accusations, and the jealous outrage are all done to make us feel responsible for the abuse.

Sadly, the ultimate goal is to break our spirits and crush our sense of autonomy and power. Why? To gain the upper hand and control.

Sexual Violence[70]

Rape and sexual assault is one of the most common crimes against women, especially young women between the ages of 20 and 24, but these acts are rarely reported. Because we have been conditioned to blame the victim, holding women in some sense responsible for their own sexual abuse, countless perpetrators of sexual assault roam our communities unpunished. When we do press charges, the justice system requires us to relive our abuse at trial and to prove that we were in fact forced against our will. Biased interrogation often suggests that we're at fault for being out too late or seeming too sexually available on account of the way we dress. This reality only encourages and entrenches the culture of sexual violence, so that rape becomes just something that women must be extra cautious about—especially Black women, whom our society so often hypersexualizes in the media and views as somehow inviting sexual control.

Reproductive Coercion[71]

Another form of partner control that is becoming commonplace in opposite sex relationships among adolescent girls and young women is contraceptive sabotage, or coerced pregnancy. Reproductive coercion occurs when men threaten, cajole, or manipulate their girlfriends and wives into having children before they're ready; birth control sabotage occurs when, unbeknownst to their partners, the men poke holes in condoms and destroy contraceptives—i.e., *"throw away birth control pills"* or *"flush pills down the toilet"*—so that the women become pregnant against their will. In 2009 alone, about one in five young women admitted that they had experienced pregnancy coercion and 15 percent said they had experienced birth control sabotage. Over half of these women said that they had experienced some type of physical or sexual violence at their partner's hands as well.

It's not hard to see how birth control sabotage can start a downward spiral. In the blink of an eye, a woman's entire world can change because her partner decided, without her permission, that he wanted her to have his baby. Plans for school, money-saving goals, career mobility, her value system—all things hoped for are put on hold when a woman has to all of sudden adjust her life around a pregnancy that she thought she had prevented.

Financial Abuse[72]

Financial abuse is one of the least commonly reported but one of the more powerful entrapment tactics in relationships. This kind of abuse can take many forms, but you should be aware that manipulating and controlling money—from giving you an allowance to ruining your credit and not letting you have your own checking or savings account is controlling. It is intentionally designed to keep you in line and dependent.

Financial abuse often compromises the lives of older Black women who are vulnerable to exploitation at the hands of their families or caregivers. A survey of both black and non-black elders over age 60 living in Pittsburgh found that nearly three times as many Blacks reported financial exploitation. This type of financial abuse can range from stealing money out of a great aunt's purse to committing fraud using grandma's bank account or social security benefits.

Lifting the Veil on Violence

The long-term effects of psychological and physical violence are endless. Most obviously, they result in preventable injuries and consequences such as sexually transmitted diseases. However, they can also leave lasting traumas that can easily develop into persistent mental health problems. Women who have undergone abuse experience a variety of psychological effects, such as depression, substance abuse, self-injurious behavior or post-traumatic stress disorder, low self-esteem, lack of trust and paranoia.

Depression and our ability to trust/love ourselves and others can impact, and in many cases, devastate our entire lives. We now know that more than 84 percent of intimate violence victims are women, yet this gender imbalance is largely ignored, not just in the judicial system, but in our communities. Emotional abuse, intimate partner abuse, sexual assault, rape, contraceptive sabotage—are all forms of violence that we need to recognize and respond to urgently.

During the late 1980s, when the Imperative began unraveling the puzzle of why so many of us were sick, depressed, and dying, we knew then that we didn't know enough about Black women's pain. So the Imperative began asking women what caused all of the heartache. The answer then was as it is now: women said that violence—physical and emotional battering, sexual abuse—was at the root of much of their suffering. Black women today must change the way we view violence, the way we talk about it, the way we excuse it, and we must speak out. We must begin sharing with our friends and with our families—especially with our daughters—and calling our partners to task. Lifting the veil on these violent acts against women will uncover the fact that our homes, where violence is all too common and takes many forms, may be less safe than we think.

Taking Control of Violence

Black women need to live in an environment where we feel safe, loved, and supported, where we know that we have not only the right to self-determination but the freedom to exercise it. There is too much silence around this issue for something that affects so many Black women so deeply.

Breaking the silence is a first step to stopping the abuse and starting the healing—violence is wrong and it's a crime. Sharing with our friends and families—especially with our daughters—and calling our boyfriends, husbands, or partners to task is certainly a first step. Telling the truth about these violent acts will reveal the fact that our homes, where violence is all too common and takes many forms, may be less safe than we think.

If you are in an abusive relationship—whether the abuse is physical or psychological — it is important to get support. Someone who batters is usually very good at getting their partner isolated from their family and friends. As a result, victims often begin to feel ashamed and alone and believe that no one would understand. Many survivors have even described feeling as if they didn't even know who they are anymore. This makes it even more difficult to survive the abuse, to sort through the feelings and to make decisions that will be best for you and/or your children

Join a support group. Besides offering shelter, support groups offer a safe place to talk about your feelings and experiences in an atmosphere free of judgment. It's also an opportunity to meet and talk with other people who have had similar experiences and gone on to claim healthy and happy lives.

Know your rights. After finding support, your next step is to find out about your rights. Knowing your rights helps prepare you for what you should expect if you decide to report the assault to the criminal justice system. Reporting is a way to empower yourself and protect others from future harm. This can be a difficult process; it requires retelling the experience and providing details you may prefer to forget. In fact you may feel that you are being victimized again.

Self-Defense: Consider Obtaining A Protective Order. A protective order (also known as a restraining order) can be issued by civil courts against anyone who is a threat to your safety. Although a protective order can be effective in reducing immediate harm, there is the reality of future harm that most women fear. Becoming aware of how to navigate the court system or reaching out to an advocate will help in removing some of the barriers to getting protective order services and enforcement.

Seek out medical care for your injuries. Make an appointment to talk privately about your situation with your health-care provider. Be aware that health-care provders routinely observe and screen patients in the emergency rooms for domestic violence; they also report their findings to the proper authorities, who can assist in finding shelter, counselor, or the police.

Call domestic violence resource agencies in your community. Or call the National Domestic Violence hotline at (800) 799-SAFE (7233). Through this hotline, a woman anywhere in the United States can be connected to resources to help her get away from her violent abuser.

Always take concrete steps to protect your safety. In any case, know that you are not alone and that the abuse is not your fault.

Resources:

Futures Without Violence
100 Montgomery Street, The Presidio
San Francisco, CA 94129
(415) 678-5500
www.futureswithoutviolence.org

Institute on Domestic Violence in the African American Community
University of Minnesota School of Social Work
1404 Gortner Avenue
290 Peters Hall
St. Paul, MN 55108
(877) 643-8222
www.idvaac.org

National Domestic Violence Hotline
(800) 799-7233
TTY (800) 787-3224
www.ndvh.org

National Sexual Assault Hotline
(800) 656-4673
www.rainn.org

National Teen Dating Abuse Helpline
(866) 331-9474
www.loveisrespect.org

Saving Promise
1425 K Street, NW Suite 350
Washington, DC 20005
(800) 774-5760
info@savingpromise.org

PART THREE

SELF-CARE
is
IMPERATIVE

Chapter 6

Healthy Body

"How many of you have ever taken off all of your clothes, stood in front of the mirror, and admired yourself?" asked Dr. Goulda Downer, assistant professor at Howard University Medical School, when she spoke to an audience of Black women at an NAACP convention.

"You should have heard the laughter," she recalls. "'Are you mad? Never! Are you crazy?' The women were coming up afterward saying, 'Can you imagine looking at me?' And they were very serious."

Black women's relationship to our bodies is complex and often vexed. We take a lot of trouble to look good, yet we don't always do the things that will keep our bodies toned and strong. We have a healthier concept of weight overall than women of other races—in that we don't subscribe to the ideal of thin-is-beautiful—yet we're more likely to be overweight than any other group, and we are disproportionately affected by weight-related diseases such as diabetes and hypertension. We have a rich cultural tradition around food, yet we often eat the wrong things for the wrong reasons, and social and economic factors make it hard for us to feed ourselves and our families well, even when we want to. We lead lives that keep us running, yet few of us get the exercise we should. We're more likely than women of other races to say we feel good about ourselves no matter what—yet, like Dr. Downer's audience, we turn away from our reflection in the mirror.

When we're this disconnected from our physical selves, we miss a lot. We miss the signs of illness. Dr. Downer worries that if women don't look at themselves, they won't notice lumps or other warnings. We miss out on the intimacy of human touch because if we can't stand to look at ourselves naked, how can our partners? Since we don't have the vitality to live to our fullest, we miss out on a lot of life's joy.

We deserve better. *You* deserve better.

In this chapter, we'll take a look at the factors that determine our physical wellness and what we can do to be healthier and happier in our bodies. Of course, our bodies come under stress from any number of sources—from smog to global warming to pharmaceutical drugs in the water supply. Here, we'll focus on the factors that are a little more within our control: namely, the food we eat and the moves we make. And we'll see how healthy eating and physical activity can, without undue strain on our part, radically transform the quality of our lives.

The Way We Eat

For some folks, just the mention of lemon-butter pound cake brings back memories of lazy Fourths of July—a family barbecue followed by a nap on a blanket under a weeping willow tree. For others, that same confection conjures up cozy, snowy Saturdays spent stirring the batter, licking the spoon, and watching the cake rise under Big Mama's loving eye. Someone else might think of the same cake as a thoughtful way to comfort a friend after a devastating loss, or as a dangerous food that she needs to avoid.

Whether we enjoy sharing it when we socialize, use it to express love to one another, or consume it to comfort ourselves on a solo Saturday night, Black women experience a complicated relationship with food. Like people of all backgrounds, we savor our favorite foods for many reasons. We know that nothing knits our family together as tightly as the ritual of breaking (corn) bread together. We are aware that the easiest way to entice the members of any Black group to a meeting is to promise that food will be served. We realize that food plays a vital role in keeping our own body and the bodies of our loved ones healthy.

The foods we eat affect every aspect of our being: our energy level, our ability to think clearly, our emotional stability, our body's ability to repair and regenerate itself, the ease with which it maintains a healthy weight. We know that food affects our children's ability to learn, sit still in school, behave appropriately at home and in public, and separate themselves from their video games for a dose of real life. Yet all too often we use food to "take care of" others or ourselves in a way that isn't healthy at all. Far too many Black women turn to food for when we feel overloaded or overwhelmed by the realities of life—especially when we aren't tending to our mental health as we should.

"We are not going to see the psychologist, the psychoanalyst, the psychotherapist, so we nurture ourselves the only way we know how—with food—and that is the bottom line," Dr.

Downer says. "The lawyer, the unemployed housewife, the jobless teenager—every single one of us, that's what we do."

"Black women deal with the hand we're given," Dr. Whitt-Glover adds. "If we're big, it's like, 'I'd like to lose weight, but if not, life's going to go on.'"

"A lot of women eat to comfort themselves from all the things that they missed—relationships, marriage, kids, jobs, money, nice clothes, nice lifestyle," agrees sex therapist and psychologist Gail Wyatt, Ph.D. "They found comfort in food and have not evolved beyond that."

Then there are times when eating healthfully just falls lower down our priority list than more pressing needs: finding a job, keeping a roof over our head, feeding our children and fending off the bill collector. Sometimes it's all we can do just to find a moment to put food in our mouths. "I have crazy hours," says one mother of six. "I might get home at twelve o'clock from getting off of work, and I might get some rib tips or pick up wings and eat and lay down on that."

What's wrong with this picture? In spite of America's overabundance of food, research[1] shows that about two-thirds of diseases in the United States are caused by poor nutrition and inadequate physical activity. Our society abounds with special interests seducing us to eat in ways that undermine our health. These forces operate in the lives of all Americans, but their impact on Black American women is particularly harmful. No matter where we live, our educational level, and our economic class, we live—and our loved ones live—in the crosshairs of social, cultural, political, and economic factors that encourage us to eat poorly. To put it bluntly, our food is making us sick. If we want to take charge of our health, we need to understand how our food affects the quality of our whole life. We need to start with a clear picture of what's taking place on our plates.

The Facts of the Food Supply

Only a few generations ago, people ate foods grown on family farms. In 1900, 40 percent of Americans lived on farms. But as folks of all races migrated from farms to cities and from the rural South and Midwest toward the East and West coasts, that number plummeted. During the 1930s, as Americans weathered the extreme poverty of the Great Depression and the Dust Bowl, the U.S. Department of Agriculture tried to insulate struggling family farmers against the ruinous fluctuations of both the weather and the market by paying them to grow certain foods. These subsidies for corn, cotton, rice, soy, and wheat continue today, and now include programs to protect sugar and dairy farmers.[2] But these days, only 2 percent of Americans live on family farms, so the subsidies are going to large-scale industrial operations. This industry, known as Big Food, produces roughly 85 percent of America's food supply. [7] Big Food gives rise to powerful lobbies dedicated to selling crops that are the healthiest for their bottom line, not necessarily for our bodies. Thanks to technological innovations such as hybrid crops and the development of fertilizers and pesticides, farms are also producing food in vastly larger amounts than ever before. Advances in processing and transportation mean that food today can be shipped around the world. Today Americans not only enjoy the lowest food prices in the industrialized world, we're also the most likely to eat foods grown outside our local area and growing season—say, strawberries shipped in from Mexico so that northerners can enjoy them in February.[4]

These technological breakthroughs are wonderful, but they come with some downsides. Big Food yields enough to feed the average woman 3,800 calories a day [5]—roughly twice the calories the average 5'4" woman's body needs.[6] To sell this excess, food companies try to move more of their products—in this case by encouraging us to eat more. While that's the nature of business, the impact on consumers is highly personal. It's no accident that America's obesity epidemic—accompanied by a host of related diseases, from diabetes and hypertension to colon and kidney cancer—emerged during the Big Food era. [7]

Processed Foods

These days, Black women, like most Americans, struggle to manage overscheduled lives and overextended budgets with meals that are the fastest and easiest—which usually means they contain highly processed foods. In contrast to "whole" foods such as fresh fruits and vegetables, nuts and seeds, beans and legumes, and whole grains. By contrast, processed foods have been altered for more convenient packaging and storing in ways that often drain them of essential nutrients. We can keep a box of macaroni and cheese in the cupboard for months (or years) and cook it up in minutes, but foods like that don't have enough nutrition for our bodies. Not all processing is bad; cooking, canning, freezing, drying, and aging foods are examples of low levels of processing. Grinding wheat into flour or a sugar beet into table sugar involves high levels of processing. Incorporating chemical additives into a processed product can render a food unrecognizable. "If it doesn't look like it looked when God made it, it's processed," says naturopath Roni DeLuz, who counsels people in making eating choices that support optimal health.

A few processed foods all by themselves won't kill you, and we don't mean to take all the pleasure out of eating. It's just a matter of making conscious choices—and to do that, you need to know what you're getting and why. Nutrients are living elements. Foods with less "life" in them are less likely to spoil, ferment, decay, or attract bugs or rodents—between the manufacturer's warehouse, the supermarket shelves, and your plate. So the longer their *shelf life* is, the more convenient they are to store, prepare, and eat and the more profitable they are to the manufacturer.

Of course, there's a trade-off: fewer nutrients mean less energy entering our body, and the food loses taste and color. To compensate, manufacturers artificially enrich and fortify processed foods with vitamins and minerals and boost their flavor with large amounts of salt, sugar, and fat (particularly unhealthy fats). They add artificial colors, preservatives, and other man-made ingredients that take a toll on the body's well-being. Manufacturers gamble that convenience will outweigh compromised quality. Processed foods have become so much a part of our lives, we forget what we're missing.

The more the manufacturing process alters a food from its natural form, the more difficulty the body has in metabolizing it. "I call highly processed foods 'plastic foods,'" says Dr. DeLuz. "The body literally doesn't know what to do with them, so it stores them away in our fat cells." These foods challenge the body in ways that lead to low energy levels and illness. For example, processed flour and sugar—the main ingredients in most cookies and cakes, breakfast cereals and salty snacks—impact the body's blood sugar: the glucose in processed ingredients enters the bloodstream more rapidly than the body can handle. Over time this can lead to weight gain, heart disease, and other serious conditions.

Eating processed foods also makes you look and feel old. "It's not so much that people are getting old, it's that their body is getting toxic," says Dr. DeLuz. "It's a choice and often we don't even know that we're making it."

Mixed Messages

Another problem is that we're getting conflicting messages about what we should or shouldn't buy and eat. Food companies increase their sales by advertising and marketing their foods, regardless of those foods' effects upon consumer's health.

In *Food Politics: How the Food Industry Influences Nutrition and Health*, Marion Nestle, Ph.D., writes:

> In this regard, food companies hardly differ from cigarette companies. They lobby Congress to eliminate regulations perceived as unfavorable; they press federal regulatory agencies not to enforce such regulations; and when they don't like regulatory decisions, they file lawsuits. Like cigarette companies, food companies co-opt food and nutrition experts by supporting professional organizations and research, and they expand sales by marketing directly to children, members of minority

groups, and people in developing countries—whether or not the products are likely to improve people's diets.[8]

Research confirms that all of us are highly influenced by advertising and marketing. And it's quite possible that Black consumers are influenced most of all. What makes us particularly susceptible to persuasion? The time we spend in front of the screen (be it TV or computer). In Nielsen Media Research's ethnic ratings, Blacks of all age groups (beginning at age two) were reported to watch more television during every time slot—from daytime to prime time to late-night—than any other racial or ethnic group.[9] Black adolescents spend about thirteen hours daily using all forms of media (some at the same time) versus eight and a half hours for white children.[10]

Studies confirm that fast foods and other high-calorie, low-nutrient foods, as well as alcoholic beverages and cigarettes, are marketed disproportionately to consumers of color, including our young people. Over the past decade advertisers have perfected marketing strategies that target people of color.[11] Sonia Grier, Ph.D., M.B.A., associate professor of marketing at American University's Kogod School of Business, describes such *ethnic marketing* as advertising "that doesn't just say, 'Here's a burger, we want you to buy it,' but instead says, 'Here's a burger that tastes like mama made it, or here's the McRib or here's sweet tea, which comes from the South and is very much related to soul food.'" In effect, advertisers take our cultural traditions and "play them back to us," she adds. "It's like 'I'm going to play back to you what you want to hear.'"

When we look around for impartial information to guide our choices, we find an environment cluttered with confusing and conflicting messages rather than consensus. This week drinking coffee is healthy; next week, it's not. One month, eggs cause high cholesterol; a few years later, they're a good source of protein.

Whom and, more importantly, what should we believe about what's healthy? It's very difficult to know, and some researchers believe it's intentional.[12] If marketers can keep us baffled about what's good for us, we are more vulnerable to being enticed by their newest product innovation.

The federal government isn't much help either: every five years the USDA issues *Dietary Guidelines for Americans*, the government's official healthy-eating advice. It can be hard to know which of its interests the agency is serving—the well-being of consumers or the business of agriculture.[13]

The USDA's detractors, including authorities at such mainstream institutions as the Harvard School of Public Health,[14] say this is a lot like asking the fox to guard the henhouse. The

2010 *Dietary Guidelines* provide a case in point. They advise Americans to eat fewer artery-clogging solid fats [15] but do not recommend that they avoid any of the products it identifies as among their top sources of saturated fat: cheese (9 percent), pizza (6 percent), or desserts made of dairy products (6 percent)—products the USDA both subsidizes and promotes.

These same dietary guidelines remind Americans to eat more fruits and vegetables, yet produce farmers do not receive any financial subsidies as meat, poultry, grain, dairy, and other food producers do. No wonder fruits and vegetables are so expensive. A single apple costs about 50 cents, but an entire fast-food meal can cost less than a dollar.

Location, Location, Location

Walk through an upscale neighborhood on a Saturday morning and you'll see shoppers sauntering through their community's farmer's market, sorting through bushels of fresh asparagus, cartons of juicy strawberries, and bins of colorful new potatoes. Drive into the parking lot of any suburban supermarket and you may literally get caught in gridlock as shoppers make their weekly grocery run. But travel through predominantly Black neighborhoods both urban and suburban and you'll be lucky to find anyplace where residents can buy fresh produce and meats and other healthy foods. Just as a home's whereabouts help determine its value, the location we live in has a tremendous effect on how well we eat. In fact, where a person lives is perhaps the most important determinant of diet. It dictates his or her ability to eat healthily, their ability to avoid gaining weight, and vulnerability to food-related chronic diseases.

The unfortunate truth is that many Black people don't have a supermarket or even a smaller grocery store—likely sources of healthy foods—in their neighborhood, only convenience stores and corner stores stocked with cans and boxes, snacks and junk food. When "white flight" to the suburbs began in the 1960s and 1970s, many supermarkets left the inner cities too. Today only 8 percent of Black people have a supermarket within a mile of their home, compared to 31 percent of whites. For many, buying produce can require a half-day crosstown excursion by bus and a struggle home with our heavy bags.

"There are no stores in the neighborhood," said one participant in the Imperative focus group in Chicago on obesity and healthy eating. This is the reality across the country: in Los Angeles, poor areas have half as many supermarkets as more affluent areas; in the low-income community of West Louisville, Kentucky, it's the same; in poor parts of Washington, D.C., it's worse. [16]

Even in well-off areas of Atlanta, White neighborhoods tend to have better grocery stores than Black areas, suggesting that race, not just income, may play a role in determining the quality of foods available to urban residents.[17] And in rural areas, too, people have limited access to markets.

The food stores that *are* present in lower-income neighborhoods tend to be higher priced and offer lower-quality items than stores in higher-income areas. "Most of the time you are shopping in the neighborhood store and spending more money than you actually would in a regular grocery store," said one focus group participant. "And they don't have quality produce or quality meat, you know. You don't have a choice." When eating healthfully is that difficult, it's no wonder so many Black women resort to feeding their loved ones the less-nourishing food that's closer at hand. While the neighborhoods we're talking about are short on supermarkets, they have disproportionate numbers of fast-food restaurants, as well as take-out joints, corner stores, liquor stores, and convenience stores.

"I was upset when I saw those [fast-food] places moving into the neighborhood," said a focus group participant. "Who told them that was what we wanted to eat? They look at our community and say, 'We can bring in what we think we want you to eat.'"

"People know that they need to do better," says Dr. Toni Yancey, professor at UCLA's Center for Public Health and author of *Instant Recess: Building a Fit Nation 10 Minutes at a Time*. "It's just very hard to do better and you have to go out of your way to do better. That's the problem."

The Paradox Of Plenty

The decline in food quality that has occurred over the past century has changed our reality in some significant ways. For the first time, we face what experts call *the paradox of plenty*: a state in which food is abundant and people eat more than their bodies need. They suffer from health problems associated with poor nutrition—tooth decay, degenerative eye diseases, diabetes, heart disease, and certain cancers, for example. The United States ships food all over the world, but more than 50 million Americans—including 17 million children—live in households where they don't have enough to eat. Households headed by single Black women suffer these problems more than any other American families: almost one-quarter of families headed by single Black women are what public health experts call *food insecure*,[18] making it difficult for the families to function and for children to grow and learn. Large numbers of people are also both heavy and hungry—a combination that theoretically should be impossible. "Americans are overfed but undernourished," says Dr. DeLuz.

Diet and Disease

Research confirms that once people begin to transition from their indigenous diet to the highly processed foods common to industrialized societies, they develop health conditions and diseases previously not experienced. Obesity, Type 2 diabetes, hypertension, stroke, and heart disease are what many experts' term *diseases of the modern diet.*

In fact, we develop these conditions at a rate that has many health experts alarmed. "We have twin epidemics of diabetes and obesity," says Constance Brown-Riggs, author of *The African American Guide to Living Well with Diabetes.* "You can superimpose the diabetes map on top of the obesity map—you see exactly the same trends." People who have diabetes have a much higher risk of diabetes-related complications—depression, loss of sexual interest, hearing and vision loss, and even amputations. They're also more likely to experience a heart attack or stroke—among Black women's leading causes of disability and death.[19]

The Weight of Beauty

In the American media and popular culture, weight is often presented as a beauty issue— the less you weigh, the smaller your frame, the more attractive you are. Whether or not you buy into this notion, the relationship between weight and beauty muddies the waters for many of us. The words *overweight* and *obese* are medical terms, not judgments on our looks. Both describe weight ranges heavier than what is healthy for a person of a given height.[20] The higher your weight climbs above the optimal range, the greater your risk of disease. Almost 80 percent of Black women over age twenty are either overweight or obese, compared to just under 60 percent of white women, and this gap exists at all educational and socioeconomic levels—it's not just the poor and uneducated who are too heavy for their health.[21]

Every person feels her best and her body functions most effectively at a certain size. Weigh too little and the body will literally digest itself so that it can carry out essential bodily functions; weigh too much and the body will struggle under the burden of excess weight. Many Black women know quite well that weight and well-being are connected; however, this message shares space with images of what's considered beautiful in pop culture—whether conveyed on the catwalk, the big screen, or in women's magazines. These beauty standards can interfere with our understanding of weight as it relates to health. Consequently, we may not take our extra weight seriously enough. Many Black women feel ambivalent at best about the belief that thin is beautiful. Research suggests that most Black women's ideal body size is curvier than their White peers. The beauty industry often equates being overweight with being less attractive; however, many Black women (and men) do not to see a conflict between being full-figured and looking good.[22]

"I've been the official weight-to-the-height ratio and it was too small for me," said one Imperative focus group participant. "I looked in the mirror and it's like, 'New, you need about five more pounds.' To me, that weight fit me more than what the chart said."

Unfortunately, though, what we casually call "healthy"—some meat on our bones—may not be medically healthy at all. Even weighing a mere 20 or 30 additional pounds above the recommended body weight can increase our health risks. Because we don't realize—or don't want to accept—that our beauty standard and the medical standard conflict with each other, we may be slow to react as our weight creeps upward. Nevertheless, the goal of the health standard is to head off a health catastrophe. "Losing ten or fifteen pounds can prevent or even delay the onset of diabetes," says Brown-Riggs. Some people don't take their weight seriously. "Part of that is cultural acceptance of being a little heavy, or what some people call 'thick'. But it's hurting us."

Measures That Work

Fortunately, there are some more objective measures of healthy weight than media messages or our own best guesses. The body mass index, or BMI, as it is often called, measures the relationship between your weight and your height to determine if you are at greater risk of disease.

A measure between 18.5 and 24 indicates normal weight; 25 to 29 indicates overweight; over 30 tips a person into being obese. A BMI over 30 often means that the person is at greater risk for many of the diseases we've been discussing. To calculate your exact BMI value, multiply your weight in pounds by 705, divide by your height in inches, then divide again by your height in inches.

In 2002 the average Black woman's BMI was 31, putting her at high risk for health problems. One in every six or seven Black women had a BMI greater than 40, which qualifies her as morbidly obese.[23] But the BMI is "not the be all and end all" of obesity measurements, Brown-Riggs says. "It's only a measure of height versus weight: it doesn't tell you how much of that is fat and how much is lean tissue"—that is, muscle and bone.

BMI can be misleadingly high in muscular people, such as athletes, overestimating the amount of body fat they have, and misleadingly low in older adults and others who have lost muscle, underestimating theirs. The BMI also tends to overestimate the amount of body fat on Black people's bodies. Brown-Riggs notes that we carry more muscle per pound than Whites, making the BMI a less accurate measure of our disease risk. (People of Asian descent often have the opposite problem—their BMI may suggest that they are not at risk when, in fact, they are.)

BODY MASS INDEX RISK LEVELS

Height	Minimal Risk (BMI under 25)	Moderate Risk (BMI 25-29.9) Overweight	High Risk (BMI 30 and above) Obese
4'10"	118 lbs. or less	119–142 lbs.	143 lbs. or more
4'11"	123 or less	124–147	148 or more
5'0"	127 or less	128–152	153 or more
5'1"	131 or less	132–157	158 or more
5'2"	135 or less	136–163	164 or more
5'3"	140 or less	141–168	169 or more
5'4"	144 or less	145–173	174 or more
5'5"	149 or less	150–179	180 or more
5'6"	154 or less	155–185	186 or more
5'7"	158 or less	159–190	191 or more
5'8"	163 or less	164–196	197 or more
5'9"	168 or less	169–202	203 or more
5'10"	173 or less	174–208	209 or more
5'11"	178 or less	179–214	215 or more
6'0"	183 or less	184–220	221 or more
6'1"	188 or less	189–226	227 or more
6'2"	193 or less	194–232	233 or more
6'3"	199 or less	200–239	240 or more
6'4"	204 or less	205–245	246 or more

Source: Adapted from Obesity Education Initiative: Clinical Guidelines on the Identification, Evaluation, and Treatment of Overweight and Obesity in Adults. Bethesda, M.D.: National Institutes of Health, National Heart, Lung, and Blood Institute, Obesity Research, 1998.

The BMI doesn't account for the positive impact of a person's activity level no matter his or her weight. Regular physical activity reduces the risk of heart disease, even for people with higher BMIs. Their diabetes risk seems to fall as well. In fact, recent research suggests that people with heart disease who are overweight but physically fit may be somewhat better off than those with heart disease who tip in on the skinny side of normal. While still controversial, this so-called *obesity paradox* [24] is giving health experts pause. Some have begun to investigate whether a little extra weight might be okay as long as you remain physically active.

The average Black woman is 5'4" tall. Her ideal weight from a medical standpoint falls between about 110 and 140 pounds; between roughly 140 and 170 pounds is overweight from a medical point of view; 170 to 227 makes her obese; and above 225 pounds she's considered morbidly obese.

Another way to assess whether weight may be jeopardizing your health is to measure the circumference of your waist. Weight that accumulates around the belly disturbs a person's metabolism and increases the risk of heart disease more than weight that accumulates on the hips, thighs, and behind. So someone whose figure is round like an apple is more likely to develop heart disease than someone who weighs the same amount but has a small waist and big hips—shaped more like a pear. A woman is considered an apple if her waist measurement is greater than 35 inches; for a man, it's more than 40 inches.

Dangerous Curves

There's a widespread notion that women who are heavy don't care about their weight, even when it is jeopardizing their health—and when this misconception is shared by the very health professionals who treat obesity-related diseases, women's care can suffer. Many Black women report being poorly treated by medical staff.

"My first neurologist couldn't seem to hide his contempt of me for not being bone thin. His staff was just as sour," says Cherie Ann Turpin of Washington, D.C.

"My gynecologist told me I was too fat and needed to lose weight," says Sylvia Forbes. "When I told him I was trying, he insisted that I was being lazy."

"When I got as fat as I could be, almost two hundred and fifty pounds, my doctor said to me, 'You look like a pin cushion,'" another woman confides.

Research bears these women out. Some studies show that almost 70 percent of overweight women experience discrimination from physicians and over half experience ongoing discrimination. Though it's hard to imagine a doctor confessing that she or he treats patients differently on account of their race or gender, some health providers openly admit that they discriminate on the basis of weight, listing obesity only after drug addiction, alcoholism, and mental illness as a condition they respond to negatively.[25]

"Overweight and obese people are commonly viewed as lazy, lacking in discipline, and noncompliant with programs and treatment for weight loss," says Rebecca M. Puhl, Ph.D., director of research and weight stigma initiatives at Yale University's Rudd Center for Food Policy & Obesity. "These stereotypes are rarely challenged in American society despite recognition of the complex causes of obesity, and often lead to prejudice that impairs quality of life for obese children and adults." [26]

Other research shows that prejudice toward overweight people is as common as the discrimination exhibited toward any other stigmatized group, including racial discrimination. Fat bias is socially acceptable, even among health-care professionals.[27]

As Sylvia Forbes experienced, some health-care providers believe that people choose to be fat because they are lazy and eat too much. Some even think that overweight people deserve whatever negative health consequences they get. One doctor has shared off the record that jokes and disparaging comments about overweight people are common—and, worse, that with heavy patients some doctors don't adhere to basic medical standards for testing and treating conditions such as high blood pressure, diabetes, and irregular hormone levels that often accompany the excess weight. "It's criminal," this doctor says.

So how can you protect yourself from fat bias in a medical setting? First, know that you are always entitled to respect from your health-care providers no matter how much you weigh or how closely you have followed your doctor's advice. Second, if you don't like how you're being treated, look for another provider. Use the girlfriend grapevine and ask people you know about their doctors, whether they like them and what it is that they like about them.

Knowing Better, Doing Better

"We know that obesity increases risk of high blood pressure, diabetes, stroke, and arthritis, but we don't understand how important our behavior is—there is a disconnect," Dr. Downer says. "When I talk to my patients about heart disease, they know what I'm talking about, they understand. But they don't connect heart disease to themselves. To them it's about somebody else, not me."

Some of us are just not willing to do what it takes to create a change for the better. We may think it's going to be all sacrifice and deprivation. Given all the things that many Black women already feel deprived of—joy, romantic relationships, money, material goods, and so on—perhaps we cling to food because we feel it's the only thing we've got.

Or perhaps we want to show that we *aren't* deprived anymore. Dr. Downer describes a highly educated woman who came to her for a nutritional consultation. When Dr. Downer suggested that she cut back on the steaks she ate for dinner every evening, the woman blew up at her: "I'm finally able in this generation to buy whatever I want to buy and eat whatever I want to eat, and now that I can afford to do so, you're telling me now that I'm not supposed to eat red meat? How dare you!"

Dr. Downer was shocked: This was a woman with diabetes, hypertension, and cholesterol through the roof. But when she clarified that she meant cut *down* on the steak, not cut it out, the woman insisted: "I can afford it and I buy it. And I want the marbled cut."

The truth is that being overweight doesn't just increase our risk of health problems, it diminishes our quality of life in countless ways. "People talk about having knee and joint pain," says Dr. DeLuz. "They don't have mental clarity or energy; they have potbellies filled with gas; they don't have a good sex life."

We Black women who are overweight are often too tired or physically uncomfortable to play with our children. We may even avoid attending our children's activities because we don't want them to get teased about their mother's appearance. We may shy away from situations where we could easily feel humiliated—whether sitting in a standard office chair or theater seat or going to the company cookout. Our intimate lives may suffer, or we may avoid sex altogether. We may lose out on personal and professional connections because we struggle in our relationships with issues of self-worth and shame. We often struggle to accomplish even our daily chores.

"When I am overweight, I feel like I am dragging a weight with me," says one woman.

But no matter what your habits have been until now, to paraphrase Dr. Maya Angelou, as soon as you know better, you can do better. Whether your waist measures 34" or 64", or you're a size 2 or a 22, no matter the current state of your health or what conditions may run in your family, you can take steps to improve your well-being. Even if you already have a health condition (think allergies or digestive ailments), a precondition (think pre-diabetes or pre-hypertension), or even a chronic disease such as diabetes or cancer, by improving the way that you care for yourself you can improve the way you look, feel, and live your life.

Many diseases we believe run in our bloodline actually run in the recipe box and lifestyle choices that we, and our family members share. While it is true that some Black people may carry a genetic predisposition to certain health conditions—say, diabetes or high cholesterol—there is a difference between being predisposed to a disease and actually developing it. "I always tell Black women that diabetes is not inherited. You don't have to get it. It's not your inheritance," says Dr. Downer. "Genetics load the gun, yes, but your lifestyle pulls that trigger." We can head off, change the course, or even reverse many diseases by the changes we make in our daily habits.

Lifestyle changes undertaken slowly and over time can have a profound impact on our health and transform our quality of life. As you make these changes your body will feel better and you'll feel better about yourself. And you can start right now.

Change Is Hard

Change is hard—there's no getting around it. And life as a Black woman—ranging from factors in our own families to mindsets in our communities—can make change especially challenging.

Those of us who are married or partnered may struggle to balance our own needs with what our loved ones want and need. "I have set goals for myself," said one woman who'd been diagnosed with diabetes. "Then my husband comes in wanting a prepared meal every day when he gets off work. What he's eating, I prepare it, and that's what we eat. I start on my goals, but I have to put them to the side."

Black cultural traditions exert their own pressures to conform. "It's a whole lifestyle, and I think it's just the way some of us were raised and brought up—that everything is centered around food," one focus group participant recalled. "I think that growing up you associate everything with food—happy, sad, depression, whatever emotion you are going through is connected to food, somehow." Then there's the old stricture against wasting food. How many of us were raised to clean our plates because there were "starving children in Africa"?

Sometimes we just get trapped in our inertia and America's couch-potato culture. "I think TV has contributed to it; I think even the radio contributes to it," one Black woman admitted. "I am up at six and when I get home and I just want to sit. I am physically exhausted. All I can think about is what is on TV."

Let's be honest: some of us don't know how to cook like people used to. Says Kristie Lancaster, R.D., Ph.D., associate professor of nutrition at New York University, "This generation doesn't know about healthy meals, and many of them think they're supposed to eat processed foods." She notes that a farmer's market in East Harlem closed because area residents weren't buying—they didn't know what to do with the fresh foods.

Changing our eating habits is an education process. From sampling foods that we've never tried before, to finding places to eat with healthy menus, to learning to cook all over again (or for the first time), taking better care of ourselves means becoming lifelong learners, including in the kitchen.

"Food is the easiest way to have fun," Lancaster believes. "Figure out who you would like to spend more time with and invite them to go grocery shopping with you and cook together. If I'm making chili for the week, it's more fun to make a big pot if there are other people around. You can share, have dinner together, and celebrate food and yourselves."

Making the Change

You've heard it all before: stop eating soul food, no more fried foods, cut out sweets. But unless you're experiencing a health crisis, there's no need to go this far.

"Food should be enjoyed and celebrated, not feared and isolated. That's my motto," says Dr. Downer. "All foods can fit—all of it! It's just how we go about it."

The answer isn't self-denial, it's eating less of the foods that are less healthful for us, or eating those foods less often, and eating more of the foods that do us good. It involves learning how to prepare some foods differently—say, doing more baking instead of deep frying—and eating a variety of foods that offer healthy choices alongside our more traditional options.

It also means seeking foods that work well for our particular body—foods that energize us, help us think clearly, that we enjoy and that help build up our family culture, from shopping and cooking together to enjoying meals in one another's company.

Learn to listen to your body. What is good for someone else may not be optimal for you. "People tell me all the time that they can't eat pork or beef—they can't digest it; they have to stick with a lighter source of protein, like fish," says Dr. DeLuz. "Some people say, 'I can't eat steak or I'm sick for two or three days.' Well, then don't eat steak. If a food makes you feel sick, don't eat it."

Pay attention to whether your energy goes up or down after eating a food. Do you feel more alert and attentive? That's a good food for you. Does it cloud your thinking, make you lethargic, or even put you to sleep? These are clues that perhaps you should avoid the food. Do you have gas, an upset stomach, headaches, constipation, or diarrhea? These are typically signs that the food doesn't agree with your body.

If you want to lose weight, remember that weight-loss diets usually don't work because the conditions they create aren't sustainable in the long term. You'll almost certainly end up gaining back whatever weight you lose—or more—and you may even alter your metabolism without realizing it. The body doesn't know that you're dieting; it believes that you're starving, so it slows your metabolism to save your life. After you go off the diet, your metabolism stays slow and you gain weight.

We also know now that calorie counting doesn't work, at least not the way we once thought. Weight-loss experts understand that the quality of the calorie is at least as important as the quantity. Whole foods—fruits, vegetables, whole grains, beans, etc.—count as quality foods.

"People think all calories are created equal, but they aren't," says Dr. DeLuz. "A glass of orange juice and a bran muffin both may have 150 calories, but the bran muffin is better for you because it has fiber and sustains the blood sugar more evenly." Many low-quality calories have been stripped of fiber, which gives you the feeling of being full and tells your body that it's time to stop eating. So if you eat processed foods while you're calorie-counting, chances are that you'll overeat. It's far better to make gradual adjustments that you enjoy, that make you feel good about yourself and that you can maintain over a long period of time—ideally, the rest of your life.

"Set small and reasonable goals," Brown-Riggs reminds us. "People become overwhelmed because they think they have to do it all and make a 180-degree turn. They think, 'Why bother?' Instead I try to get them to look at it from a reasonable perspective. I encourage them to set SMART goals: Specific, Measurable, Achievable, Relevant, and Timely."

"But if you want to have a piece of candy, have it and keep moving," says Dr. Downer. "When you have diets that are too restrictive, nobody wants them."

If you can, try getting some additional support for your change: talk with a nutritionist to discuss strategies for success. Once you have a healthy eating plan, begin monitoring what you eat and what's going on when you eat it. Ask yourself questions like:

- How much of this meal am I eating for health and good nutrition and how much am I eating for comfort or pleasure?

- Am I eating in response to some form of stress, such as worry, depression, anxiety, or something else?

- Am I eating mindlessly and relapsing into behaviors that I'm trying to outgrow?

- Am I eating under the influence of peer pressure because I don't have the knowledge or willpower to explain what I'm doing and stick with it no matter what my loved ones say?

Healthy Eating

So, when we get right down to it, how *should* we eat?

"The most important thing goes back to thinking about what your mother taught you," says Brown-Riggs. "Eat sensibly: fresh fruit . . . and vegetables—as close to nature as possible."

Bite by bite, step by step, try organizing your diet around the following time-tested tips.

Consume Less of These

Sugar. Sugars come in two types: those that occur naturally in foods such as fruit—and even bread and milk—and sugars that are added to foods during processing or cooking or at the table. These *added sugars* can range from the high-fructose corn syrup mixed in at the manufacturing plant to the table sugar and honey that we often stir in at home. Most people can healthily consume naturally occurring sugars in moderation (if you have pre-diabetes or diabetes, follow your dietitian's advice); however, too much added sugar increases your risk of health hazards.

"Think of glucose like sandpaper rubbing against the fine, delicate skin of the blood vessels—I often use the analogy that it's like

---

STEALTH SUGARS

Picking out the sugar on a food's ingredient label isn't always easy. If any of these items appears in the first five ingredients, the food is sweetened to an unhealthy degree. Consider leaving it in the store and making a different selection.

- Agave nectar
- Brown sugar
- Cane crystals
- Cane sugar
- Corn sweetener
- Corn syrup
- Crystalline fructose
- Dextrose
- Evaporated cane juice
- Fructose
- Fruit juice concentrates
- Glucose
- High-fructose corn syrup
- Honey
- Invert sugar
- Lactose
- Maltose
- Malt syrup
- Molasses
- Raw sugar
- Sucrose
- Sugar
- Syrup

Source: Harvard School of Public Health, The Nutrition Source.

a baby's bottom. It's very tender and going to become irritated, then end up with breakages, and you get damage to the kidneys, to the blood vessels, eyes, and all," Brown-Riggs says.

High-fructose corn syrup, a sweetener often found in soft drinks and baked goods, is widely agreed to be so hazardous to human health that lawmakers from New York to California have attempted to prohibit its sale. In fact, an increasingly vocal group of experts regards added sugar not only as something for us to cut back on, but as downright dangerous.[28]

You can protect your health by drastically cutting back your consumption of soda pop, sweetened teas, juice drinks, and juice beverages. When you buy packaged foods, read the nutrition facts on the label and look for no more than about 5 grams of sugar per serving. In the list of ingredients, sugar should be no higher than fifth on the list. Also, reduce the amount of sugar of any type that you add to your cereal, coffee, tea, iced tea, and desserts— including honey, whether processed or raw—especially if your body is experiencing any difficulty in processing sugar, or if you suffer from a metabolic disorder, pre-diabetes, or diabetes. Even agave nectar, which enters the bloodstream more slowly than other sweeteners, is still processed and should be used judiciously.

The bottom line? "Limit cookies, cakes, candies—the foods your mother said to wait until you finish your dinner to eat," Brown-Riggs advises. "If you do that, you'll basically stay out of trouble."

Sodium. The average woman consumes 3,300 milligrams (mg) of sodium per day, but experts advise Black folks, who tend to be more salt sensitive, as well as anyone with diabetes and or high blood pressure, to consume no more than 1,500 mg[29]. This includes table salt, one of the many forms of sodium. For most people, though, sodium in their diet comes mainly from prepackaged foods, not from what they add at the table.

"Stay away from the rice mixtures and rice bowls, roll-up biscuits, canned soups and croutons—they're loaded with sodium," Brown-Riggs suggests. In fact, many processed foods contain so much sodium that you can consume 1,500 grams in just one or two meals.

But how do you lose your taste for salt? Start by switching to lower-salt foods, then begin to cut back on the stove and at the table. Decrease gradually; instead of three shakes, use two shakes, then one. As you stay away from salt, your sense of taste will sharpen, and eventually anything with salt in it will taste too salty to you. In place of salt, season instead with herbs and spices, including lemon, lime, vinegar, oregano, onion, cilantro, ginger, garlic, parsley, and salt-free seasonings. As you transition toward more natural foods, you can worry less about how much sodium you eat—you're unlikely to get to 1,500 unless you're eating processed foods.

Saturated fat. This type of oil or fat turns solid at room temperature—think butter, meat fat, bacon grease, shortening, and lard. So back off of the butter *and* margarine, toss out the bacon grease, shortening, lard, and palm oil, and go light on the baked goods—whether you make them yourself, buy them at the store, or eat so-called low-fat options.

We've been hearing a lot lately about *trans* fats or trans fatty acids. Trans fats are considered by some doctors to be the worst type of fat; unlike other fats, they both raise your "bad" (LDL) cholesterol and lower your "good" (HDL) cholesterol. Another name for *trans* fats is "hydrogenated" or "partially hydrogenated" oils. Look for these on the ingredient list on food packages.

Alcoholic beverages. Deciding whether and how much to drink is a personal decision. For someone who doesn't have an alcohol addiction, drinking a moderate amount—say, a glass or two of red wine each day—may help reduce your risk of heart disease. If your body is showing any signs of struggling to process sugar—you have pre-diabetes, diabetes, metabolic syndrome, or insulin resistance—you should eliminate even social drinking, since alcohol can impact blood sugar, interfere with diabetes medications, and increase blood pressure and levels of triglycerides (fats in the blood). Bottom line: if you don't drink regularly, it's best not to start.

Consume More of These

Water. Although our bodies seem to be solid, they're actually composed primarily of water. In fact, the brain itself is 75 percent water, the blood 83 percent, and the heart 80 to 90 percent.[30] Get too dehydrated and you'll feel tired, hungry, and foggy headed. You may also feel hungry, so when you're hungry, try drinking water first and see if that does the trick.

The average adult woman needs about 64 ounces of water daily from all beverages, including caffeinated beverages. The bulk of our fluids, though, should come from plain water. Experts advise drinking it between meals, not with food: drinking with meals dilutes digestive enzymes that should be hard at work.

Healthy carbohydrates. Carbohydrates are the body's main source of energy; the healthiest sources include whole grains, fruits and vegetables, and beans. Even though carbs are often vilified, we can't live without them. But most Americans eat too many processed carbs and not enough whole grains and fruits and vegetables.

Over time, phase out processed carbs, such as products made with white flour, and phase in more whole foods in their place. "From a quality perspective, whole grains are best," says Brown-Riggs. "But does that mean you can't have a piece of white bread from time to time? No."

It's like Dr. Downer says: all foods can fit.

Fruits and vegetables. Messages about what we should and shouldn't eat seem to be changing all the time, but what never changes is "Eat more fruits and veggies." Black people don't eat enough fruit and tend to eat too little fiber—the part of the carbohydrate that we can't digest, which helps removes toxins from the body. We also get inadequate amounts of key nutrients like potassium and folate, probably because we eat fewer fruits and vegetables.

At each meal, plan to make half your plate colorful, fresh fruits and veggies.[31] Try to pick foods from each color group—from white (onions and garlic) to yellow (corn and summer squash) to orange (oranges and carrots) to red (tomatoes and strawberries) to green (bell peppers and greens) to violet (red onions and eggplant). Each color indicates the presence of a different set of antioxidants, and cancer-fighting ingredients.

When possible, get your fruit in its original form, not in the form of fruit juice. Because the body can't easily manage fruit sugar separated from its fiber, fruit juice may be the single most fattening food in the American diet.[32] "People think that orange juice is healthy, but the way your body will use it, you're going to gain weight," Dr. DeLuz says.

Fiber. If you up your intake of fruits, vegetables, and whole grains, you'll also increase the amount of fiber you consume. Fiber makes us feel full sooner and slows sugar's release into the bloodstream, keeping blood sugar from spiking and then crashing. It also removes toxins and keeps your bowel movements regular. Processing strips many foods of their fiber, which also makes them take longer to move through your system, contributing to digestive problems, including gas, constipation, and diverticulitis. Eating plenty of naturally high-fiber whole-grain foods, fruits, and vegetables will also reduce your risk of developing heart disease and Type 2 diabetes.[33]

Healthy protein. Nobody knows the exact amount of protein that's needed for a healthy diet. What we do know is that all protein isn't alike. Some contains unhealthy levels of saturated fat, such as the fat on a piece of meat. Better to focus on low-fat sources of protein, including some types of fish, poultry, nuts, and beans. If you enjoy red meat, choose the leanest cuts and eat small portions, and avoid processed varieties of meat—including bacon, sausage, lunch meat, and hot dogs, which contain cancer-causing nitrates and excess salts.[34] Also, if you drink whole milk, try switching to low-fat or skim.

An important caveat about eating fish: tuna and other big fish often contain high amounts of mercury, so it's best to limit your consumption or avoid them altogether, particularly if you're pregnant.[35] Instead, eat more salmon, mackerel, herring, lake trout, and sardines: they contain less mercury and are high in omega-3 fatty acids, which support our metabolism of glucose and our body's ability to reduce inflammation.

Vegans and vegetarians should meet with a dietitian to ensure they get enough high-quality protein. "I have a lot of clients who are sick vegetarians," says Dr. DeLuz. "I can't get them to eat enough protein."

If you can afford it, choose organic, pasture-raised and grass-fed meats. Chicken and beef grown on industrial farms are fed on corn, causing their bodies to carry more fat and more omega-6 oils, which contribute to inflammation.

Calcium. Many Black women believe incorrectly that Black folks don't get osteoporosis, the bone-breaking disease that plagues many white and Asian women. Although Black women get osteoporosis less often than others, our risk remains significant—particularly if we smoke. Because we tend to underestimate our risk, we may not pay enough attention to building and preserving calcium or exercising, which also protects bones. Most doctors recommend calcium supplementation, and you can also eat calcium-rich foods such as yogurt and dark leafy greens.

How Much Is Enough?

For many of us, how much we eat is almost as important as what we eat. If cravings or overeating pose a problem for you, talk to a nutritionist about ways to manage your desire for more food than your body really needs. Reducing refined and processed sugars and carbs helps many people keep their joints under control. Left unchecked, these foods release too much glucose into the bloodstream and do it quickly, causing your energy to spike, then crash and leave you with strong cravings. White bread, pasta, rice, low-fiber cereals, and baked goods burden your bloodstream with amounts of glucose that the body has a hard time managing. Fruits, vegetables, whole grains, and some beans release glucose into your bloodstream more slowly and help you eat less.

Pay attention to the size of your portions. Culture-wide, they're bigger than they've ever been: today's bagel is twice as big as the bagel of 20 years ago. Manufacturers sell foods in bigger packages, which can make it difficult to figure out the number of servings you're eating. Restaurants, too, serve ever-larger portions of food. Even plates have gotten larger. So it's easy to lose track of how much you've eaten.

A good rule of thumb is to think of your plate as a pie chart. Fill at least half of your plate with fruits and vegetables, one-quarter with whole grains and one-quarter with protein. This is the visual—known as MyPlate.

Healthy Body: Part II

Keep It Moving

Let's face it: as much as we admire Michelle Obama's arms, many of us know that we don't stand a snowball's chance in hell of getting them. It's best just to make do with what we have. Maybe next lifetime, as Erykah Badu croons.

Then again, maybe not. Because many of the ideas about being physically active that may have traumatized you in the past—wearing that 1980s Jane Fonda thong, being the only fat lady at the gym, working out until you're gasping for your last breath—have actually gone the way of the boom box and the leotard.

We now know that you can improve your quality of life by doing something as simple as standing instead of sitting. You can exercise for ten minutes at a time while wearing your street clothes—well, you do need to take off your cute shoes—without even setting your big toe in a gym.

These changes are tremendously important for Black women. In the short term, keeping your body in motion will help to improve your mood, make you feel better in general, think more clearly, and feel less stress. It can also help to lower your blood pressure and control your blood sugar. Incorporate exercise into your daily routine and, over time, you reduce your risk of a catastrophic illness that could destroy your health and your life.

In today's world, physical activity is no longer a "nice-to-do" for a Black woman's health—we need to reprioritize it to our "must-do" list as an essential part of caring for our bodies and putting our health first.

Yet just thinking about exercise can make our blood pressure go up when it should go down. "When in the world am I going to squeeze that into my schedule? I need to rest, not work harder. Where am I going to get the money for a gym membership? And after I work out, what am I going to do with my hair?" These are some of the many thoughts that run through our heads.

Are You Physically Fit?

Why is it so important for the human body to be physically active? To answer this, let's consider that our primitive ancestors spent most of their time searching for, killing or harvesting, and preparing their food. Many walked from place to place, searching for meals and grazing on whatever they found; others planted and cultivated and harvested; still others sprinted after—and ran *from*—animals. Our ancestors carried and played with their children, prepared meals, then went back to walking and working.

"We weren't sitting around in groups; we were doing a lot of moving as hunter-gatherers for ninety nine percent of our history," says Toni Yancey, M.D. You ate what you killed, what you grew, what you gathered or caught. If you didn't catch anything, or if the crop failed, you didn't eat—plain and simple. Your body automatically slowed its metabolism to allow you to subsist on little to no food. (This is why weight-loss dieting doesn't work.) Women's bodies naturally stored fat in their midsections so that if they were pregnant the fetus could be nourished no matter what.

Clearly our bodies were designed to burn energy. Nobody was picking up the phone and ordering from Domino's. The movements they made every day—walking, sprinting, bending, lifting, pulling—have been fundamental to humans' survival for millennia.

In the 21st century, science allows us to understand better how these movements are essential to human life. Among other benefits, they cause our muscles to contract and release. These basic muscle activities—including the beating of the heart, which is a muscle—squeeze and milk the veins and arteries, propelling oxygen- and nutrient-filled blood to the cells and recirculating used blood to the heart. This can't happen as effectively when we spend the afternoon on the sofa glued to reruns or HGTV.

So while popular culture tells us physical activity can give us great legs and a tight behind, and doctors tell us it can help prevent heart disease and stroke, its benefits are much more fundamental than that. Don't move enough and blood and other fluids will pool in your body; don't move enough and your sex drive goes down; don't move enough and toxins will build up in your tissues. No wonder we feel so poorly sometimes.

Why Exercise?

There's at least one other benefit to getting physically active that's essential to the survival of the species. "Immediately you feel a little bit better so you don't want to kill your kids," says Dr. Yancey, who has spent much of her career helping people of color and low-income people get healthier. Stress reduction is the very first benefit that she shares with mothers when she encourages them to become more active.

"It clears my head so I can breathe," says 24-year-old Althea, a mother of two who is taking classes at a community college and struggling to pay her tuition bill. "It helps to just walk to a bus stop that's farther away than the one I'd usually get on. Sometimes I just have to start running. I run and cry at the same time. It makes me feel better."

"When you don't know the 'why' behind physical activity, you may or may not do it," says Dr. Whitt-Glover, Ph.D., who works closely with Dr. Yancey. "It's interesting to watch women 'get it' and say, 'Oh my gosh! Why didn't I know this before?' Sometimes they become so angry that nobody explained it before. They ask, 'Why didn't they tell me?' "

Here's what these women are seeing when that lightbulb goes on: expending energy gives us more energy. All of the nutrients, oxygen, and hormones that our movement spread around the body help us to solve problems, reduce stress, get a good night's sleep and feel better about ourselves. Being active can also help you tone your body without losing your curves.

Physical activity can lower your blood pressure, improve your cholesterol, help you lose weight, and reduce inflammation in your body. Because it helps to change both your body weight and your body composition, it indirectly protects against other conditions as well, including fatty liver, many cancers, sleep apnea, low-back pain, gout, and more.[36] Staying in motion increases longevity and lowers your risk of developing heart disease, stroke, hypertension, and Type 2 diabetes—all conditions that disproportionately affect Black women.

Vigorous physical activity (as long as it's not related to work) has also lowered the risk of depression in Black women.[37] Being active also strengthens your heart, which makes life much easier all the way around. Just ask anyone who's out of shape how hard it is to do even the simplest things, such as walking back upstairs to get your keys or your purse.

Getting active strengthens our bones, too. Even though they seem rock solid, bones are living tissues, and any weight-bearing activity—meaning any activity that requires you to resist or support weight,[38] including walking—strengthens them. (Other weight-bearing activities include lifting weights, using resistance bands, and some forms of yoga.) After our twenties we typically start to lose bone density and strength; consistent exercise prevents bone loss, which is important because, no matter what your girlfriend told you, osteoporosis *does* affect Black women. It's never too late to start: becoming physically active supports our bones at any age, and also improves flexibility and balance, which can help keep us from falling and breaking a hip or some other bone in our senior years.[39]

Couch Potatoes by Choice?

Americans just don't exercise enough, period. It isn't a "Black thing," it's a "thing" that affects women of all backgrounds.

Unfortunately, Black women sit on our blessed assurances more than almost anyone else. In one study, more than half of Black women reported that they were physically inactive—meaning that they participated in no physical activity at all in their personal time.[40] The numbers vary from study to study, but the message is the same: we don't move as much as we should. And the harder up we are, the harder it is. It's been found that women whose family income is about $45,000 for a family of four are twice as likely to meet the federal government's guidelines for physical activity than women who make roughly $11,000 per year.[41]

Even when we know better—and most of us do know—it's hard to make it happen. Nikki, a 28-year-old former welfare recipient, takes three buses from her apartment in Camden, New Jersey, to her job as a custodian at a mall in the suburbs, then three buses back home at the end of the day. The round trip can take as long as four hours. "I do my best to study when I'm riding the bus. But I want somebody to tell me when I am supposed to work out," she says. "Someone please tell me how I'm supposed to work this little raggedy job I have, take care of my daughter, go to school, study, and go to the gym. Please, somebody, tell me how to do that."

Just as our environment sometimes holds us back when we try to eat healthfully, the neighborhoods Black women tend to live in often place us at a disadvantage for exercise. Not only do our stomping grounds tend to lack gyms, community centers, parks and trails, but we are more likely to live in high-crime neighborhoods. Too often women and girls face street harassment and a wide variety of physical dangers, from decaying sidewalks to shootouts. In the suburbs, walking can be unsafe for a different reason—suburbs that lack sidewalks, forcing people to walk in the street.

It takes creativity to overcome such obstacles: some women succeed by using the gym at work, walking at lunchtime or on breaks, joining together to walk in groups, walking with a dog, or exercising early in the morning when the streets are quieter. "One mom's child is in a lot of different sports, so she spends a lot of time waiting," says Dr. Whitt-Glover. "Now when she drops her child off, she goes and walks."

Black women have told researchers that they didn't have physical activity role models growing up and didn't participate in many physical activities themselves. What's more, Black parents often don't raise their children to be active in their leisure time. So Black girls don't get into the habit of exercising when they're young.

For younger women who are childless, getting moving may be easier. Once we have children and life gets complicated, being physically active becomes more complicated, too. With competing responsibilities, low motivation, no energy to work out, and no space to do it, exercise often drops to the bottom of our to-do list.

A woman who's been at work all day may not want to take her kids to day care or take time out to recharge because it's not fair to the rest of her family. We don't want to disappoint people, so we sacrifice ourselves.

"Black women can tell you all sorts of nice things they do for other people, but when they have to think about what they have done for themselves, the number of women who break down and cry just even thinking about it says that there's a lot that we have to unpack," Dr. Whitt-Glover observes. "Black women are not used to caring for themselves."

Interestingly, though, once they get their children out of the house, some Black women do much better than younger women on the physical activity front. "They are actually counseling the younger women in the group, 'Girl, don't let these people run you crazy; you have got to take time out for yourself. I know where you are; I've been there.'"

As one Imperative focus group member in Philadelphia put it: "You just say no, but you've got to mean it. You've got to say no and mean it."

Getting a Move On

It's important to get moving in a way that works for you, one where you won't risk an injury or otherwise weaken yourself—particularly if you've never exercised before, if you carry excess weight, or if you already have a health problem. Avoid activities that generate a lot of wear and tear on your body. Running and tennis, for example, can overextend the body's ability to repair itself. What good is getting active if it just lands you back on the sofa? Talk to your doctor before you start an exercise regimen if you're new to exercise or very overweight, to make sure you're healthy enough and find out if you need to take any precautions.

Now let's look at ways to get different levels of activity into your life. "Physical activity" describes any bodily movements that work your muscles and expend more energy than you use when you are resting.[42] Light physical activities include common chores and everyday actions—ironing, cooking, housecleaning, walking slowly, and standing. You're engaging in this kind of low-intensity physical activity when you choose to stand in a meeting rather than sit, get up to change the channel rather than using the remote, tend to your children around the house, and park at the far end of the parking lot. None of these activities require a gym membership, are embarrassing, or mess up your hair. But they're not to be dismissed either—they can go a long way toward shifting you out of couch-potato mode.

Moderate physical activity uses the large muscles of the legs and arms; it's the equivalent of a brisk walk. It might mean taking that brisk walk or riding your bike at a comfortable pace, but many everyday activities fall under this heading too: pushing a stroller, weeding the garden, raking leaves, and wheeling yourself in a wheelchair.[43]

High-intensity physical activity includes jogging or running, hiking, playing tennis, biking vigorously, or swimming. Both moderate and high-intensity physical activity can also include structured forms of exercise, such as lifting weights or taking an aerobics class.[44]

The federal government recommends that adults get this amount of physical activity every week:[45]

> 2 hours and 30 minutes (150 minutes) of moderate-intensity activity *and* muscle-strengthening activities on two or more days to work all of the major muscle groups (legs, hips, back, abdomen, chest, shoulders, and arms);

> *– OR –*

> 1 hour and 15 minutes (75 minutes) of high-intensity activity *and* muscle-strengthening activities on two or more days to work all of the major muscle groups (legs, hips, back, abdomen, chest, shoulders and arms);

> *– OR –*

> An equivalent mix of moderate- and high-intensity aerobic activity *and* muscle-strengthening activities on two or more days to work all of the major muscle groups (legs, hips, back, abdomen, chest, shoulders and arms).

Can't spare two and a half hours at a time? Few of us can. Fortunately, we don't have to. "Physical activity means getting at least ten minutes at a time of at least moderate-intensity activity, defined as walking at a three- to four-mile-per-hour pace—that's getting enough activity at once," says Dr. Yancey. In fact, it's better for your health if you move around more frequently, especially if most of your day is spent sedentary. "People think, 'I need to go to the gym for an hour a day,' but you're not doing the best you can for yourself because you need to break up long periods of sitting even if you do get in that hour at the gym."

Every Body's Different

Not every person has the same natural energy level. Everybody—literally every body—is unique and allocates energy differently. Some bodies naturally direct more energy to muscles, while other bodies direct more energy to cells that store energy as fat. This is why some people naturally have more energy while other people naturally have less energy. If your body directs more calories—energy—to your muscles, you probably can't stop yourself from fidgeting or moving around. People whose bodies direct more energy to their fat cells have a harder time getting moving.[46]

Both genetic and environmental components affect how the body directs energy. Our food choices, toxins in the environment, hormonal changes, and damage to our pancreas and other organs can also affect this delicate balance. For example, a person who is exposed to a toxic substance, or who has eaten a lot of sweets over many years, may unwittingly exhaust their pancreas. Even a person who is naturally energetic may lose steam if, because of a medication's adverse effect, her body begins to redirect more energy to her fat cells instead of to her muscles. For those of us struggling with blood-sugar issues, the fact that the sugar can't get into our cells means that our body will feel tired and will convert some of that blood sugar— which would otherwise have been used to create energy—to fat. These factors—the fact that you have less energy and the fact that you carry more weight—make it harder to work out: a Catch-22 if we ever saw one. The person who's struggling with exercise may internalize this "failure" and feel like it's her fault, when, in fact, it's beyond her control. Nevertheless, she must reckon with it, one way or another, either now or later.

Active Couch Potatoes

On top of feeling poorly and having low energy levels because of inadequate self-care, we live in a culture that thrives on passive entertainment. In this distracted state we either don't see or don't mobilize ourselves to respond to the way our community is coming undone. Black people watch more television and movies than anyone else,[47] and our screen time grows exponentially once you add cell phones and computers to the mix. Could it be that we're numbing ourselves out?

But you can be a couch potato even if you're physically active. Carey, a very active young woman, exercises for about an hour three to seven days a week, depending on how well she's doing with her self-care. In between workouts she returns to her sedentary work on the computer as a writer. This makes her what is called an "active couch potato," meaning that while she gets many of the benefits of exercise, she also experiences some of the risks that come with sitting on her behind.

In an attempt to compensate, Carrie does yoga stretches periodically throughout the day and switches between her standard desk and a stand-up desk she bought at Ikea for $120, since even the shifting around that she does when she's standing helps to keep her body in motion. We can all find ways to do this: standing when we're on the phone or in meetings, drinking our coffee upright at the coffee-shop counter instead of settling into a chair, getting up and walking to the TV before we use the remote, running to do our close-by errands instead of hopping in the car, parking at the far end of the lot at work or the mall, and taking the stairs.

So what's our goal when we exercise? In the broadest sense, we want to improve our body's capacity to withstand, recover from, and adapt to the challenges it faces, whether we're talking about viruses, workplace stress, or aging. We want to improve our fitness in several ways.[48]

Flexibility

Bending over to pick up a pencil, tying our shoes, reaching for something on the top shelf all refer to flexibility—how far and how easily we can move our joints. Flexibility is important because it helps us do the practical things that we take for granted until we can't do them. Our flexibility becomes particularly important as we age, entering a time of life when regular physical activity is one of the most critical things we can do for our health. Flexibility can prevent many of the health problems that seem to come with age. It also helps our muscles grow stronger so we can keep doing our day-to-day activities without becoming dependent on others.

Working on flexibility might mean signing up for a yoga class—there are special classes for first-timers, but any good teacher should help you feel at ease and learn the basics safely if you're new to the practice. Or it might just mean getting up from your desk a few times a day for five minutes of gentle stretching.

Try: Stretching, yoga, using resistance bands and exercise balls.

Aerobic Fitness

Moderate-intensity activities that raise your heart rate all count and challenge our heart and lungs, whether brisk walking, dancing, water aerobics, bike riding, or mowing the lawn. So are vigorous exercises such as jogging, swimming laps, bike riding on hills, or playing tennis. Boosting your aerobic capacity is what helps you walk up long flights of stairs and run for the bus.

In fact, walking, the least expensive activity around—is one of the best ways to add movement to your life. Walking and talking can be a no-cost way to reduce stress and share time with family and friends. If you can afford it, buy a pedometer so you can count your steps each day ($12 and up). Shoot for 10,000 steps per day, but if it's a stretch for you to get to 5,000 steps, celebrate that—just keep it moving.

Dancing counts as exercise; in fact, it's an excellent way to get your heart pumping. So go line dancing, take a salsa class, or try the latest rage—Zumba, a dance-fitness class combining hip-hop, samba, reggae, and belly dancing with lunges, squats, and martial-arts moves.

What's best exercise? The one that you're actually going to do. Whatever you do, move it before you lose it.

Try: Walking, bike riding, swimming, Zumba, salsa, or African dance classes.

Muscle Strengthening

Weight lifting, weight training, strength training, resistance training—whatever you call it, it's building your muscle strength. These activities strengthen your heart muscle and your bones, reducing the likelihood that you'll break a bone or develop osteoporosis. They will also help you carry your own weight, pull, move, and lift things—whether you're lifting your children or a ten-pound bag of rice.

Core strengthening is an essential component of weight training. Core muscles run the length of the torso, and allow us to stand upright and move on two feet. They also stabilize our spine, help make us feel solid and balanced, help us shift our body weight so that we can move in any direction, and give us a solid base of support. When our core is strong, we are less likely to trip and fall, we have control of our movements, and our posture looks downright regal. We also experience less lower back pain[49]—a benefit that's particularly important since so many of us spend our lives hunched over a computer.

The shocking truth is that women who don't exercise lose 30 to 40 percent of their muscle strength by the time they reach age 65, a loss that starts slowly but accelerates after menopause. By age 74 over two-thirds of women can't even lift more than ten pounds. This means we will struggle not only to carry our groceries, but also to get up from the sofa, step on and off the bus, and lift ourselves up and down off the toilet. This loss of strength is not a natural consequence of aging; it's a consequence of spending too much time sitting. We can protect ourselves by starting to build our strength today, and it's never too late to start. Strength training offsets and can even reverse bone loss. It also raises the rate of our metabolism—the amount of calories we burn even when we are resting.

Try: Weight lifting, resistance bands, old-fashioned push-ups and sit-ups, and yoga classes that require you to do postures that support your own body weight.

Losing It

Often when Black women get active it's because they want to lose weight or they've gotten a wake-up call from their doctor that they need to hop on that right now. Exercising will help you in many ways, including losing weight; however, it's just one part of the equation.

We don't gain our weight all at once, so we shouldn't try to lose it all at once either. Instead, make a lifestyle change that you can sustain over time. In fact, some experts suggest that we not even focus on weight, but on how we feel and whether we can perform our daily activities.

So integrate physical activity into your lifestyle slowly, starting with 10- or 15-minute sessions, rather than 30 minutes one day but then none for a week as you recover. "That doesn't help you," Dr. Whitt-Glover says. "We focus on consistency. Be consistent."

If you can't do exercises standing up when you first get active, do them sitting down until you're strong enough to stand. And whether you take a class or pop in a DVD, don't worry about following every movement, just keep your body moving.

The biggest challenge is to exercise consistently. Answer the hard question: how many days this week did you do it?

This is important for several reasons. First, when people start exercising, sometimes they also start eating more. Or they believe that they can get away with eating a "treat" because they are working out. And it doesn't help that we often fool ourselves about how much we're doing. Women think they're being physically active, but after two minutes they say, "Hasn't it been ten minutes yet?"

Then there's the problem of the ways we reward ourselves: many women reward themselves by either doing something sedentary like going to a movie or eating out. Either way, we're not burning the energy necessary to lose weight. Then we get frustrated because we're exercising but the weight's not coming off. The best solution is to build toward an active, healthy lifestyle.

Take a Ten-Minute Recess

You don't have to buy a gym membership, wear spandex, or invest in a lot of equipment to get fit. You don't have to sweat for an hour every day. Whether at home, at work, or in between, try breaking your exercise regimen into 10-minute increments: say, ten minutes in the morning, ten during your break, and ten in the evening, and you're done!

"Ten minutes of moderate intensity activity won't create a problem for most people," says Dr. Yancey, whose book *Instant Recess* has turned many people on to the quick-hit workout.

"It will allow most people to get their activity and break it up into the segments of the day, since a lot of us as Black women have more responsibility in terms of family."

Ten-minute exercise breaks are gaining in popularity because they're doable. Walking the stairs at work, jumping rope, or walking and dancing on a rebounder are all great ten-minute exercise breaks. The ten-minute habit can rapidly blossom into a new love of movement that we can actually sustain.

Ten-minute breaks work especially well for very overweight and obese women. For one thing, it helps us get over the physical discomfort of getting started if we don't have a lot of experience with being physically active. Also, because we can take a ten-minute recess wherever we are, we don't have to go to a gym or some other public place where we will feel embarrassed if we can't keep up.

Dr. Whitt-Glover recalls one very obese woman who worked at a local Y, where she had a free membership but never worked out. She tried a ten-minute instant exercise break right there in her chair, behind her desk. She lifted her arms above her head as much as she could and then pushed her legs out to stretch before completing her ten minutes with foot bounces—lifting her heels in time to music. "When the ten minutes was over, she said, 'That felt good. Was that it? I can do this.' Then she started using her membership."

What to Wear

You can exercise almost anywhere you are; just make sure you're dressed for the part. The single most important piece of gear is a good pair of shoes, and we don't mean the cute heels that match your outfit. Wearing the right shoe supports your whole frame and can spare you the knee, ankle, hip, foot, and even back pain that often results without that support. Don't buy your workout shoes off the rack; go to a good sporting-goods store where they can suggest a brand based on your foot type, your gait, and your needs. Don't exercise in heels, slides, or flat tennis shoes with no support—an unstable foundation sets you up for an injury.

Second only to the shoes is a good sports bra, particularly if your breasts are larger. A sports bra will not only give you the support you need, it will also make you feel more comfortable. A good sports bra has wide straps and comes in cup and band sizes; shelf bras and the kind you pull over your head don't provide enough support. Get fitted at a department store or sporting-goods store, and pass up the 2-for-$12 special—plan to spend about $30. Wash your bra by hand and hang it to dry to help it last longer.

There's one exercise obstacle that we can't overlook. Not wanting to sweat out our hair sits at the top of the list. Black women of all ages worry about "my hair," although older women seem to find it more problematic than younger women do.

"This is a real issue for a lot of women, especially in corporate America, where wearing natural styles won't get them promoted or as widely accepted," says Dr. Yancey.

"That's why I'm happy to keep it nappy," says one 31-year-old Brooklyn, New York, resident who works in a more creative profession and alternates between twisted styles and an "Angela Davis–style bush." "I can exercise, go swimming, take a walk in the rain. It's so sad what Black women give up because they don't want to have natural hair. What they don't realize is that in exchange for that relaxed look and Friday nights at the salon, they are giving up their lives—they are missing out on really living."

"Well, the reason I relax my hair is because it helps me exercise," her best friend responds. "I don't feel like I'm giving up my life. I can wash my hair easily or just snatch it back into a ponytail if it starts looking too crazy. That's where the problem lies—with women who don't want to snatch it back. Just go on and get your exercise on, then snatch it back, girl!"

Let's get real and acknowledge that figuring out what to do with your hair has to be part of your wellness plan if you wish to succeed. Since we want our body to look as good as our hair, here are some tips that may help keep the "do" while getting that body moving:

Wrap It Up. If you have short or medium hair, wrap a cotton or silk scarf around it. But keep in mind that you don't have to cover your entire head. You can place a cotton bandana over your head and tie it at the nape of your neck, or you can just wrap the scarf around your hairline, leaving the crown exposed, and keep the volume or curl without flattening your 'do. Cotton is not usually recommended for workout wear, but worn on your head, it can absorb perspiration and keep it from getting onto your face.

Style a Ponytail. If you have longer hair, try pulling it back into a ponytail, ideally a high one that doesn't sit against your neck. This will not only keep your hair out of the way, but give you the chance to match a headband or other hair accessories to your exercise outfit.

Braid It. If your hair is long enough, braid it. You can then wrap it with a scarf or pin the braid or braids up. After your workout, unbraid your hair for a wavy look.

Wear It Natural. Natural hair is the easiest to deal with at the gym—naturally. But if natural doesn't suit your lifestyle, you can still get a lower-maintenance style by using a texturizer instead of fully straightening it. With semi-relaxed hair, you can shake it out and go, or wash and go without too much effort.

Putting Your Body's Health First

In this chapter, we've seen some of the factors in Black women's lives that make it hard for us take care of our bodies—social inequities that leave us more vulnerable to unhealthy eating and make regular exercise seem beyond our reach. Yet it's crucial to remember that the health effects they create are *preventable*. Our disadvantages are real, and they call for large-scale change, but there are personal changes that we can make right now to improve our bodies' health.

Black women, both individually and collectively, must take the resources we *do* have and use them, both to educate and to challenge ourselves and each other to take greater care with what we put in our bodies. If you take one thing away from this chapter, make it this message: *you can do this.* Healthy eating and exercising do not have to be complicated undertakings that only financially privileged people can experience. You don't have to shop exclusively at the farmer's market and belong to a glitzy gym in order to be healthy. Being more conscientious of your portions throughout your meals; eating only when you're hungry and not out of stress, sadness, or boredom or because of the advertisements you see; drinking at least eight glasses of water per day; minimizing your salt and sugar intake; avoiding escalators and elevators when you can take the stairs; doing desk exercises while you're at work or standing longer than you sit—all are ways to champion a healthy body with the resources at hand. Putting your health first doesn't have to be expensive—it's about making the decision to love and respect your body so you can have the healthy quality of life that you deserve.

Chapter 7

Healthy
Mind

———————————————————————■———————————————————————

No matter where you live, what you wear, how many degrees you have, and whether you are happily married or stressfully single, just live a little and sooner or later you're likely to experience a challenge that makes you feel like you're losing your mind.

Are you? Probably not—but that common expression reveals a telling truth. Many of us, when we think about mental health, tend to think first of mental *illness*. And such a narrow perspective makes it harder for us to be our healthiest on any level, whether mentally, physically, or spiritually.

By any measure, emotional wellness is essential to a truly healthy life. Take a look at America's "official" definition, offered from the viewpoint of conventional medical practitioners and public-health experts, in the 1999 Surgeon General's report on mental health:[1]

> Mental health is a state of successful performance of mental function, resulting in productive activities, fulfilling relationships with other people, and the ability to adapt to change and to cope with adversity. Mental health is indispensable to personal well-being, family and interpersonal relationships, and contribution to community or society. It is easy to overlook the value of mental health until problems surface. Yet from early childhood until death, mental health is the springboard of thinking and communication skills, learning, emotional growth, resilience, and self-esteem. These are the ingredients of each individual's successful contribution to community and society.

From a more holistic perspective, we may use a different language to frame the same core truth: that well-being in mind is a foundation for well-being overall. Washington, D.C.-based naturopath Andrea Sullivan, N.D., Ph.D., offers this description in *A Path to Healing: A Guide to Wellness for Body, Mind and Soul*. When we enjoy emotional wellness:

> We are aware of being part of a greater whole. Our behavior is likely to be productive and fruitful. We pursue goals of health, happiness, wealth and love. We encourage others to do the same. We have selfless creativity for others and ourselves. When we are well, we can give freely of ourselves, from the overflow of who we are. When we are well, it hurts not to give.[2]

So while many of us don't think about our mental health until it's in jeopardy, it plays an integral role in creating good health and a high quality of life. "Our mental health is in the background in a way that we really don't give it a lot of credit, but it's as much a part of us as anything else," says psychologist Argie Allen, Ph.D., director of clinical training at Drexel University's couple and family therapy program.

It's interesting to note that when you ask Black women to identify the most important ingredients of a healthy lifestyle, more than half of their answers pertain to their mental and emotional well-being. At the top of their list are maintaining emotional wellness (75 percent), managing stress (74 percent), allocating personal time for oneself (73 percent), maintaining spiritual wellness (70 percent), feeling self-confident (69 percent), and maintaining work/life balance (64 percent).[3] Yet when it comes to putting these aims into practice, it's clear that although we aspire to them, many of us don't get to experience them as often as we'd like. If we know our emotional health is so important, why don't we take care of ourselves in this way—and how can we care for ourselves better?

To answer these questions, we will need to get real about Black women's traditional approach to mental and emotional well-being. It typically includes "soldiering" through our difficulties, neglecting our own needs while we take care of others, taking our troubles to the Lord or our pastor (and thinking that's enough even when it isn't), dismissing the role that professional treatment can play, and being far too slow to ask for help.

Let's be honest: many times we know that *we're not really okay*. And being honest about where we are and what we're dealing with empowers us to take steps that will actually address our problems, rather than just shoving them under the bed because company's coming.

In this chapter, we will start to reframe our outlook. We'll talk about the relationship between our mind, our body, and our spirit. We'll ask what it means to be emotionally healthy in a world that challenges our peace of mind at every turn. We'll take a hard look at what we need to do to restore and preserve our well-being—and we'll help you answer the question "Are you okay?"

The Mind-Body-Spirit Connection

All of the processes that take place in our bodies and the activities that take place in our daily lives—whether our moods or our dance moves, our ability to savor chocolate or to commune with Spirit—are controlled by the three-pound organ inside of our skull that's known as the human brain. While nobody understands exactly how the brain works, we do know that it depends on an exceedingly complex network of physical structures, biochemical reactions, and pathways of information. Anything that alters the brain's structure or functioning, for better or worse—exercising more, experiencing a bout of insomnia, having a baby, taking medication, getting a concussion—also alters how we think, feel, and behave, and sometimes all three at once.[4]

If the workings of the physical brain are hard to fathom, the concept of mind is even more elusive. The world of technology gives us an easy way to think of the difference between the two. Think of the brain as the hardware (like a mainframe computer, or your desktop, laptop, or smart phone) and the mind as the operating system that runs all the programs—that is, our memory, our ability to concentrate, the things we think about, the way we express ourselves, the intensity of our feelings, our choices and actions, the amount of willpower we possess, how we perceive and interact with the world, and more. All these dimensions of our being constitute different aspects of our mental and emotional health.

Through them we experience the profound mind/body/spirit connection—our body's miraculous ability to communicate back and forth across these realms. Here's a typical example: say you experience anxious thoughts. You might also feel your heart start to race, you may break out into a nervous sweat, or have a hard time sleeping come bedtime. And many believe that prayer—communication between the physical and spiritual realms—not only can calm the mind, but may even help sick people heal from illness.

Just as many aspects of the brain lie beyond science's ability to understand them, our mind/body/spirit connection is so profound that researchers haven't probed it deeply either. But it is tangible and very real—and fundamental to a healthy life. When our mind, body, and spirit operate in synchrony, we experience optimal health on every level. When we take care of one aspect of our self, we take care of our whole self. Wellness in one area helps to create wellness in another. Similarly, poor health in one area undermines our health in another. So when our mental health declines—when we feel overwhelmed, when we're overtired, when we can't concentrate—other aspects of our health decline as well.

Chronic stress, for example, inhibits the production of growth hormones, so that our body can't regenerate itself as effectively. We may see this manifested in the slow growth of our hair and nails or even hair loss. Chronic stress also depresses our immune system, making us susceptible to colds and more serious illnesses; decreases blood flow to our digestive system, causing us to lose our appetite; and reduces blood flow to the reproductive organs as well, reducing our interest in sex. When we're overwhelmed, we may isolate ourselves and become lonely—and loneliness, too, depresses our immune system's functioning.[5]

"If you're not straight in your head, nothing is right," says Dr. Achong. "If a woman is not settled or the stresses of life are overwhelming her, it doesn't matter how strong her body is because it won't stay strong; it doesn't matter how beautiful she is because she won't stay beautiful; it doesn't matter how good her relationships seemingly are because they'll deteriorate."

Trouble In Mind

Every human being goes through times, be they hours, days, weeks, months or even years, when we are too stressed to be blessed. And for many Black women, those high levels of stress often seem unrelenting. As one single mother of two teenagers in Baltimore put it, "I see myself as a strong black woman because I've been through a whole lot of things that would have taken the average person down."

There's a long list of factors that can disturb our healthy brain activity: genetic makeup, everyday stressors, life-changing events, shifts in our brain chemistry, nutritional imbalances, hormonal changes, physical illnesses, changes in the environment, and more. These periods of mental or emotional imbalance are common—most of us are far more likely to get "out of balance" than we are to suffer from a serious mental disorder—but their effect on our lives is profound: such shifts can alter our thoughts, feelings, and moods and disrupt our ability to function and relate to others. Our thinking may become distorted in ways that keep us from living our best life—unless we identify the problem and do something to bring ourselves back into balance.[6] (Refer to the box below to check a list of common "cognitive distortions" and see if you recognize yourself.) We become particularly vulnerable when we don't take the time to nurture ourselves physically, mentally, and spiritually, as all of us experience at one point or another.

The Historical Yardstick: Mental Health And Black Women

For Black women—and particularly for those of us who were born in the United States—the combination of stressors in American culture and the intergenerational legacy of being enslaved and terrorized weighs strongly against good health of all types, including mental and emotional.

STINKIN' THINKIN'

Cognitive distortions are ways that our thinking becomes twisted, convincing us that things are true when they really are not, undermining our relationships, and leading us to make decisions that don't serve us well. Do any of these negative-thinking tendencies sound familiar?

1. *Filtering.* We magnify and focus on the negative in a given situation and minimize or filter out the positive.

2. *Polarized thinking.* We see things in black and white, as either/or, with none of the shades of gray that characterize healthier thinking.

3. *Overgeneralization.* We reach a conclusion based on one incident or very limited evidence.

4. *Jumping to conclusions.* We think we know what people are feeling and why they behave in the way they do, without doing them the courtesy of letting them tell us themselves.

5. *Catastrophizing.* We expect the worst, no matter what.

6. *Personalization.* We believe that everything people say or do is in reaction to us.

7. *Control fallacies.* We feel controlled by outside circumstances—helpless victims of fate.

8. *Fallacy of fairness.* We consistently feel bad because life isn't fair.

9. *Blaming.* We blame someone for every problem—if not other people, then ourselves.

10. *Shoulds.* We have ironclad rules for how we, and others, ought to behave.

11. *Emotional reasoning.* We think our unhealthy feelings reflect how things really are.

12. *Fallacy of change.* We think people will change if we just convince them or pressure them enough.

13. *Global labeling.* In this extreme form of generalizing, we turn a single quality or incident into a global judgment about ourselves or others ("I'm a failure").

14. *Always being right.* We're constantly trying to prove that our ideas and actions are correct.

15. *Heaven's reward fallacy.* We expect our self-denial to pay off, then feel bitter when the reward doesn't come.

"We come from a long lineage of brilliance but also traumas," says psychologist Ruth King, author of *Healing Rage: Women Making Inner Peace Possible.* "I don't think that we can deny the fact that we have been a part of historic traumas, cultural genocide, environmental traumas, mental traumas, traumas from the health-care system, traumas that have been the result of internalized oppression. At some point there has to be the acknowledgement of ourselves as emotional beings who have been wounded by this generational historic impact."

In fact, many experts agree that a degree of mental and emotional ill health is intrinsic to today's Black culture. In her book *Post Traumatic Slave Syndrome: America's Legacy of Enduring Injury and Healing*, Joy DeGruy, Ph.D. explores the lasting impact of that historical legacy. "In addition to chattel slavery, we have experienced 246 years of trauma, with no Dr. Phil to help us. Tell me when the healing took place?" she asks. "It's not plausible that we did not develop certain stress-related illnesses that became embedded in what we now call culture."

People with Post Traumatic Slavery Syndrome (PTSS), Dr. DeGruy explains, may demonstrate a lack of self-value and self-worth or persistent anger, adopt racist socialization such as White prejudices or standards of beauty, persistently gossip about other people, or fall into a "crabs in a barrel" mindset. Even though we have not experienced the trauma of slavery firsthand, we are learning "broken" behavior "because collectively we didn't unlearn it, so we pass that along," Dr. DeGruy believes. "None of us is undefeated."

There's no shortage of present-day pressures to erode our mental well-being either. High levels of economic insecurity, physical illness, and disability, combined with a lack of social support, cause many Black women to be plagued by anxiety, worry, and fear. We are far more likely than other women to struggle with economic insecurity. The poverty rate for Black women is 25 percent, more than twice the rate among White women, according to the latest statistics from the U.S. Census Bureau. In addition, according to the latest census, 44 percent of Black families are maintained by women with no spouse present.

And emotional pressures are not confined to low-income women. Black women with higher incomes often become overwhelmed by the pursuit of perfectionism, the drive to meet goals, the need to mediate family conflicts, and the challenge of meeting the criticisms and doubts of others. In the workplace, too many Black women believe that they are being treated as if they do not deserve to be there, and as a result they feel the constant pressure to be "twice as good" as their White peers just to gain acceptance. "I had to be at the top of my class," said one such Black woman who was always feeling not good enough. "I was always seeing myself being compared and competing with this white ghost. These issues play out in the lives of Black folk. It is impacting how they feel about themselves and it is impacting their physical and mental health." Blacks regularly receive this message that they are inferior to other people. Charisse Jones and Dr. Kumea Shorter-Gooden, authors of *Shifting: The Double Lives of Black Women in America*, poignantly portray the routine struggles of Black women trying to disprove this untruth, "often going to great lengths simply to demonstrate that they are as intelligent, competent, trustworthy, and reliable as their non Black friends, associates, and coworkers." [7]

Post Traumatic Stress

What's more, Black women and girls are particularly vulnerable to trauma related to community violence. "Every day in the African-American community, there may be violence that causes people to experience post-traumatic-stress disorder, where they will relive that traumatic experience, or have flashbacks, or have difficulty sleeping, or have nightmares," says Dr. Annelle Primm, medical director for the American Psychiatric Association. "People with PTSD are very easy to startle—maybe loud noises or something could make them very jumpy. Some people may experience emotional numbing. It's not limited to combat or combat exposure. Even disaster can trigger PTSD, like Hurricane Katrina."

In *Post Traumatic Slavery Syndrome,* Dr. Leary identifies many ways in which Black people have internalized our oppression and continue to take it out on ourselves and each other.

"The work is about basically parceling out the poison from the cookies," she says. "Because we've got a lot of poison embedded in what we call culture. At the same time we've got some incredible brilliant material that we continue to build upon—the strengths of our ancestors and our own familial strengths."

For this reason alone it's particularly important that Black women tend to our mental and emotional well-being and seek help quickly when our thoughts and emotions go awry. Unfortunately, there is a long tradition of Black women neglecting their mental and emotional self-care. Far too many of us experiencing emotional problems, particularly depression, do not seek help or medical treatment.

Distress Or Disorder?

Everyone experiences periods when they feel blue, when people have plucked on their last nerve, or when days go so badly that we joke about wanting to jump off a building. These stressful times come and go. We know that this, too, will pass. "These are common responses to life stressors and various life events," says Dr. Primm. "If something sad happens, to be sad about it is just a response. Nobody can go around being happy all the time, because things that happen to us may make us experience the whole spectrum of typical emotions."

But sometimes the human brain comes under so much strain—whether genetic or brought on by, say, a nutritional imbalance or a high level of stress—that it has difficulty functioning well. Such individuals may suffer from major depression or schizophrenia. When such a condition exists, we say that the person is mentally ill. According to the surgeon general's report:

> Mental illness is the term that refers collectively to all diagnosable mental disorders. Mental disorders are health conditions that are characterized by alterations in thinking, mood, or behavior (or some combination thereof) associated with distress and/or impaired functioning.[8]

Dr. Primm explains what the surgeon general means by "diagnosable mental disorder," which is different from the garden-variety periods of distress we all encounter. "An illness or a disease is defined by a specific cluster of symptoms," she says. "You have to have a group of symptoms in order to reach a diagnosis of an illness, as opposed to the individual symptoms, which are sort of the building blocks to an illness. If you have one symptom in isolation— like you feel bad one day—it doesn't mean that you have the illness of depression. You need a cluster of symptoms, and you have to exhibit them over a period of time."

For example, to be diagnosed with dysthymia, a chronic but less debilitating form of depression, you must have experienced a low mood most of the time for at least two years and have at least two of the following symptoms: a poor appetite or overeating, insomnia or excessive sleep, low energy or fatigue, low self-esteem, poor concentration or indecisiveness, and hopelessness.[9]

Some mental illnesses are more serious than others; for example, many experts consider dysthymia and anxiety disorders, such as seasonal affective disorder and generalized anxiety disorder, to fall at the less severe end of the spectrum. Counseling alone often helps remedy these less severe forms of mental illness. More serious illnesses respond better to a combination of counseling, prescription medication, and other support systems.

Fortunately, just as there are steps you'd take to clear up a sinus infection or to manage hypertension, there are steps we can take to treat mental disorders and illnesses. Not only are these legitimate medical conditions, they are also highly treatable, and help is available for every level of mental imbalance—even if you are in poor physical health. Mental illnesses are common, often ignored, but treatable. And unlike in the past, when being diagnosed with a mental illness meant being labeled as deficient forever, today even people with serious mental illnesses can recover and return to a normal life.

How Common Is Mental Illness?

Every year about one in four American adults suffers from a diagnosable mental illness—that's some 58 million people. Of those, 25 percent are suffering from a serious mental illness. About 4 percent of Black people, and 6 percent of people of mixed race and 6 percent of women, have developed a serious mental illness, such as bipolar disorder or schizophrenia, within the past year.[10, 11, 12]

Out of all of the mental illnesses, depression is one of the most common, affecting about 13 percent of the population during any given year. In fact, about one in ten women and 6 percent of Black people experienced a significant episode of depression in 2006, the most recent year for which data is available.[13] And the actual incidence is probably higher still. "Mental illness goes underreported for sure because nobody's acknowledging it to themselves," Dr. Allen says.

In particular, there's reason to believe that the rate of depression among Black women may be considerably higher. Many of them feel hopeless about the state of their relationships and family life. "Young women are despondent because there's no one to date," says therapist Pamela Freeman. "A lot of the depression I see among young women is, 'I'm getting these skills, but for what?' They're struggling

> ## SIGNS AND SYMPTOMS OF MENTAL ILLNESS
>
> The signs of mental disorders vary depending upon the condition and range from mental and emotional to physical symptoms. They include:
>
> - Feeling sad or "blue"
> - Confused thinking
> - Excessive fears or worries
> - Withdrawing from friends and activities
> - Difficulty sleeping
> - Detachment from reality, delusions, or hallucinations
> - Inability to cope with daily problems or stress
> - Alcohol or drug abuse
> - Significant changes in eating habits
> - Changes in sex drive
> - Excessive anger, hostility, or violence
> - Suicidal thinking
> - Fatigue
> - Back or chest pain
> - Digestive problems
> - Dry mouth
> - Headache
> - Sweating
> - Weight gain or weight loss
> - Rapid heart rate or palpitations
> - Dizziness
>
> *Source: Adapted from MayoClinic.com.*

with this and their families are offering them no comfort. Middle-class Black women have one or zero children. They need to see that even though things are hard, people can have full, rewarding lives without getting beaten up every weekend or spending all their money at Target."

The stress of trying to make ends meet, find meaningful relationships, and also give back to family and community may translate directly into Black women having a higher rate of depression than previously known.

Seeing the Signs

As common as mental disorders are, many people misunderstand them—and there's often a stigma attached to them—so people of all backgrounds tend to be slow to seek help. To complicate matters, in many cases there's no easy way to tell when we cross over the line between going through a difficult time and actually having a disorder. Many Black women experience "this fallout that manifests itself in ambiguous ways," says Dr. Allen. "For example, either we're really angry and others catch our wrath or we experience the balls start to drop all around us and are not sure what's going on."

Even when symptoms clearly meet the standard for a mental disorder or illness, we often miss or ignore the signs. Some experts believe that depression, for example, may pass for normal in certain families and communities. A Black woman who grew up in a household or community with people who were depressed may see that behavior as the baseline, because she doesn't have any other model for how she should be. They think "My mother suffered. My grandmother suffered. It's just the lot of Black women in America." But Dr. Allen explains, "It doesn't have to be that way."

Sometimes we and our practitioners fail to recognize the signs of a mental disorder because it doesn't fit the textbook description or the symptoms we find on the Internet. "Often African-American women present differently," said Allesa English, M.D., an assistant professor of psychiatry at the University of Tennessee, Memphis Center for Health Science, and director of its psychiatry residency program at a continuing medical education program there, as reported in *Psychiatric News*. "They may not use words like 'depressed' or 'sad' but rather complain that they are tired or have nonspecific back pain."[14] Compounding matters, because we disproportionately lack health insurance and often don't have a regular health-care provider, many Black people seek primary care from the emergency room, where doctors and other personnel often miss diagnoses of depression.[15] And sometimes it's overlooked because we just hide it too well. "If we work every day and we dress well, then it's very difficult for people who don't know African Americans to see distress because it isn't always visible," Dr. Gail Wyatt says. "If you're disheveled and you can't get out of bed, that's easier to see."

Stopping the Suffering

Just as a physical disease can get worse when we fail to address it, if we don't seek help for our mental health problems, they tend to increase over time, and we start to see the fallout in all areas of our lives. An untreated mental disorder can lead someone to develop an addiction, lose a job, become disabled, lose a home, waste years of a life, or even reach the point of suicide. Rates of smoking and drug use run significantly higher among people who have been depressed in the last year than among those who haven't been, though no evidence exists to say that smoking or drinking causes depression.[16] The sooner we seek help, the sooner the treatment will ease our pain, improve our quality of life, and prevent the condition from becoming worse.

"When you get to the point where you're having difficulty with certain thoughts, your thoughts are very scary, you're having nightmares and you ruminate—you keep thinking about things and you can't get them out of your mind—and that goes on for a while, then there's a need to find out what that is and to address it," says Dr. Gail Wyatt, sex therapist and psychologist.

"If it's affecting the person and keeping them from accomplishing their goals or their roles, than that's something worth looking at," says Dr. Primm.

Perhaps even worse than the impact upon ourselves, when we fail to get the help we need, we harm our children too. Not only do we expose them to our issues, we model unhealthy habits of self-care (or lack thereof). What's more, we can't support them in the ways that *they* need to achieve their full potential in life. Children, Dr. DeGruy says, develop their sense of themselves "through their appraisals of the significant people in their environment. That is: I am not who I think I am, and I am not who you think I am. I am who I think that you think that I am. So it becomes very critical that all of us are clear about who we are, because we transmit that unwittingly to our children."

Ultimately, when we let our mental and emotional pain go untreated, we miss out on the joyful and meaningful life we desire on every level. "So many of us believe the door is locked when it's not," says Dr. DeGruy. "We don't believe that we can open it anyway."

The Strong Black Woman Syndrome: Getting The Help We Need

Black women are notorious for looking good in public and claiming that we're doing well, then going home and falling apart. If we keep pretending that we're doing well, how can we ever get the help we need to live a better life? It's a challenge, because the roots of this tendency run deep in our culture. In the process of caring for everyone else, as so many of us are hardwired to do, we—and the people around us—may lose sight of the fact that we need nurturing ourselves. In some quarters of the Black community, it's almost as if "self-care" is a synonym for "selfish."

"Because most people still consider mental health and mental illness to be very separate from mind/body health, they often don't want to accept the fact that their mental status is something they've got to monitor and nurture and go to the doctor for, just like any other part of the body," says Dr. Wyatt.

"Sometimes you don't give yourself enough time. You look out for everybody else and you don't have time to look out for yourself," said Bebe, 42. "That's my problem. I'm looking out for everybody else, but I don't look out for myself."

"Oftentimes we're so busy taking care of everyone else that people don't hear us because we've sort of silenced ourselves in terms of saying what we need," Dr. Allen says. "Then there's an implicit message that there's no space for you to ask for help, or no space for you to express your needs. So we don't speak it, we don't ask for it, we just say we're okay when we're not."

In fact, the Black woman's lexicon is filled with slang that puts this reality into stark words: *Keep it moving, get to stepping, get over it, or die of it.* But we don't have a corresponding language to talk about what's challenging us. We can talk about getting a grip, but not getting healthy or getting help. And it's not only because our culture says we shouldn't need it, though that message is powerful indeed. Here are several other reasons that Black women may find themselves reluctant to speak up when they're troubled.

Fear of Stigma

"I had a diagnosis when I was a child and I don't want my own daughter to receive a diagnosis," says Cheyenne, 23, who has attempted suicide three times in the last four years. "I spent much of my life in foster care and group homes. I know what happens when you get labeled as crazy. I don't want that for her."

Often, when Black women don't seek help, it's for reasons like Cheyenne's: we fear we might hurt our family, or ruin our career, or we feel we can't afford to appear weak, or we're ashamed. In other words: people might think we're crazy.

Mental health stigma—defined as unconstructive attitudes, beliefs, views, and behaviors that affect the person or society, causing fear, rejection, avoidance, prejudice, and discrimination against individuals with mental disorders—causes many of us who are afflicted to become trapped in our illness or avoid treatment until our problems incapacitate us.[17]

There are two types of stigma: public stigma and self-stigma. Public stigma is based on other people's beliefs that those with mental disorders are weak, incompetent, or even dangerous. Self-stigma comes into play when we believe about ourselves the negative things that others believe—or that we fear they believe—about us. We may think, *I'm already Black and female; I don't want to be "crazy" too!*

These concerns are certainly understandable. Many of us have had legitimate experiences with labels being wielded against us or our loved ones, costing us opportunities and causing us to lose control over our lives. So perhaps it shouldn't surprise us that when we're distressed, the majority of Black folks seek help from informal sources—for example, friends, family, and untrained clergy—rather than mental health professionals.[18] But relying on untrained resources when we are dealing with serious issues often keeps us from getting to the root of the problem so that we can solve it. In fact, it can make our emotional problems even worse.

"If it doesn't come out in the wash, it's coming out in the rinse, and that means it's coming out," says Dr. Smith. "Our stories and our pain and our trauma and our suffering have to come out somewhere. And when they can't find a safe place to escape, then they come out in non-safe places, simply because they have to come out. So sometimes we have nervous breakdowns; sometimes we physically harm people; sometimes we harm ourselves. Because no matter how fast we think we can run, we can never outrun the truth."

Lack of Health Insurance

Even when we want to take care of our mental and emotional selves, we don't always have the means to do it. As with any professional service, counseling can be expensive, running between $75 and $150 an hour in many areas where Black women live, although low-cost group sessions are often available and some providers offer sessions on a sliding scale.

And because Americans consider mental health a lower priority than physical health, not all employers include mental health benefits in their plans, so even those with health insurance may not have mental health coverage, or its deductible may be high or its cap on covered expenses low. In fact, a 2009 study found that two-thirds of primary care physicians were unable to obtain mental health-care for their patients who needed it, largely because their patients lacked insurance coverage or the barriers to using—such as high deductibles and low caps on the number of visits allowed—were prohibitive.[19]

Mistrust of "The Man"

Call it the "ghosts of Tuskegee," or chalk it up to firsthand experiences with less-than-respectful medical professionals. Either way, many Black women remain wary of the medical establishment, so we are slow to seek out care, and particularly a mental health diagnosis.

When we do decide to seek help, we may struggle to find a mental health provider whom we can trust. According to the Department of Health and Human Services, Blacks make up only 4 percent of social workers, 2 percent of psychologists, and 2 percent of psychiatrists, and practitioners of other backgrounds are typically not required to obtain training in "cultural competence"—the skills and awareness needed to serve a patient within the context of her own culture's beliefs and practices. So many of us don't hold out much hope of finding such a person and we may take the position that, as Dr. Allen puts it, "I'm not gonna tell someone 'downtown' about my story because they just wouldn't understand."

And since no longstanding tradition of mental health-care exists in Black communities, some of us find ourselves in a vicious cycle, not exploring our options because we don't know that we actually have options to explore.

"I had heard about counseling—this was before Oprah started talking about it—and felt like I needed whatever it offered, although I wasn't exactly certain what that was because I didn't really know anyone who went," says 47-year-old Sarah. "Since I didn't know anyone Black who went, I asked one of my white girlfriends from work who had no problems telling people that she had been going for twenty years. I didn't know why anyone could possibly need twenty years of therapy, but I liked and trusted her. So I asked her to ask her therapist, who was a white man, if he knew of any Black women therapists. He did, and I saw that woman for four years."

Praying It Away

You'd see an accountant to help you with your taxes or call a plumber if your sink got stopped up, wouldn't you? Yet some of us, when we face a challenge in our mental health, don't schedule an appointment with a practitioner—we prefer to rely solely upon our Higher Power.[20]

To be clear, Spirit is a powerful source of support to draw on for our well-being and we'll devote a whole chapter to it later on. But some Black women think they should turn to their pastor in place of a psychologist—the implication being that there's nothing wrong with them that prayer alone won't fix. And unfortunately, their pastor may feel the same way. One survey of 99 African-American pastors found that while 62 percent thought mental illness was caused by biological factors, just as many described "stunted spiritual growth or unconfessed sin" as contributing factors. And only 25 percent said they had ever referred their parishioners to a mental health practitioner. Some members of the clergy may even disparage or discourage it.

We don't need to limit ourselves to an either/or scenario. Pastoral care can occur alongside mental health treatment, and many therapists assist their patients within a spiritual context. "It was such a relief to know that I could talk about spiritual stuff with my therapist," says Bertha, age 38. "For some reason I didn't think it would be okay, but she 'got' it and supported me even though I attend a traditional and conservative church, and over time it became clear that she was very spiritual also. For some reason I just assumed that she wouldn't be as spiritual as I am."

The New Strong Black Woman

Black women value characteristics like mental toughness, self-reliance, and being in control. So if we sense that we're lacking in any of these areas, we may equate asking for help with being weak and attempt to cover up what we wrongly see as our failure.

"The 'strong Black woman' dynamic keeps us from talking about what's really going on with us," says Gloria, age 37. "We function as if there's no pain because we've got to get it done."

"It's like we've all agreed not to betray the 'Sisterhood of the Stiff Upper Lip,'" agrees Sasha, age 45. "Like if one woman 'fesses up to how she is really feeling, then the whole house of cards is gonna crumble and everyone in the room is going to start crying and our mascara and concealer—don't the names of our makeup really say a lot?—are going to come all off and we're going to have to take off our five-inch stilettos—because who the heck can cry in some five-inch stilettos?— and we'll all be exposed for faking like everything's okay. Then what? That's the problem. We 'fake it 'til we make it,' but never really figure out how to make it."

When we project our image of the "strong Black woman" to the world, to our family, to our friends, to ourselves, we deny the assault that is taking place on our mental health. We deny that we don't get respect, that we don't receive equal pay, that things hurt us, that people abuse or betray us. We deny our disappointments, our sorrow, and our pain—and we deny ourselves any chance to heal.

But we have a choice: we can choose not to buy into any of the cultural myths about strong Black women being the pillars of the community. We can shed those images and set that baggage down. It's time for us to redefine what it is to be a strong Black woman. Being strong doesn't mean never needing help; on the contrary, asking for help is a sign of our strength.

What's more, the world won't grind to a halt if we aren't doing it all as we've been accustomed to. Our loved ones will survive—and maybe even surprise us. "I had to stop one night and call people in and just say, 'Listen, this is what is going to have to be, because I have issues that I have to address,'" says Diane, age 35. "And believe it or not, people really did fall into place."

Forms Of Treatment

"Nobody's walking around if they have a broken arm and saying, 'I'm not gonna do anything about it; I'll just let it swing until it falls off,'" says Dr. Allen. "But we're saying, 'I'm gonna walk around with depression, because I don't really know what it is.'" Once you decide to seek professional help for your mental health, you open the door to new understanding and the prospect of real change.

From talk therapy to pharmaceuticals to regimens that combine both, mental health-care can help to liberate us from the life-limiting consequences of mental and emotional disturbances, freeing us to experience the joyful, fulfilling, and loving lives that God intended us to have. Whether we suffer from a minor anxiety disorder or a serious mental illness, it's possible not just to improve but even to recover from any type of mental imbalance. As little as a generation ago, that possibility didn't exist, in part because mental health wasn't openly talked about in our community.

Yet fewer than one-third of adults with a diagnosable mental illness (and even fewer children) receive mental health treatment during any given year. While the effectiveness of treatment varies depending upon the individual, their condition and their demographic group, any treatment is better than no treatment at all,[21] and every new piece of knowledge is a step in the right direction. "You can't heal what you don't understand," says Dr. DeGruy.

How do we embark upon this process of self-discovery?

Psychotherapy

Commonly known as "talk therapy" or simply "therapy," "mental health counseling" or just "counseling," psychotherapy is a highly effective learning process that helps people deal with the challenges they're facing in their lives and/or navigate stressful life transitions, such as losing a loved one or changing careers, more effectively.[22] Although three styles of therapy dominate—psychodynamic, behavioral, and humanistic—there are many different treatment philosophies out there, most of which focus on problem-solving and achieving the client's goals.

Therapists have various forms of training and credentialing; you might work with a clinical psychologist, a social worker, a licensed marriage and family therapist, or a pastoral counselor, just to name a few. To find a therapist, you can get a word-of-mouth referral from your circle of friends, family, or acquaintances; request a guide from your insurer that provides a listing of therapists; or, if you feel comfortable, you can research trusted websites on the Internet. (See chapter 9 for a little more on finding online information you can trust.) Some websites even let current patients post reviews of a health-care provider's services, which may help you get a sense of the therapist's style and personality.

Therapy sessions are typically 50 minutes, usually weekly or biweekly, and a course of treatment may last a couple of months or extend over years. You can go to therapy as an individual, with a spouse or family members, or as part of a group of people working collectively to heal from similar issues, such as grief or abuse.

Some Black people may resist counseling because we "don't want people telling us what to do," but therapy doesn't work that way. When counseling starts, you and the therapist agree upon the changes you want to make in your life, a realistic timeframe for achieving them, and how success will be measured. Then you begin working together toward achieving these changes. You won't have to lie on a couch unless you want to (you're more likely to sit in a chair), and your therapist probably won't resemble the caricature of a bearded shrink dissecting your dreams. "You've got a person who is committed to and invested in helping you—based on your history and what's going on with you or the people you're in relationships with—navigate where you've been, where you are, and where you're going and come up with appropriate or best strategies and steps to help you to shift," says Dr. Allen. "Therapy really is, in essence, about making a shift."

This may sound something like talking to a good friend—and indeed, talking to a friend can be valuable and healthy. But it may also go the other way, if your friend is turning the conversation in a negative direction, or focusing on how bad off you are so *she* can feel good, or just being warm and supportive but not challenging your thinking or behavior. A trained therapist can guide you into the places where difficult truths are concealed and help you bring them into the light in a safe and productive way.

"When you look at what you are hiding, you will begin to find where some of your injuries are," says Dr. Smith. "Now, I didn't say you go put your 'business' out in the street. What I am saying is that you want to know the truth—at least yourself. And you want to have a safe place to take that injury so that it can be in the light and receive attention and care. You don't put a Band-Aid on a gunshot wound and expect that you will be healed."

Therapy may not mean digging around in your childhood for the answers to all today's problems, but it does often involve examining aspects of your past. "If you go to a medical doctor, right after they get your insurance they're going to ask you your history. If you go to a mental health professional they're going to ask you your history also. So looking at history in relationship to healing is not a new thing; it's necessary in order for you to heal," Dr. DeGruy says.

"What was the message? How did it land here?" asks Dr. Allen. "If we can figure that out, we can come up with ways—if you are willing to roll up your sleeves and do the necessary work, and you have a therapist who is willing to roll up their sleeves, and you become partners in the process of healing—to propel you to a place that is much more fulfilled."

Medication

As we've said, there are a number of different therapies that can bring relief to people who are suffering with mental health conditions. In addition to talk therapy, a whole arsenal of pharmaceutical treatments has been developed in recent decades—sophisticated medications designed to directly target the neurochemical factors that may be at work in disorders such as depression. Your health-care provider can advise you about what treatment might work best in your particular situation and whether medication is a good option for you. As in any medical treatment, it's critical that you follow your provider's recommendations. And don't ever take medication that's been prescribed for someone else—it can do more harm than good. Use only those medications that a doctor has prescribed specifically for you.

The Look Of Love: Signs Of A Healthy Mind

In seeking to understand and treat any condition, it helps to have a baseline in mind— what the body part or process we're treating should look like in its healthy state. And here we come up against a strange obstacle in our quest for emotional well-being: not only does American culture teach us that our mental and emotional health is secondary to our physical health, but it discourages us from even understanding what mental health *is*.

Popular culture tends to stereotype and stigmatize what it looks like when, say, a life event, nutritional deficiency, or chemical imbalance unsettles us. From the nightly news to reality shows to movies and magazines, the media exploits obvious examples of women struggling with their mental wellness—those who live in "clutter houses," go "psycho," or develop "fatal attractions." We don't hear much about the more mild ways that we swing out of balance mentally, ways that cause us to drop balls we used to juggle, obsess about our problems, take our anger out on others, ache all over or want to sleep all the time, and just get sick and tired of feeling sick and tired.

As a result, when most of us think about mental wellness, we often think first of mental illness, but such a narrow perspective makes it hard for us to optimize our health on any level—mentally, emotionally, physically, or spiritually. If we're to recover from our bouts of mental and emotional pain—and keep them from recurring, so that we can create and sustain joy in our lives—we need to know how to fix what's wrong. To do that, we need to know what it means for things to go right.

People whose minds work in a healthy way think, feel, and behave in ways that affirm and support themselves and other human beings. What does it look like when a Black woman lives this way?

"It looks like love," says Dr. Allen. "And how does one love one's self first? Be kind to yourself, but not just in your actions. I'm not talking about what you put on your body, what you buy; I'm not talking about all that external stuff that the hype has taught us to pay attention to. It's really about talking with yourself in a loving and kind and generous way. And if you're a spiritual person and really believe that God loves you, subsequently that love spills outside of you into your relationships."

So let's look at some of the hallmarks of good mental health.

High Self-Esteem

Black women who demonstrate high self-esteem take care of themselves body, mind, and spirit. Their lifestyle include communing with the Higher Power of their understanding, eating in ways that support good health, engaging in physical activity, paying attention to their own needs and wants, engaging in activities they enjoy, making use of their natural talents and abilities, spending time with people who make them feel good about themselves, investing in their own growth and development, and treating others well.

Importantly, they don't buy into the hype and distortions that pop culture perpetuates Dr. Allen says: "That if you're not the right complexion; your hair is not the right type or the right length; or your body parts aren't the way the newspapers or the magazines or the television say they need to be; or you're not in the right relationship; or you're not married, you're single; or you don't have the right job; or you don't have the right stuff—that somehow there's something wrong with you. That's not being loving toward yourself. You're valuable because you're here!"

"I have never had the curvaceous figure that many Black people consider beautiful," says Daphne Washington. "I have been called a toothpick; I've been told that I'm built like a White girl; I've been described as having more of a boyish figure. People can call me what they want; I really like how I'm built. I'm tall, I'm slender, and my body is strong. In our culture people think of curves as hips, booties, and breasts—and that's fine. But I like the curves of my muscles."

Good Connections

People who are strong in mind have successful relationships with others, enjoy the company of other people, support them, and receive support. They communicate their wants and needs and talk about the issues that face them instead of keeping them to themselves.

"When the recession came on, I knew I might be in trouble since I'm single and self-employed. So I called my family and my closest friends and laid out my entire financial situation—no secrets, no shame," says freelance writer Kelly Dumas of northern Virginia. "I had come up with several plans depending upon how the economic situation went down, and I asked for their feedback on all my options. My brother and sister told me that I could always come stay with them if I reached the point where I had to bail, which was wonderful. And several people offered me money, which I appreciated a lot. But I didn't want their money unless it was absolutely necessary because I needed to develop the muscles to work this out myself. Knowing that they were all in my corner made all the difference in the world, though. Having their support helped me make it."

They also avoid people who take from them without giving back. "There are a lot of people who dump their trials and tribulations and you are saddled and laden with it," says Dr. Goulda Downer. "Sometimes when people come to tell you their stuff, step away."

Philadelphia-based therapist Pamela Freeman, who has been counseling Black women for over 30 years, goes a step further, recommending that women let go of relationships with anyone who doesn't have their best interests at heart—and that they evaluate those relationships with integrity and a strong sense of their own value. "Recently when we were having an argument, my husband told me that I was stupid and ugly and not worth anything," says Kendra, 36, a mother of three. "He came to me almost crying and apologizing the next day and saying that he didn't mean it. But I don't care about his tears—I know I'm not stupid. And while I may not be the best looking woman, I know I'm not ugly—especially in my spirit. I love my husband, but you can't talk to me like that. I'm eight years into my marriage and I have three wonderful young children, but I've been thinking about leaving ever since."

Self-Awareness and Self-Control

People who do well in this area are aware of their thoughts and feelings, learn how to identify and address the reasons behind their reactions (particularly difficult emotions such as disappointment, sadness, frustration, anger, and grief), express their feelings in appropriate ways, and think before they act. They do not allow their negative emotions to build up so much that they then feel entitled to "go off" on other people, take their anger out on them, gossip, or talk about others in unhealthy ways. Those modes of relating "destroy your own mental health, and they contribute to the destruction of other people's mental health," Freeman warns.

Often, mental health difficulties can trigger other problems that negatively impact our physical health. For example, we may use food as a means of coping with stressful situations. People who are mentally healthy do not eat to stuff their emotions. While the brain's craving for a certain food is satisfied after three mouthfuls, Dr. Downer's patients tell her that they're downing the whole bag of chips or tub of ice cream in a sitting. "If you're eating more, you just want it because it's there—neurologically, the brain has been satisfied," she says. "Until we know what is eating us, we will continue eating the way we are and nothing can stop it."

Self-Care and Seeking Help

Rather than suffering in silence and keeping their struggles to themselves, emotionally healthy people know when to ramp up their self-care and how to ask others for help. "When you're wounded, caring for yourself really is important to be in the mix on the top priorities of your life," says Ruth King, author of *Healing Rage: Women Making Inner Peace Possible.* "That includes caring for your emotional well-being, your health, your capacity to love and so on."

Knowing how to care for ourselves also means knowing when we should seek help from a doctor or a counselor. "If a person has a great deal of difficulty in nurturing their mind in the morning, and through the day they have difficult and very unhappy days, and that's a pattern that repeats itself over time, they really need to go and talk to someone like a mental health professional, who can help them to sort out if they have something going on in their lives that's getting in the way of having quality of life," says Dr. Wyatt. "It's just that important."

Standing Up and Speaking Out

Healthy people also respond to unfairness and injustice, whether it involves them directly or not. "If the environment becomes toxic and you're healthy, then you start feeling like I've either got to speak on this, I've got to stop this, or I've got to get out of here. Something you're feeling on the inside is going to compel you to respond," says Dr. Allen. Conversely, when a person's mental state is less healthy and "the building is on fire or the community is on fire, then you might be likely to sit there," she adds. "You might stay in that misery, stay in that pain, stay in that hot space."

When some young people started dealing drugs in her Detroit neighborhood, Mary Brown and her neighbors came together to try to keep the situation from undermining their quality of life. "For about a year we tried to find ways to develop relationships and mentor the young men, since some of them had grown up in the neighborhood and we knew them.

When that didn't work, we had honest conversations with some of their moms, who were at work all day and couldn't control their kids—in fact, one of the mothers was a cop. But when a shootout happened at one of the houses after a party, we had to take control. We met with the police on a regular basis and provided them detailed information about what was going on." Within a year the drug houses were shut down and the neighborhood was much safer.

Cultivating Good Mental Health

We must accept the fact that there are some forces beyond our control—from political realities to painful budget cuts—creating stressors that undermine our mental and emotional health. These facts of life we cannot change. But we can control our responses to these situations, including committing ourselves to protect and build upon our emotional well-being and to restore our psyche when it succumbs to an assault.

Just as our physical bodies require focused attention to optimize our physical well-being, our mental and emotional selves also need care. And when we make this kind of self-care a regular part of our life, we create an environment where the mind/body/spirit connection can really kick in.

Here are some principles and practices you may want to try in your own life—some working from the inside out, others from the outside in, all designed to keep your emotional self in balance and your mind at peace.

Eat, Sleep, and Move

Knowing what we know about the intricate interconnections between our mind and body, we shouldn't be surprised to learn that taking care of ourselves physically can enhance our mental well-being powerfully. We'll devote the whole next chapter to ways of caring for your physical health, so for now, let's just look at a few important ways in which the body supports the mind.

Nutrition

When we're feeling down, we're often quick to reach for comfort foods, but that soul-soothing chocolate bar is ultimately undermining your energy and your mood. Sweet foods can leave you dragging once you come down from your sugar high; salty snacks dehydrate the body and brain, leaving you fatigued; and high-fat meals increase your stress hormone levels. Foods in their most natural state are less likely to contain artificial ingredients that alter the brain's chemistry. Eating a balanced diet that's high in fruits, vegetables, whole grains, and high-quality forms of protein—such as fish and lean meats—and low in processed, refined, and "junk" foods can help you stay balanced. It's also important to make sure that you consume foods containing B vitamins, which help maintain nerves and brain cells and help the body manage stress. Get them from bananas, dark leafy greens, avocados, fish, or chicken, or take a vitamin B supplement.[23]

The human body is mostly water, and every system in the body depends on having enough of it. Getting dehydrated—even just a little—makes it more difficult for our brain to function, for nutrients to get to our cells, and for toxins and waste to be released from our body. As a goal, try to drink eight 8-ounce glasses of water a day. Your urine should be slightly yellow or almost clear (unless you're taking a multivitamin; then excess riboflavin may turn it brighter yellow).[24] When it comes to other choices, use a bit of caution.

Rest

While everyone experiences a too short or restless night from time to time, a long-term lack of adequate sleep makes you more likely to gain weight and develop high blood pressure. Inadequate sleep can also cause your immune system to weaken and leave you too tired and irritable to do things you enjoy. Proper sleep is absolutely critical to good physical and mental health, and research has revealed that Black women often don't get enough. In fact, Black women, who average about six and a half hours of sleep per night, get less sleep than any other Americans.[25]

So how can you get a proper night's rest? There are whole books written on the subject, but some of the soundest wisdom is simply good self-care. A nightly glass of red wine to relax you can be good for your heart, but it can also disrupt your sleep and act as a depressant. Drinking coffee and other types of caffeinated drinks may give you the pep that you need to help you get through the day—especially if you're tired from lack of sleep!—but too much can backfire and prevent you from sleeping well that night. Some experts say you shouldn't watch the news before bed; others suggest keeping your bedroom dedicated to bed (no TV, no home office in the corner). One thing that's known to improve sleep is regular physical activity. Getting your body moving during the day can help you get a good night's sleep so that your body can rejuvenate itself.

Physical Activity

The human body was created to be in constant motion. Not only does movement propel blood around the body and help us to clean out toxins, but it also helps to clear excess glucose from the bloodstream, reducing the damage it can do when it is unable to enter our cells.

Physical activity can affect your mental health in other ways, too. Results from research suggest a connection between physical activity, depression, and anxiety: it's thought that physical activity may improve mood because it leads to the production of chemicals in the brain—called neurotransmitters and endorphins—that help you feel good. Physical activity may also help to lift your mood by *decreasing* the presence of chemicals that make depression worse.

There are other emotional benefits, too. Setting and meeting goals for exercise can boost your confidence. Getting to the gym or a yoga class can connect you with other people and serve as a healthy distraction, focusing your attention on other things besides worries or negative thoughts. Of course, even though physical activity can help to alleviate a depressed mood or feelings of anxiety, it's important to keep up with any treatment you're getting—therapy or medications. Don't stop going to sessions or taking your medication just because you feel better—at least until you get the green light from your health-care provider.

Reduce Multitasking

Emotional well-being means being able to quiet our minds when we need to. It's essential for our focus, our balance, and our peace. But in our world it's hard for anyone to turn down the volume—and stillness may be especially hard for Black women to come by. "It's not in African American culture," says Pamela Freeman. "Since we arrived in the United States, we've been bred for work. But it's important to be still instead of always multitasking. Multitasking is the worst thing for good mental health."

Though we think we're being productive and efficient by doing a lot of things at once, research shows that shifting mental gears is actually an inefficient process—it makes whatever we're doing take longer in the end.[26] And, in the moment, we're getting ourselves wound up tighter and tighter.

Uvena, 41, described a typical morning: "I had gotten to work early so I could get started and was sitting at my desk, feeling overwhelmed. I started thinking through a project, then realized I could let my computer start up while I was thinking, so I turned my computer on. Then I thought that while that was happening, I should leave voice mails for some of my colleagues who hadn't come in yet so they'd get them as soon as they arrived. Then that made me think about starting on *another* thing. When I looked back at my notebook, I remembered I was supposed to be thinking about my project. I realized that I was like a hamster on a wheel. All these things were going on but I was going nowhere,"

Human beings are intended to be in relationship with each other. Unfortunately, thanks to that same modern society that has us multitasking like hamsters on a wheel, we're all too likely to find ourselves in relationship with the cell phone we text on, the car we commute in, the MP3 player we zone out with on the bus, or the computer we use at our job. This makes it hard for us to do the healthy things we've just discussed. It also keeps us from giving and getting the support we all need.

"We are so accustomed to being silent about our health issues and challenges, what we feel about and think about stuff, and our own experiences that it hurts us," says Pamela Freeman. "We don't form community to talk to each other. Not talking about something hurts us spiritually, and it leads to a level of denial or shame that doesn't have to be there and isn't great to be walking around with."

Discover Yourself

Many Black women find that good mental health is grounded in their relationship with a Higher Power, however they understand it. Their connection to God gives them a sense of purpose and helps to sustain them during difficult times.

One powerful way to come into God's presence is to explore and express our God-given gifts. Some of us get so used to putting other people's needs ahead of our own that we start to lose touch with those gifts—if we ever identified them in the first place—and sometimes we feel resentful of others for having what they want in their lives. All human beings deserve to know who they are.

"I come from a family of eight; I'm the oldest; I raised them practically all my life and I don't want to do it anymore," said one BWHI focus group participant. "I'm just discovering who I am."

That's when we know we need to get better acquainted with ourselves.

It needn't cost a lot of money to discover who you really are. If there's something you are drawn to, something you loved to do as a child or have always wanted to try, then of course you can do it in a formal way—take piano lessons or tap dancing or acting classes. You can also start right where you are with whatever you have. Create a scrapbook out of your favorite things. Write a song or a poem in a notebook, or create art with a pencil or paints.

Or just sit still and listen to what thoughts bubble up—not just typical day-to-day thoughts, but the new ideas that start to break through. "I don't quite know how to describe it, but these thoughts have a different quality to them," said one woman participating in a meditation group for people of color. If you pay attention, you may find that from some-place deep within, your self is speaking to you.

Five Strategies to Support Your Mental Health

The more you learn to value your true self, the better able you'll be to make choices that support your emotional well-being. That doesn't mean it will always be easy, especially when obstacles get in the way (and they will!). Here are five strategies that can help you stay on the path of good self-care.

Trust Your Intuition

Your intuition is your inner intelligence, a voice that guides you in the right direction—even when logic would lead you elsewhere. Thus, in order to access your intuition, you must be connected with your self. You must be able to trust that you have access to the answers you need for your life. If you don't have a sense of peace about a decision, don't feel compelled to move forward. Inner turmoil is often a message to be still or move in a different direction. Gather the information you need to make intelligent choices for your life, but accept your intuition as an important source of guidance too.

Listen to Your Emotions Selectively

Emotions are real, and they offer important messages. They are not necessarily the truth, though, and for this reason, it's not wise to make decisions based on them. Emotions are based in the moment, ever-changing, influenced by insecurities, and often illogical. You *can*, however, use your emotions as a guide to teach you more about yourself.

If you are angry or irritated on a regular basis, explore the reasons why and think about ways to resolve the issue. If you are feeling overwhelmed, read that as a sign that you may be trying to do too much too fast or without enough support, and adjust accordingly. Anytime you feel a strong emotion, negative or positive, take time to ask, "What is this emotion trying to tell me?" Then allow yourself time to come down from your emotional "high" (yes, even a negative emotion is a kind of "high") before acting on it.

Solve Your Problems Honestly

Some Black women spend more time focusing on a problem than they ever spend trying to solve it. Make a decision to look at every problem or challenge as being solvable—or not. If it is a solvable problem, then focus on the solution. If the problem isn't solvable, then let the problem go. In this way, you'll be able to focus more of your time and energy on the people and things that matter most to you. Rather than becoming seduced by drama and sucked into worry, you'll be taking responsibility for solving problems and creating a healthy life.

Face Your Fears

Many Black women never consider the possibility that they could actually have the life they dream of because they are afraid. Fear stops them from moving forward because they don't want to take risks that will result in failure, rejection, or regret. The truth is that every choice has its share of risk. Whatever it is that you fear, ask yourself, "How can I reduce my anxiety or fear of failure in this situation?" Brainstorm with others; open your mind to options you may not previously have considered. Then stop asking, "What if I fail? What if I don't have what it takes?" and start asking, "What do I have to do to ensure my success?"

Ask for Help

We've already explored the downside to being a "strong Black woman," so you know now (if you haven't learned it firsthand in your own life—and you probably have) that it's not possible to carry a heavy load indefinitely without heavy consequences. To create and preserve good emotional health, establish limits for what you can do alone.

Honor your own humanity by admitting when you need help. Whether it is as simple as teaching your children to help with household chores or standing up for yourself when your spouse owes child support, expect those around you who benefit from your efforts to also help lighten your load. Ask for help and expect to receive it—from someone who can actually provide it. Honor yourself by admitting when you need a break, and then arrange for one. Schedule a real vacation once a year. You don't have to go far or spend much—just give yourself a few days to lay your burden down.

Chapter 8

Healthy Spirit

---◼---

For most Black people, any definition of health must include spiritual health—no matter what spirit may mean in our individual lives. That meaning, of course, is both personal and elusive. As Gloria Wade Gayles, Ph.D., writes in *My Soul Is a Witness: African-American Women's Spirituality,* "Spirit, or spirituality, defies definition—a fact that speaks to its power as much as it reflects its mystery. Like the wind, it cannot be seen, and yet, like the wind, it is surely there, and we bear witness to its presence, its power. We cannot hold it in our hands and put it on a scale, but we feel the weight, the force, of its influence in our lives. We cannot hear it, but we hear ourselves speaking and singing and testifying because it moves, inspires and directs us to do so."

For Black Women spirituality reflects the imprint of our race, gender, and culture. It is the unspoken wind beneath our wings that can offer the direction necessary to claim a truly healthy life. "For so many people," says Annelle Primm, M.D., MPH, deputy medical director for the American Psychiatric Association, "without the spiritual component almost nothing is possible, including healing." If we're to transform ourselves from women who are literally killing ourselves to take care of others, and into women who love ourselves enough to tend to our own health first, we will have to tap into our Higher Power.

We know that this Power exists. A deep and abiding spirituality resides at the heart of Black people's existence in America. Our ancestors clung to it as they endured the Middle Passage. Our enslaved forebears rooted in it as they stood on auction blocks, endured back-breaking labor, and had their children taken away from them, yet survived. Our parents and grandparents used it to summon the courage to orchestrate the Civil Rights movement, the most powerful liberation movement in the history of humankind—one led by courageous Black women, from Rosa Parks to Dr. Dorothy I. Height to Fannie Lou Hamer—and that continues to be emulated all around the world.

Now *our* time has come.

Unlike times past when we've asked for the strength to make it to the other side of a situation, the 21st century requires that we muster the strength to stand up and lead a change. This means we must first create change within ourselves.

In this chapter we explore how we can call upon our spirituality not just for our survival, but rather as an invaluable working tool that can help us free ourselves from habits that no longer serve us. A healthy spirit can allow us to define who we are as conscious, strong, and well Black women, create joy in our lives, and navigate our own destinies. Spirituality takes many forms; Dr. Wade Gayles says that "the Spirit speaks in the voice of, sings the songs of, dresses in the symbols of, wears the face of and moves in the rhythm of the people who receive it."[1] So we will leave it up to you to define Spirit in whatever way you understand it—as God, Creator, Higher Power, or simply the power of the universe expressing itself through you.

"We are whole people; there's nothing in our lives and in life itself that's not spiritual," says Rev. Monica Coleman, Ph.D., an associate professor of constructive theology and African American religions at Claremont College in Southern California and an ordained elder in the A.M.E. church. "In light of that we need to ask ourselves, what does it mean to be healthy and whole, and how do we get there?"

"It means acknowledging our divinity, our interconnectedness, and our preciousness," says Rev. Emilie Townes, D.Min., Ph.D., a professor of African American religion and theology at Yale University's Divinity School. "It means recognizing that you bring something unique and unprecedented to the world."

Exploring and expressing our natural gifts and talents is an important way to discover the power of the indwelling God. Every human being has been endowed with a unique combination of abilities that no human being has ever had or ever will. Many people who follow a spiritual path find that these gifts, their experiences, interests, and passions, give them a sense of purpose. But American society does not teach this. Just the opposite: our socialization inhibits us from learning who we are.

Perhaps some of the lack of joy among middle-aged Black women can be traced back to not having an opportunity to discover who they really are, what makes them happy, and what they have to offer. Many of us hold jobs that leave us feeling unfulfilled. Others of us are putting off living today in hopes of having a better life after retirement. But if we make it there, what kind of shape will we be in? Black women too often struggle to claim happiness. When are Black women going to give themselves permission to seek spiritual satisfaction?

Joining in Strength

"My greatest hope is for Black women to awaken a spiritual and social consciousness within ourselves," says Rev. Marcia Dyson, a political strategist and social entrepreneur and an affiliate at Georgetown University's Center for Social Justice and Policy. There's nothing paradoxical about this pairing: our spirituality is what connects us to the universe and to other living beings. As we learn and grow, we change our consciousness to reflect the larger reality that we depend on one another for survival.

The closer you move to your inner truth, the more you connect to your soul, and the more powerful you become. "I have lived my life on the basis of following a call," says Dr. Townes. "It has made me one of the happiest people I know among those I work with or work for. I'm not second-guessing what should I be doing or if there is something else. I am content and that alone helps you live a better life. If you can be content in yourself and your work, that's worth its weight in gold." That means, for example, that you don't spend ten hours a day at your job, hating what you do for a living but pretending you enjoy it. Such an inner conflict can make you crazy. Yet large numbers of Black women do this, mistakenly thinking that's how they have to live.

"Being afraid of letting go is part of the very process of finding your call," says Dr. Townes. "I think, to our detriment, we try to be fearless. I don't think that's the point; I don't even think that's healthy. I think trying to live lives of courage bolsters our health and kicks us into more creative possibility of who we can be."

Living as Witness

On the journey to spiritual empowerment, we change the way we see the world, and the world changes the way it sees us. We give out a different kind of energy as our spirit evolves. We are changing, and the path to the person we want to be can become very clear now. As beings in transformation, we must expect others to understand that we're not the same people we were before we started becoming empowered. We understand others in a new way, too. Instead of blaming ourselves for their misgivings or shortcomings, we perceive the barriers that keep them from growing.

"Our lives should be the living witness," says Dr. Dyson. "I think of the scripture that we are the living epistles. Our lives in the way we are living should demonstrate something holy and wonderful and God's presence within us."

"The more I understand what I have to offer the world, the more secure I feel," says Amaya Mason, a 37-year-old middle-school history teacher. Amaya thought that a career as an educator would mean she'd always have secure employment; now she is realizing that's no longer the case. "That is not to say that I don't feel financially vulnerable; I do. But the more I explore my natural interests, the more I really start to 'get' the fact that I have something that belongs to me that no one can take away."

Tending To Our Spiritual Health

Looking back to the question Dr. Coleman posed earlier in this chapter, we ask ourselves: what *does* it mean to be spiritually healthy and whole? How *do* we get there? How can we tend to our spiritual health so that empowerment will take root?

"I grew up in Black churches that were socially active but didn't teach how to maintain or nurture one's relationship with God," Dr. Coleman says. "You're supposed to come to church and to Bible study, but when you're at home what do you do?"

Most Black Americans are raised to be Christian. In fact, about 85 percent say they are Christian, and almost 60 percent go to historically Black churches; 2 percent practice other religions, mostly Islam (1 percent); only 12 percent don't affiliate with any religion at all.[2] While many of us go to church, however, there's a big difference between following the rules of our respective religions and being spiritually healthy—witness all the Black women who run themselves ragged overextending themselves in a weekly marathon of church community service in a misguided effort to be "good enough" for God.

We'd like to propose that spiritual health means honoring Spirit in all of its manifestations—from treasuring nature to treasuring other human beings to treasuring ourselves. And since every human being consists of many dimensions, including a body, a mind, and a spirit, being spiritually healthy involves proactively caring for all aspects of ourselves. Although Western thought typically considers these three to be separate entities, African-descended people typically believe that the body is connected to the mind, which is connected to the spirit.

As a mobile revolves above an infant's crib, touch one aspect of a person and you put all the other aspects of her into motion. Our physical selves are intricately intertwined with our spiritual selves, so we cannot be healthy physically if we're not spiritually healthy as well. And being spiritually healthy also requires that we take care of our physical body, which Christians call the temple of the Holy Spirit and others know as the seat of the soul.

SAYING YES TO YOUR LIFE

Women living in the new millennium know they must have a deeper connection to their spirits. While we have inherited certain ancestral memories and cellular programming from our foremothers, we recognize the importance of affirming and nurturing self, the mind, body, and spirit. We also understand that the true path to self and life satisfaction is a function of choice. Women today know that we must choose to take care of ourselves if we are to live longer, healthier lives. We must choose to honor our own needs, if we are to receive the fruits of our efforts and labor.

As difficult as it may be to believe, women are not genetically predisposed to take care of others. We are, however, conditioned to believe that doing so is the path to satisfaction.

Soul satisfaction for women today is no longer intrinsically connected to what we can do, should do, or must do for others. Instead, it is a function of understanding our behavior patterns and choosing new ones that are life giving and life affirming. While we may know each of these statements to be true, the challenge becomes doing what we know is required, doing what will lead us to a longer, more satisfying life experience. It is a function of choosing *me* over *we*, with the understanding that I cannot give you what I do not give myself. It is the choice of *I* over *you*, with the recognition that the better I am, the more I can offer you.

As the first caregivers, teachers, and sources of inspiration, women are not made aware that *affirming self does not equate to selfishness*. The fully realized and honored self of every woman gives those around her permission to be their best selves.

Spiritual satisfaction for a woman is a function of being "self-full." We must be full of self-knowledge, self-trust, self-acceptance, self-value, self-worth, and self-love in order to give the best of who we are to the world. We must choose to reprioritize our lives, learning to give from the overflow of our time, energy, and resources, keeping what's in the cup for ourselves. In order to live and age gracefully, we must begin to live consciously through every stage of our lives. We must also identify the sources of stress and overwhelm, making every effort to eliminate them. We must rediscover the sources of our joy and peace.

In order to realize the fullness of self and spiritual satisfaction, we must acquire the tools and develop the skills to keep our heads and hearts clear. In some cases this may be as simple as learning to say no without guilt. Or taking a day off without pay. In extreme cases, it may require that we let go of beliefs, situations, and sometimes people. It may also mean that we run the risk of upsetting people we have always put first. When you put yourself first, somebody else may get upset. Trust yourself to know what is right for you. Also trust they will get over it.

Most of us know exactly what it is that we do that does not affirm, sustain, or advance our spirit. We know but we are not sure what to do about it, or how to do it differently.

Every one of life's moments is precious. It must be filled with joy and peace. Every moment is an opportunity to make a statement to ourselves and the world that we are grateful to be alive, awake, and aware. In our aliveness, we must seek and find soul satisfaction. In our awakeness, we must pay attention to ourselves first and take others as they come. In our awareness, we must make moment-by-moment shifts and changes to be better, feel better, and live fully.

One of my daughter Gemmia's therapists made a very astute observation. He told her, "If you do not enjoy your life, cancer will." She took that to heart. May I offer that the very same is true of being stressed, overworked, overwhelmed, and taking care of others? It is up to each of us to choose who or what will live our lives."

—Iyanla Vanzant

10 Contemplations: Self-Care From the Inside Out

We are blessed with a unique gift of consciousness that allows us to learn who we are, to recognize our personal truths and to understand our relationship to others. Knowing how to stay healthy is not enough, we must apply what we know so we actually get good results. So if you are taking care of everyone else and neglecting your needs, you can lose sight of what the priority should be—a healthier you. Our spiritual self-care is essential because it demands that we go inside and make time for ourselves.

Iyanla Vanzant offers us the 10 Contemplations as our spiritual homework.[3] These healing words challenge us on our journey to becoming a Health-Wise woman and support our transformation from the inside out. Reflect on the following affirmations as an intention for your daily prayers or use them as inspirations for your journal work. Invite Spirit to help you to see and be all that you are.

IYANLA VANZANT'S 10 CONTEMPLATIONS

I take the time to deal with unpleasant memories.

Until today, you may not have realized that you were angry or understood why. Just for today, set the intention to heal any unexpressed anger that may be present in your life. Then, ask the Holy Spirit to transform that anger into a passion for life.

When I withhold the truth of who I am, I cannot receive the truth of what I want.

Until today, you may not have realized that the thing you want is the thing you most resist. Just for today, be willing to be honest about who you are, what you feel, and what you want in every situation.

I know that I don't have to know.

Until today, you may have believed that it was your duty and responsibility to know everything. Just for today, be willing to admit that you don't know it all. Open yourself to receiving new information from expected and unexpected sources.

I have permission to spend time with myself.

Until today, you may have been totally absorbed by the people, duties, responsibilities, and obligations in your life. Just for today, absorb yourself in yourself.

What I tell myself I am . . . I am.

Until today, you may not have realized that you have the power to reshape and redefine any experience, no matter how devastating it seems. Just for today, look at your experiences and ask the Holy Spirit to show you how to use them for your good.

The ways I give and receive love . . . may not be loving at all.

Until today, you may not have realized that love is simple. You make love hard with your trappings, expectations, and demands. Just for today, give consideration to your beliefs about love. Are you really being loved, loving, and lovable?

When I do not open up, I set myself up to explode.

Until today, you may have been holding on to secret thoughts and feelings. You may have been afraid to open yourself up to self-examination or outside scrutiny. Just for today, be willing to release those things stored in your heart and mind that are causing you discomfort.

I am learning to forgive myself.

Until today, you may have found it difficult to forgive yourself for certain behaviors you have engaged in. Just for today, be willing to grow, learn, and heal yourself with forgiveness.

I accept that things are the way they need to be.

Until today, you may have held perfection as the standard that you needed to live up to or achieve. Just for today, accept that you are perfect just as you are.

Love is the voice of God whispering to you from within.

Until today, you may not have realized that the voice of love is God's voice calling out to you. Just for today, listen closely to the voice of love calling out to you from within, and you'll find it everywhere.

Self-Care as Salvation

"Salvation comes from the word *salve*, which means 'health,'" Dr. Coleman explains. "To be saved is to be healthy, not to get into some locked spiritual community." So taking good care of our bodies can and should be intensely spiritual. How can you care for your family, enjoy your life, live a purposeful life to your full potential, if you are living with a body that doesn't function optimally, or worse, if you're trapped inside one that's deteriorating with you in it?

"Far too many of us are dying far too young because of stress-related illnesses, not taking time to replenish our spirits and our souls," says Dr. Townes. "And if we're not doing that, we're also not doing it with our bodies. It's all one piece; it's not body or spirit. I don't separate spiritual health from physical health; it's all one fabric."

"We need to expand to include care for our self as an act of salvation," Dr. Coleman agrees. "We're used to thinking that salvation is important and we're to share the gospel so that people can be saved. But what does it mean to be healthy? What is the Good News then?" She adds: "Health is a place where salvation happens even though the acknowledgement of God isn't as specific."

What does it look like to care for yourself as a spiritual act? Melicia Whitt-Glover, Ph.D., is a community-based researcher whose work includes helping communities of faith integrate health programs into their ministries. She explains: "In faith-based communities, our whole program is centered around questions of 'What are you on earth for? What does the bible say about taking care of self?'"

Dr. Whitt-Glover challenges the participants in her programs to consider their physical activity within a spiritual context. "If you believe your role on earth is to further God's work or to manifest God's kingdom here on earth, how can you do that work if you're hollering, 'Oh, my knee!'" When she puts it that way, she says, "People stop and say, 'Huh!'"

She encourages women to think about why they are here. "Then once women figure that out, we talk about the body being God's temple. If you are going to be a witness and talking about how good God is, but you're all broke down, what would make someone want what you have?" The more we empower our spiritual selves, the better we are able to impart our insights and inspire others—leading through example.

Spiritual Hygiene

Our mothers and grandmothers taught us to engage in physical hygiene so that our bodies would be clean and presentable. Just as they used to ask us if we'd brushed our teeth and washed "down there" and were leaving the house wearing clean underwear, we need to start asking ourselves whether we've attended to our spiritual hygiene—intentional practices in which we prepare our minds and our spirits to encounter the challenges of the day. These are ways to cultivate the soil of our spirits, water our hopes and dreams, and then cleanse our spirits of the debris of the day so that we can restore ourselves with a good night's sleep.

These spiritual practices can be as unique as each of us. "I could be walking down the street and see the wind on a leaf and see how that leaf is connecting with me, and I'm connecting with it," says Zamiyah Johnson, 42, a nurse. "Being in that moment, not walking down the street thinking I don't have money for this; I'm worried about my children; I had this argument with my husband. I'm being in that moment, and that is healthy."

"Sometimes things that are immediately gratifying are spiritual, like cooking," Dr. Coleman says of her own "spiritual hygiene." "Riding my bike is a really spiritual process—the endorphins make you feel more spiritual—and the time I spend with my headphones on. We can have a broader understanding of what spiritual disciplines are, outside the classical ones. If it brings us closer to what's holy and what's human, it can become a spiritual discipline."

We often think of the word discipline's negative connotations—the strictness and rules that we may have experienced during our youth. But discipline can also be thought of as a way to create structure, the foundation upon which to build a healthy and prosperous life. The walls of a house can't stand strong until its frame is built with systematic care; spiritual discipline, when practiced faithfully and regularly, can open us up to what God is saying to us in ways that haphazard spiritual practices can't. Engaging in spiritual disciplines teaches us how to cope with this world, how to care of ourselves, and how to recognize and listen to our own voice so that it isn't drowned out by the noisy world around us.

The Inside Job

When we practice disciplines that allow us to turn our attention toward our often-neglected insides, we get the opportunity to search our souls. This is a chance to examine our thoughts and to experience insights that can help us live more joyful, satisfying, and healthier lives and make necessary changes to ourselves, our families and our communities.

"We need to ask questions of ourselves internally," says Rev. Dyson. "We've relegated so much of our lives to other people and other things that we need to sit and become our own ministers.

"We wouldn't see the lack of power that we see in the streets if people were being fueled up within the church, the sanctuary, the lodge," she adds. When we minister to ourselves, we begin to claim our power so that we direct it toward our self-care and appropriate care for our loved ones and our communities.

Prayer

Many of us wouldn't be here if our forebears had not recognized the power of prayer—communicating and communing with God, the Creator, or whatever spiritual force we acknowledge. Sometimes, though, as we rush out of bed, tend to our partner, and scramble to get ourselves and our children out the door on time, we may skimp on or even miss entirely the opportunity to bend our knees before God.

Of course, we can talk to Spirit anywhere, anytime, and we don't have to literally get down on our knees to start the conversation. However, many women find that setting time aside for morning prayer helps them align themselves with their Higher Power and get their heads straight for whatever the day may bring. If you think you couldn't find a moment in your morning to utter a single "Amen," you're not alone—but you *can* almost always find one moment, and that may be all you need. For example, decide to pray for the first five minutes after you get out of bed (or even before you get out of bed!). If you can't take five minutes, begin with two. You may find, paradoxically, that devoting this time to connecting with the Divine starts to free up *more* time, so that your morning feels less pressured and everything, including your prayer practice, fits in with greater ease.

There are any number of ways to make prayer work for you. Some of us find comfort in the ritual of bedtime prayers we learned in childhood, and some of us prefer to pray moment to moment as we move through an ordinary day. On those occasions when we give ourselves over fully to prayer, we often find it deeply restorative, even transformative—a source of both grounding and inspiration. If you can, consider doing your own "prayer retreat" in which you pray without ceasing for an entire day. At day's end, write down what you experienced and how you felt as the day unfolded.

Meditation

Even if we pray every day, in our busyness we often forget to listen for the answers to our requests. As part of our daily prayer time, it's important to take 5, 10 or 15 minutes or more to be still and quiet—to stop *talking to* God and start to *listen*. What are we listening for? A voice, ideas, feelings, visions, and gentle urgings that come not from our home, our family, or whatever worries we may have that day, but that provide pieces of genuine answers to the questions we're asking.

For some people, the idea of meditating puts a bad taste in their mouths. Some Christians fear meditating because of its association with Eastern religions. In reality, meditation is part of many spiritual traditions. Every major religion encourages us to set ourselves apart from the world for periods of time so we can receive divine inspiration.

"Meditation is a form of spiritual discipline for Christians. It is a process of listening, deep listening," Dr. Townes affirms. "During our waking hours we need to take time in our days to stop—to unplug from whatever tasks we're doing and seek even as little as ten to fifteen minutes of centering ourselves with listening deep within and outside of us. For me it would be listening for God, for others it might be listening to a Higher Power or a Higher Force. Regardless of what we call it, taking time to pray and meditate can provide just the peace that often eludes us."

Some Black women have been taught that if they stop their own thoughts, the devil will jump in. Even if this belief were true, though, very few meditators, even seasoned ones, can actually stop their thoughts, so there's no danger of that happening for most folks. Rather, many describe meditating as a process of just observing their thoughts as they go by, like watching them from a passing train.

Again, meditation is a spiritual discipline that allows us to be intentional about how we shape our thoughts and our communion with the Spirit. "You don't always have to react to thoughts," says Ruth King. "You can start to say, 'Oh, yeah, that's me hating myself. Oh, yeah, that's me wishing this. I'm wishing; I'm wanting; I'm hungry; I'm not hungry.'"

We can meditate alone or in a community of friends as a part of our process of spiritual growth and restoration. "Who knows what we may find?" says Dr. Townes. "But fearing what we may find is probably the very reason why we need to stop and do it."

Spiritual Study

Many Black women go to church, but fewer of us actually read or deeply study the Bible, Koran, or another sacred text or spiritual readings that speak to our higher self.

"Bible study is important, but it should be what I call 'fearless Bible study,'" says Dr. Townes. "The Bible is full of scriptures that challenge our comfort zones. We tend not to deal with them. We tend to sell the Bible short. We don't ask it tough questions."

"Crucifixion, for Christ, wasn't pretty," notes Dr. Dyson. "The flood wasn't pretty. Exodus wasn't pretty. None of those things was pretty, but in all of those horrific stories of somebody's body being sacrificed or mutilated or isolated, as in the case of Moses, there's a

TROUBLE DON'T LAST ALWAYS

When I was 22 and fresh out of college, I was working in a residential facility for emotionally disturbed children. One evening I was charged with keeping one of my clients up overnight so that she could have a procedure done in the morning. At around 4 AM, I was lost in my own thoughts: I had a good job, a reliable car, had just been accepted to graduate school and was in love. In spite of that, I was singing "woe is me," feeling self-doubt, self-pity, self-loathing, hopelessness and like my life was meaningless. Out of nowhere that 14-year-old child said to me, "Trouble don't last always."

You can only imagine my initial reaction. After a few minutes, once the words truly penetrated me, I realized that she was right. If I could just get beyond this moment, I would be okay. I was supposed to be on a life's journey to discover and answer the question: "Who is Tamara Unise Carey?" My life was changed forever.

My personal journey has taken me to places of self-discovery and introspection. I have learned so many things about myself that make me appreciate who I was divinely created to be. Some things have made me cry, some have made me laugh or smile, and ultimately love deeper.

As I pulled my head out of the sand and learned how to get out of my own way, I realized that other women and sister friends were on or attempting to get on their own life's journey. My vision was born: my business Journey To Self, which offers retreats and services to help women tap into their greatness and explore their vision in a safe and nurturing environment.

I will always remember and be grateful to that 14-year-old girl. She was that butterfly that landed and put a poem in my heart, and life has been forever changed because of her.

—Tamara Carey, LSW, Age 38, Philadelphia

lesson in life. All the Bible is, is life lessons and stories that ancient people decided to tell for our hope and promise for today."

We can study these hope-giving spiritual readings alone or in a group. Finding a space, text, or community that empowers our *whole* selves is what's key to finding spiritual fulfillment. While traditional scripts of spirituality can be helpful especially in fostering community, it's the inner wisdom that truly elevates our spirit more than any other outside source or element. It's impossible to prescribe one way to engage our spiritual hygiene. Just as we seek out specific types of deodorants for our physical hygiene, finding the one that works best for us, we must experiment in finding our spiritual path. It's a personalized journey that must be met with authenticity—meeting us where we are and challenging us to tap into the connectivity of the universe to reach our divine selves. If you're working with others, try listening to each woman's perspective, challenging each other to practice the ideas in your lives and sharing and offering feedback on how these higher ideas help to transform your life.

Journaling

Sometimes we become so caught up in our worries, our fears, our to-do lists, and the thoughts that swirl around in our heads that we lose our objectivity and can't figure out which way to move. Journaling gives us an opportunity to air out our cluttered thoughts on the openness of a clean white page. Through writing, many Black women finally find a place to express the thoughts and feelings that don't have a place in other aspects of their life. Writing often helps us become clearer about what we think and offers us a private world where we can explore our secrets, dreams, and deepest longings in a way that's never yet been heard.

When you journal, the things you write don't have to make sense. You may simply find yourself downloading your to-dos and other worries, which can clear your mind and help you sleep better. While some women purchase fancy decorative journals, you may find that a spiral-bound notebook serves your purpose just fine. As an experiment, try turning in half an hour early at night and giving yourself some time to wind down by expressing your thoughts on the page. Do this every day for a month and see if you don't feel clearer and have greater peace of mind.

Fasting and Cleansing

Living in a culture that encourages us to have a dysfunctional relationship with food, fasting is often the last thing we want to do. "I have never been able to pull that off; I love food too much," admits Dr. Townes. Yet many women find that they feel more peaceful and mentally clear as they remove less healthy ingredients and add more healthy foods to their daily diet. It's not uncommon for a faster to experience a spiritual breakthrough, attaining a level of peace and clarity she could never reach before.

Many indigenous cultures practice regular periods of fasting and cleansings, whether by increasing consumption of vegetables or scheduling days to stay home and drink a laxative tea. Even in our food-driven culture, from time to time it's healthy to turn down your plate—whether for a day, a long weekend, or for longer than that. This gives your body the opportunity to rest and to cleanse itself of many of the toxic ingredients that we consume in many of the fast and "junk" foods we eat, as well as those that enter our bodies through the environment. It also allows us to cleanse ourselves of the emotions that have backed up inside of us, which we have stuffed down with food instead of expressing them.

Nature

"Sometimes you just need to sit with the Universe and really humble yourself," says Micelle, age 32. Communing with Spirit in nature can be a powerful way for us to refresh our own spirits. Cycles of birth, growth, maturity, death, and renewal play out in the natural environment, and by observing them we can learn about their power in our own lives. How often are we awed when a whiteout shuts down America's largest cities and most sophisticated technologies, or when we notice how the soothing sounds of rain against our window can serenade us to sleep?

Too many Black women live in environments where we aren't exposed to nature—like inner-city streets where the only trees you see are growing from cracks in the sidewalk—or where we learn to fear it because we believe it poses a threat to us. Spending deliberate time observing nature's wonders, large and small, can help us take stock of our place in the scheme of Creation. Taking a walk in a park with a friend, sitting quietly on the bank of a river, cultivating a garden—these are all ways we can reconnect with the power that surrounds and supports our daily living.

Micelle often travels from Phoenix to the spiritual center of Sedona, Arizona, where she sits among the area's famous red rocks and reflects upon the timelessness of the scene before her. "People talk about the 'spiritual vortexes' there, and I don't really know what that means," she says. "But what I do know is that the beauty of nature can just bring me to my knees. I have been through a lot of things in my life, but when I look at what God can create, sometimes I just sit there and cry."

Silence

Women who don't choose to pursue a formal meditation practice can find the benefits of stillness in other ways—such as the quiet time in nature that we mentioned above. Some people decide to go hours, days, and even weeks without talking on religious or meditative retreats, but often silence is just a matter of tuning out the noise that fills our days.

Practicing silence doesn't merely mean that we don't talk. It means that we turn off the radio, the television, our iPod so that we can actually hear the urgings of the still, small voice within. In fact, people who practice silence often may experience a calming of their thoughts, and greater peace along with it, and find that the still small voice actually becomes a very insistent and loud one. To test this out for yourself, try going all morning without speaking, listening to any form of media, or going on the Internet.

Turning Outward

Ministering to ourselves in prayer or stillness or study can tune us in to God and help us hear our own voices more clearly too. As Dr. Townes reminds us, we're called to honor Spirit in all its manifestations, in ourselves and around us, and part of that process means sharing our gifts with the world. So we can also practice disciplines in which we turn our efforts outward to focus on the needs of others—not in the same I'll-take-care-of-everyone-but-me way that so many of us are used to, but in a way that supports our own spiritual health.

Service

In a world that's focused on "me, me, me," many people find it fulfilling to do for others. Through service we not only share what we have, we also learn firsthand from the people we serve that we have value to them and something important to offer. We recognize the danger in telling overworked and overextended Black women, whose culture already teaches them to sacrifice themselves, that they should serve others *more*. However, this is a different type of service from the (often) thankless serving we do for our family and friends.

Service undertaken from a spiritual perspective can be a particularly powerful tool for Black women who have low self-esteem, who feel undervalued in their personal lives or at work, or who have not found a place in life to express their gifts and talents. If you feel unappreciated at work, you can demonstrate your natural propensity to organize or manage or lead at your church, at a local nonprofit organization, for a political campaign, or in another capacity where those skills will be valued.

Surrender

Many of us, when we hear the word *surrender*, associate it with giving up. The true meaning is far from it: surrender does involve a sort of giving up, but it's giving up our ideas about how things should be done, along with (often) our controlling nature, and allowing a process to unfold that's orchestrated by our Higher Power and greater than the one that we can imagine ourselves.

"Being control freaks has not gotten us very far," Dr. Townes points out, either in our work lives or in our personal lives. "I think it's healthier to really pay attention to where we're being led and to trust that if we do let go we're not going to drop off the face of the earth." Susan Taylor, emeritus editor-in-chief of *Essence* magazine, reminds us in her book *In the Spirit* that to bring about new beginnings, we must leave behind the things that compromise our wholeness. This highlights how important it is to surrender our pain and frustrations with the realization that the intentions of the Spirit are designed to propel us in a direction of peace. When we operate with this consciousness, that our existence is for a divine purpose, then we will be much more likely to focus ourselves and powerful energy on the positive instead of being distracted by the things that we can't control. If we practice submission in that spirit of trust, we may be surprised at where it leads us. One place to start: letting go of something or someone that isn't serving you or moving you toward your goals and dreams.

Sacrifice

We practice sacrifice to give up our mistaken belief that we provide our own security. Rather, we remind ourselves that we find lasting security in our relationship with both the aspect of God that resides within us and that aspect that surrounds us and indwells all others. Our goal when we practice sacrifice is to intentionally place ourselves outside of our comfort zone and out in the desert, where we must rely on God's goodness.

There are different levels of sacrifice. On one end of the scale, we can sacrifice our morning latte, which will not only improve our cash flow and health (less caffeine and sugar); it may also force us to deal with the reality that we need to get more sleep. A bit farther along the spectrum, we can give up our Saturdays at the mall, also saving money, but now raising the issue of how we deal with our emotions if we don't get "retail therapy," and what we do with that time—perhaps enriching our lives by becoming a mentor to a younger girl or a granddaughter to someone left alone in a nursing home, volunteering for a meaningful cause, or working on our goals and dreams.

Some people sacrifice financially by being generous with their surplus. This isn't to say that we should give away only what we won't miss; rather, think in terms of skipping that Saturday shopping in order to donate what you would have spent to a charity or your church. If you do this, it's important that you meet your real financial commitments first— it is not spiritual to be irresponsible or pass over a previous agreement in favor of a "good cause." You can increase your impact by getting others involved: consider pulling together some women graduates of your high school or college to start a college fund or creating a book scholarship for college students in your community.

Spirit in Community

In modern America, cultural values tend to skew toward self rather than society, emphasizing individualism, privacy, and autonomy. African-descended people have roots in a much more communal world, but today even Black Americans lack the sense of community that previous generations had, especially now that many of us live across the country from our loved ones and families. Too many Black women live emotionally isolated lives, working all day and returning to a home where they have no one to share their hearts, souls and lives with—even though they may live in a house full of people.

Yet we are stronger when we share our lives with each other. There is synergy in community. And as author Sobonfu Somé writes in *Welcoming Spirit Home: Ancient African Teachings to Celebrate Children and Community*, our inner self and our outer world can go hand in hand and enrich each other deeply. In some traditional African societies, Somé explains—including the Dagara tribe in her native Burkina Faso, West Africa—children are born into a village that understands that each person has a purpose, and the community's job is to help to cultivate each person's gifts and give them a place to express those gifts for the benefit of all. In places like this, the philosophy of *ubuntu*—the notion that the way a person experiences her personhood is through her relationships with other people—still prevails.

Somé defines a community as an environment "where a group of people are empowered by one another, by spirit, and by the ancestors to be themselves, carry out their purpose, and use their power responsibly." Its goal, she says, "is to form a diverse body of people with common goals and empower them to embrace their own gifts, selves, and nature. Community holds a space for all its members to work at becoming as close to their true selves as possible."

It's true that this isn't the way most of us live today—Somé actually writes that the ideal of community she describes isn't possible in Western culture—but we can bring some of this support and sustenance into our own lives by coming together with "a group of people we trust and can count on with Spirit's blessings." The disciplines here are ways to connect with God in the company of others.

Worship

Who doesn't know the power of Sunday mornings spent in spiritual communion with others—the pews rocking, the choirs exalting, and the minister inspiring us with a good preached word?

"When you listen to and read religious teachings, and when you hear and participate in religious services and rituals, there's something about them, some stability and balance and comfort that I think is important for health," says Dr. Primm. "People have been studying the connection between spirituality and religious observance, and they've seen some health benefits and mental health benefits for people that have strong religious beliefs and patience."

Fellowship

For a fresh perspective, try going to a worship service in a tradition or religion that's different from your own. Remember that the church, mosque, temple, or spiritual center isn't the only place we can worship together. You might find communion sitting in a park and experiencing the wonder of nature, marveling at the beauty of a flower, or gazing into a baby's eyes—with cherished friends.

Fellowship denotes the activity of doing something together that aligns with God's will for us. Lots of us share fellowship over coffee or breakfast after church. We can enjoy fellowship as a family when we come together to celebrate a young person's rite of passage and socialize our children about how we expect them to behave. We promote fellowship as a community when we join forces to solve a problem facing our neighborhood or to create something together, such as a community garden or park. We can also experience fellowship with others as we work toward our goals and dreams.

"It's important to have a group of people with similar values to hold us accountable and remind us of the importance of courage, as well as love, and other grand words that we need to be living our lives by," says Dr. Townes. "We don't try to do this alone—that happens too much. We think spirituality is an alone act, but it's not."

Celebration

Sometimes we're so busy running from pillar to post that we skip over the good things that happen to us. It's important to celebrate our milestones and accomplishments, to formally acknowledge what we've achieved, to receive kudos from our friends, family, and neighbors, and to set a foundation for our continued growth. Celebrations can be as predictable as a party, a dinner with friends at a special place, a day trip to a location that is special to you or that get-away vacation you've been dreaming about. Or they can be simple and spontaneous—a spur-of-the-moment gathering or a warm hug to greet good news.

Chapter 9

Self-Care Now

When Jada needs time to herself, she no longer gives a hoot what else is going on in her household. She heads to her bathroom, draws a nice tub of hot water, pours in some lavender oil, lights her favorite scented candles, grabs her journal and a novel, then performs the most important act of all—locks the door. The 40-year-old accounting supervisor and mother of three—ages 5, 7, and 17—rarely gets time to herself even though her husband parents actively. When she schedules some "me time," she asks him to handle everything and promises that she won't criticize any decision he makes in her absence. Whether the children whine, get in an argument, or start crying, she keeps her backside in the water and her nose in her book. When one of them makes the mistake of calling her, she asks only one question: "Is anybody bleeding?" If not, she stays in the tub.

Renee, 55, celebrates her birthday each year by gifting herself with some "health love." First she schedules all of her annual medical appointments in the two months before her birthday so she enters each New Year knowing she's in good health. Then she also schedules "away" time. When she was more flush with cash, the Memphis resident went away to the islands; these days, she either schedules a morning at a day spa or swaps houses for the weekend with a friend who lives in the country but likes city life. But no matter how she enters her new year, she spends it consciously paying attention to herself.

How do *you* take care of yourself? Now that you have learned in previous chapters how to reduce your vulnerability to the Top Ten Health Risks, and how to tend to your body, mind, and spirit, it's time to blueprint your own strategy for self-care. Through practicing self-care you can empower yourself to become what the Imperative calls a Health-Wise

---

Woman—a woman who is an informed master of her own health, both for her own sake and for her community. This healthy self-possession can take many different forms, ranging from committing to daily physical activity to creating the most vibrant life possible even if you are living with a chronic illness.

What is Self-Care?

First, let's get clear about what self-care is and what it's not. Engaging in self-care means doing what you can to assess the state of your health; learning what it takes to attain and maintain good health; knowing available health-care options from both conventional Western or allopathic medicine and complementary and alternative medicine (CAM); understanding how to assess the information and resources you need; making informed decisions; and assembling your own health-care advocacy team.

Self-care *does not* involve getting rid of your doctors or other health-care providers, or throwing conventional medicine out the window. It means knowing who to see for what and accepting that when you are properly in tune with your body, mind, and spirit—no one knows the whole you better than you. By developing your skills in a variety of self-care practices, you will gradually learn which strategies work best for you. There are many paths along the journey to becoming a Health-Wise Woman; these steps will start you on your way.

Know your body. No one could or should ever be expected to know your body better than you do, and this includes knowing how you feel during your happiest and healthiest moments. Take note of any sensation that deviates from however you feel best. Any mood that isn't a good mood; anything in or on our body that does not look or feel right; any new sensations, aches, or pains that we may have—all are signs that we need to slow down. Take a moment to listen and assess what's going on. Depending upon your stress level or risk factors for the Top 10 Health Risks, your symptoms may flash red signal lights alerting you to make an appointment or speak with a health-care provider.

One of the best ways to learn about your health history is to shake your family tree. The next time your family gathers for Sunday dinner, a birthday party, Thanksgiving, or a funeral, start a conversation about your family's health history. By sharing information and creating your family's "health" family tree, you'll learn what conditions, illnesses, or diseases you may be at personal risk for based on your heredity, family culture, lifestyle, and habits.

Another critical aspect of knowing your body involves what health practitioners' call "knowing and monitoring your numbers," the key measures of health. Talk with your doctor to make sure you know what your targets should be and what to do if you're not measuring up to healthy numbers. Also request the results of your lab tests.

Health Factors	Goal for Your Number	
Total Cholesterol	Less than 200 mg/dL	
LDL ("Bad") Cholesterol	LDL cholesterol goals vary.	
	– Less than 100 mg/dL	...Optimal
	– 100 to 129 mg/dL	...Near Optimal/Above Optimal
	– 130 to 159 mg/dL	...Borderline High
	– 160 to 189 mg/dL	...High
	– 190 mg/dL and above	...Very High
HDL ("Good") Cholesterol	50 mg/dL or higher	
Triglycerides (Lipid fat)	<150 mg/dL	
Blood Pressure	<120/80 mmHg	
Fasting Glucose	<100 mg/dL	
Body Mass Index (BMI)	<25 Kg/m	
Waist Circumference	<35 inches	

Assess your health. At the beginning of each new season—spring, summer, fall, and winter—stop and take stock of your quality of life. One way to do this is to spend just a few moments examining your lifestyle by answering the Health Self-Assessment questions below, then working on making adjustments as necessary.

1. What is my blood pressure? What has been the trend over the past five years? What does it mean, and what do I need to do about it?

2. What are my cholesterol numbers? (These include total cholesterol, LDL, HDL, and triglycerides, a type of fat found in the blood and food.) What has been the trend over the past five years? What do they mean, and what do I need to do about them?

3. What is my blood sugar level? Is it borderline or high? What has been the trend over the past five years? What does it mean, and what do I need to do about it?

4. What are my body mass indexes (BMI) and waist measurements? Do they put me at risk? If so, how can I reduce my risk?

5. Am I physically fit? If not, what is my plan to increase my physical activity level?

6. Am I at risk for diabetes? Heart disease? Stroke? HIV/AIDS? What steps can I take to know and reduce my risk?

7. Do I smoke? If I do, what help do I need and what steps am I willing to take to quit right now?

8. How many hours of sleep do I get each night? If I am not sleeping seven hours a night, what can I do to get more sleep consistently?

9. Have I completed all of the recommended screenings for my life stage?

10. Am I spirituality connected? If not, what steps am I willing to take to grow my spirit?

Commit to taking care of yourself—body, mind, and spirit. Once you know your risk for certain health conditions, it's time to make a decision. Will you take care of yourself so that you can be a Health-Wise Black woman, or will you let inertia take its course? You can make no better investment in yourself than to take control of your health. There are things you can't control, such as your age and family history. But certain decisions you can take charge of: deciding not to smoke, to eat healthier, and to move more. These types of choices can make you healthier now and reduce your risk of developing health problems in the future.

Whether you choose to eat more fresh fruits and vegetables or to begin walking three days a week, make sure that the commitments you make fit the realities of your life. If you're just beginning, you may want to start with small and achieveable goals and build on them. If you've missed a few days, don't feel as though you're a failure. Simply start over again. Making and keeping your agreements to take care of yourself is an important form of self love. When you love yourself, you value yourself and want to protect your health and wellness. That means not just knowing the right thing to do, but actually *doing* it.

Find the best health-care provider and partner with the provider to achieve good health. You wouldn't take your car to just any mechanic, and you shouldn't entrust your health to someone you don't completely trust. Your goal over time is to collaborate with your doctor to prevent illness, create and maintain good health, and treat any symptoms, conditions, or diseases you develop. This requires good communication and some effort on your part.

"You would be well advised to vet and investigate any physician you're seeing as well as you can, especially if you're doing something surgical," says Dr. M. Natalie Achong, obstetrician and gynecologist. However, this is easier said than done, especially for patients whose health insurance limits the doctors whom they can see. Dr. Achong suggests using both word of mouth and the Internet, asking a lot of questions of potential providers and asking for and checking references. When you call a new doctor's office, start by asking what services they provide and what they think about patients participating in their treatment decisions. If the staff looks at you sideways, don't be surprised. Your questions may seem unusual, since most people just accept whatever their doctor dishes out—good, bad, or indifferent. Their response will tell you a lot about the practice and the way that you will be treated.

Before you make an appointment for the first time, read the Primary Care Primer below to help you learn about different kinds of primary-health-care providers. Then think through your reason for calling, write down any symptoms you're experiencing, and develop a short list of questions about your symptoms that you can ask over the phone (different from the more extensive questions you'll ask in person). This first conversation will help both you and the physician's office ensure that you've contacted the right type of doctor and determine whether you need to schedule an appointment or if they can help you over the phone.

A PRIMARY CARE PRIMER

The insurance industry uses the term primary care provider (PCP) to describe a physician whom either you choose (or an insurer assigns to you) to conduct your basic examinations and act as the gatekeeper controlling your access to other health services and specialists. If you've never had a doctor before, the first doctor you see will be a PCP. Insurance plans differ on the types of health practitioners that can serve as PCPs. Here are some related terms you should know:

- The term "generalist" often refers to medical doctors (MDs) or osteopathic doctors (DO) who specialize in internal medicine, family practice, or pediatrics.

- OB/GYNs are doctors who specialize in obstetrics and gynecology, including women's health-care, wellness, and prenatal care. Many women use an OB/GYN as their primary care provider.

- Nurse practitioners (NPs) are nurses with graduate training. They can serve as primary care providers in family medicine (FNP), pediatrics (PNP), adult care (ANP), or geriatrics (GNP). Others are trained to address women's health-care (common concerns and routine screenings) and family planning. In some states NPs can prescribe medications.

- A physician's assistant (PA) can provide a wide range of services in collaboration with a Doctor of Medicine (MD) or Osteopathy (DO).

Once you make an appointment, don't feel slighted if a nurse practitioner or physician's assistant sees you instead of the doctor. To curtail rising health-care costs, many practices are incorporating licensed health-care professionals who are trained to take your history, conduct your physical, order and interpret diagnostic tests, make diagnoses, and even prescribe medication. They work closely with and communicate with your doctor and can answer many of your questions. Many are also highly trained in prevention, wellness, and patient education,[1] and they may have much better people skills and more gracious bedside manners than some medical doctors.

Know your rights. You have rights as a patient and a consumer of health-care services. As you prepare to navigate the health-care system, know what they are. Key among them:

- Considerate, respectful, and compassionate care in an environment that is physically and emotionally safe, no matter your age, gender, race, national origin, religion, sexual orientation, gender identity, or level of ability;

- Treatment and care in a safe space free from all forms of abuse, neglect, or mistreatment;

- Being treated with dignity and called by your proper name;

- Being told the name of each person who is examining or treating you;

- Receiving up-to-date information about your diagnosis, treatment, and possible outcomes, communicated in language that you understand;

- Working with your providers to decide what treatment plan is best for you;

- Sharing your concerns, complaints, and questions about your care and expecting that they will be heard and respected;

- Your provider being on time for your appointment.

Doctors should run on time or close to it—although it seems not to happen consistently in many practices. "One time I was in the waiting room where they put you almost until they were closing. They had forgotten about me," said one older Black woman.

Often long office waits reflect the pressures that doctors face as a result of the demands that insurance companies place upon them; sometimes they reflect poor management practices; other times they indicate that doctors are treating and showing compassion for patients who are disproportionately ill, have unexpected health and personal issues, and may need to be seen urgently. No matter—you should never be treated rudely, dismissed, or forgotten about.

If your doctor is running more than 15 to 20 minutes late, you should receive an explanation and an apology. If it happens consistently, explain nicely that your time is as valuable as the doctor's and you expect to be treated that way. Then ask if the staff they will work with you—for example, see if you can call ahead to get an update on how the doctor's running so you can plan your arrival accordingly. If you're really dissatisfied, consider looking for another doctor.

After waiting routinely for no less than one hour and on several occasions for as long as two hours to see her doctor, Geraldine spoke with her doctor's office. On one occasion she asked the practice to pay her parking ticket. Eventually she changed doctors.

Our Role As Patients

Not only should we know our rights, we should also understand and then fulfill our own responsibilities as patients and consumers of health-care services. We must be able to communicate our expectations for medical treatment and care to our health-care providers. We can start with the following:

Know what preventive screenings and diagnostic services are available through both your health insurance plan and the Patient Protection and Affordable Care Act. In a significant victory for women and girls, the Department of Health and Human Services released new insurance rules under the 2010 Affordable Care Act requiring all new private health plans to cover several evidence-based preventive services. This includes mammograms, colonoscopies, blood pressure checks, depression screenings and prenatal tests, without charging a copayment, deductible or coinsurance. The Affordable Care Act (ACA) also made recommended preventive services free for people on Medicare.[2]

Beginning on or after August 1, 2012, all new insurance plans will be required to cover eight essential preventive services and treatments to help women improve their health immediately and over the long run—all without requiring you to open your purse for co-pays:

1. Annual well-woman preventive care visits for adult women to obtain the recommended preventive services that are age and developmentally appropriate, including preconception and prenatal care;

2. Screening for gestational diabetes in pregnant women between 24 and 28 weeks of gestation and at the first prenatal visit for pregnant women identified to be at high risk for diabetes;

3. Screening for human papillomavirus (HPV) DNA testing for high-risk women 30 years and older with normal cytology results should occur no more frequently than every three years;

4 Annual counseling and screening for human immune-deficiency virus (HIV) infection for all sexually active women;

5. All FDA-approved contraceptive methods, counseling, sterilization procedures, and patient education for all women with reproductive capacity. Group health plans sponsored by certain religious employers, and group health insurance coverage in connection with such plans, are exempt from the requirement to cover contraceptive services;

6. Annual screening and counseling for interpersonal and domestic violence;

7. Comprehensive lactation (breastfeeding) support and counseling by a trained provider during pregnancy and/or in the postpartum period, and costs for renting breastfeeding equipment in conjunction with each birth;

8. Sexually transmitted infection counseling for all sexually active women.

Do your homework before your appointment. The Internet abounds with patient-information sites, from the award-winning WebMD.com to MayoClinic.com, the website of the world-renowned Mayo Clinic, to BlackWomensHealth.org, the website of the Black Women's Health Imperative. Research your health condition or disease on HON code certified health and medical websites. Then arm yourself with a list of questions and issues you'd like to discuss when you speak with your health-care provider.

Just remember that when you visit a site for the first time—especially if it's not run by a mainstream organization—it's important to assess how reliable it is. Some sites present information that is inaccurate or misleading, including some "Astroturf" organizations—interest groups made up of citizens who appear to come from the grassroots but are actually organized or funded by corporations, industry associations, or public-relations firms. Always examine:

- Who funds and runs the website? Reliable sites make it easy to learn who's behind the scenes. This information can often be found in the About Us or Sponsor Information sections.

- Where does its information come from? Many sites post information collected from other websites or sources. If the person or organization in charge of the site did not create the information, the original source should be clearly labeled.

- Is the information current? Health websites should be reviewed and updated regularly. It is particularly important that medical information be current—outdated content can be misleading or even dangerous.

- It's easy to get alarmed when the "symptom checker" tells you that your sniffles could be due to either the common cold or a rare form of brain cancer. Read other people's anecdotal experiences e.g., posts in forums—cautiously. Some of that info can scare the life out of you, or misdirect your further research. Avoid a case of "a little bit of knowledge becoming a dangerous thing."

- Can you interact with the site operators? You should always be able to reach out to the site owner if you run across problems or have questions or feedback. You can often find this information in a section labeled Contact Us. If the site hosts chat rooms or other online discussion areas, it should clearly state the terms of using this service.

Arrive at your appointment prepared. Doctors who take health insurance experience tremendous pressure to see about 25 patients per day. Doctors who don't take insurance often see fewer patients and spend more time with each one. This means that your appointment could likely last about ten minutes from the time your doctor walks in the door until the time he or she moves on to the next person. Some will spend more, but some may spend less. You need to make a plan for how to spend that time.

Many mainstream health websites contain lists of questions to ask at your doctor's office. They often include:

- What do you think is causing my problem?

- Is there more than one condition (disease) that could be causing my problem?

- Could any medications I'm taking be causing or contributing to my symptoms? (Ask the same about any herbs or supplements you may be taking.)

- What tests will you do to diagnose the problem and which of the conditions is present?

- How good are the tests for diagnosing the problem and the conditions?

- How safe are the tests?

Also, list any symptoms or problems you're experiencing. Prioritize both your questions and the symptoms. What is so important that you cannot leave your doctor's office without having an answer? Start there in case you run out of time. "When I go to the doctor I have to write down everything that I want to say, but I don't have enough time to say it," said one focus group participant in Philadelphia. That's real.

A couple of days before your appointment, so you don't have to rush, write down the names of any medications and the ingredients and dosages for any supplements (including vitamins, herbs, and protein powders) you are taking—or bring the package or pill bottle with you. Consider bringing a family member or friend to your appointments, particularly if you are feeling intimidated or going through a tough time. Ask your companion to take notes, help you ask questions, and make sure that you understand the answers.

Don't be afraid to ask questions until you understand. Sometimes comprehending what a health-care provider is saying can be almost as difficult as reading a doctor's handwriting. This can be particularly hard if you're on the receiving end of bad news. Alex Brown had accompanied her mother on a doctor's visit on the day that her mother's doctor explained to her what it meant that she had Stage 4 breast cancer—the most advanced stage. Alex watched her mother go into shock and become unable to understand a word her doctor said.

If your provider is using technical terms or big words that go over your head, ask her to explain it to you in a simpler language. Importantly, never leave your appointment without knowing what your condition is called, the range of treatment options, and the pros and cons of each.

If you still don't "get it" when your appointment time is up, ask to speak with a nurse practitioner or other health professional who can explain it to you. If you can't squeeze all of your questions in, ask if you can schedule a telephone call to ask any additional questions.

Always tell the truth about the reason for your visit. "Often when women go to the ob/gyn, they put up a front and say that they're coming in for one thing but they're really coming in for something else," says Dr. Achong. But to get the most out of the brief time spent with any doctor, we have to be willing to be completely forthright, even if our real problem is difficult to talk about.

"I'm a person who believes in having open communication with your doctor, and I know a lot of people, not just Black women but people in general, sometimes are intimidated by doctors because they feel like the doctor should tell them what's wrong with them," says Lena, age 30. "Actually, it should be the other way around. The patient should feel like they can tell the doctor what's bothering them, even sometimes beyond the medical things. They should be able to talk to their doctor about stuff."

"Wasting time posturing and being dishonest is not helping anybody," says Dr. Achong. If you spend the precious minutes of your appointment covering up something you're embarrassed about, that leaves little time to ask important questions or to receive help. A word to the wise: many times doctors know when we're hiding something because what we're telling them doesn't add up. Remember, these interactions and conversations are unfamiliar to us, but doctors have them all day.

Always seek a second, third, and even fourth opinion for serious medical problems and important procedures or treatment protocols such as surgery or chemotherapy. Don't worry; you're not being rude. This request is a good health education practice and literally a standard operating procedure; it shouldn't offend your doctor. In fact, many doctors welcome their colleagues' perspectives and insights. Rehearse your inquiry if you need to. Say something like "I appreciate your diagnosis (or recommendation) and will spend some time educating myself. I would also like to get a second opinion. Is there another doctor or medical center that you'd recommend?" Always remember to check your insurance coverage in advance to see if you are covered for second opinions.

You don't have to undergo any test you don't want to. The doctor is the medical expert, but you are the expert on your body. Listen to it and decide accordingly—just make sure it's your body speaking and not your pride, your fear or your denial. Ask yourself, *"Why do I feel this test is not right for me right now?"* It may be something you can do without altogether—or it may be something you'll decide to schedule for another time when you feel more comfortable.

Ask to have the results of lab and other diagnostic tests sent directly to you as well as to your doctor. At the end of any major diagnostic appointment, request a copy of your medical test results. Your doctor should not be the only one who has your medical records. These documents describe your body, and you should have them in your hands. You in consultation with your doctor must take responsibility for tracking the results of your diagnostic tests.

Is your blood pressure or blood sugar trending upward? If you have your test results, you may figure this out before your doctor does, and then you can start the conversation about solutions. Chronic diseases like hypertension and diabetes generally often take ten years to develop. Don't put off making lifestyle changes or settle for watching and waiting until you're in the danger zone. Get an early jump on things so that you have time to change your habits gradually.

Exam gowns are for exams; conversations about your health should happen while you're wearing your clothing. Explain to your health provider that you'd like to speak with her or him after you've put your clothes on, not while your behind's peeking out. This alone may make you feel less vulnerable and help to change the doctor patient power imbalance that exists in the exam room. Many doctors appreciate this and may suggest it before you do—"When you're dressed, let's speak in my office."

Take your medication as directed. Many Black women go off their meds because they experience adverse reactions—not surprising, since very few meds were created or tested with either Black people or women in mind. If you experience uncomfortable or adverse side effects, tell your doctor so she or he can adjust your dosage or change you to another medication. Avoid the temptation to stop taking your meds as soon as you start to feel better. In some cases, such as with antibiotics, this can set you up for more problems. Talk to your provider first.

Follow your doctor's self-care recommendations; if you can't, tell the doctor honestly so she or he can make suggestions that work better for you. Whether you see a medical doctor or a complementary and alternative medicine (CAM) practitioner, you are responsible for your own health. The doctor can help you even more if you are committed to helping yourself. If you can't or are unable to follow your doctor's prescription or advice, just 'fess up so that your health provider can make an adjustment for you.

Knowing how to stay healthy is not enough; we must apply what we know so we actually get good results.

If you know that something's wrong with your body, but your doctor can't detect it, insist that she or he look again. The doctor is the medical expert, but you are the expert on you. Monica's mother felt a slight burning sensation in her breast for six months before a mammogram detected the presence of cancerous cells. Thanks to her insistence that something was wrong and her refusal to accept the doctor's assurance that everything looked normal, her cancer was detected early, while it was treatable.

One Imperative focus group member from Philadelphia kept complaining to her doctor that something was hanging in her throat. But each time she went to the doctor, the doctor said he couldn't see it. After the third trip, she stood firm that she needed a referral to an ear, nose, and throat specialist. When her doctor balked, she said, "Hold it. If you don't refer me to an ear, nose, and throat specialist, I'm going to go to another doctor, because I said there's something wrong." Her doctor wrote the referral, and the specialist discovered a polyp—an abnormal tissue growth—the circumference of an orange.

"When I went back to Dr. Jones after everything was over, I said, 'See, that's why I told you I know what's wrong with me. You need to learn how to listen when I tell you what's wrong with me because you're not me. If I'm telling you my symptoms, I'm telling you how I feel. You can't tell me how I feel.' "

Or as another focus group participant put it: "Doctors are educated guessers. They can only tell you what's wrong with you according to what you tell them. I mean, they can diagnose and everything, but you're the one who knows something's wrong with you."[4]

Let the church say amen!

True Wellness

We are all powerful beings, and it is this power that connects us to the universe—the same power that promotes healing and transformation within us. To tap into this power requires examining ourselves and drawing deeply on our inner strength. We are blessed with a unique gift of consciousness that allows us to learn who we are, to understand our relationship to others, and to recognize our personal truths. This self-awareness is the essential condition of empowerment, and as we become empowered, we recognize the importance of self-*love*—the kind of love that means we care about ourselves enough to put ourselves first in our lives and teach others by example.

Through years of engaging Black women in self-help groups and analyzing the process they use to make changes in their lives, the Black Women's Health Imperative has asked, "What does it mean to be healthy and happy and whole and how do we get there?" many times. We've identified five strategic steps to self-empowerment that makes true wellness possible: awareness, coalescing, taking control, transformation, and maintenance.

Awareness

Learning who you are is the first step toward personal healing. It requires you to be brave, to entertain thoughts you have never had or acknowledged before and not be afraid of them.

Gaining awareness means letting truths about your life come to light. Let's say you're living in an abusive relationship and have thought of leaving, but haven't been able to take the necessary steps to free yourself. You can become aware that you are participating in domestic violence: even though you're the oppressed, not the oppressor. You can seek out information about the issue that troubles you, raising your awareness of the problem and your options. You can confront the beliefs, justifications, and fears that keep you stuck—a crucial step in awareness.

Awareness means that you give attention to a thought and hold it up to the light to examine its truthfulness. Awareness of self means bringing the same attention to your own spirit.

Coalescing

We all have good times, and we all have problems. It's important to realize that the problems we struggle with are also the problems of many others. We are not the only ones. But there's a conspiracy of silence that often keeps us from grasping this truth and the power it can give us. In one focus group, a Black woman said she thought only White women were victims of domestic violence because they were the only ones she ever heard talk about it. Many of us turn a deaf ear to screams from the house next door, as we may have blocked out the screams we heard from our mothers when we were children. By exchanging experiences, problems, and solutions with one another, we come together to forge a common bond, share a common struggle, and get affirmation that we can do something to change our lives. "Sharing our stories or consciousness-raising is an essential form of healing that dates back to the early days of the women's movement," says Byllye Avery, founder of the Imperative.

Taking Control

Personal growth is measured by our ability to take charge of our thoughts and behaviors at every level. When our body, mind, and spirit act in concert with each other, what we say, what we think, and what we do are in alignment. Our lives unfold more smoothly and more joyfully, and we start to feel more powerful with each act that moves us toward our goal. Every step is important, large or small: for instance, telling someone you want to stop smoking becomes significant as you continue on your road to health. The simple act of opening a savings account and making monthly deposits means you're actively engaged in taking control of your well-being.

The more you face your fears, the more powerful you become. "It wasn't my goal or intention—but my life was a lie," says Hilary of her early career. "For day after day, I woke up at a time I didn't want to get up; I put my square-toed feet in pointed-toed shoes and pretended all day that I loved what I was doing and that I wanted to spend my life there. Most of the time I liked my corporate job and sometimes I loved it, but I knew it wasn't 'me.' I had to shove 'me' aside to interest myself in things I didn't have any passion about, and the pretending just became too much. At one time I reached a point where I thought I was going to get sick or go crazy. Of course I was dressed to the nines as I felt like this."

Even though she didn't know anyone else who had left a "good" job to follow her dreams, Hilary knew that she had to develop an escape plan. She dreamed of becoming a novelist, but she felt fearful of leaving the security her job seemed to offer. That fear, she realized, was letting her know that she needed to grow. "So I created a personal development plan, where I would stretch my faith just like I stretched myself at work," she says. "My big thing was to ask myself how I could walk on water in my own life."

Transformation

On the journey to personal empowerment, we change the way we see the world, and the world changes the way it sees us. We give out a different kind of energy as we evolve. We are changing, and the path to the person we want to be can become very clear now. As beings in transformation, we must expect others to understand that we're not the same people we were before we started becoming empowered. We understand others in a new way, too. Instead of blaming ourselves or others for their misgivings or shortcomings, we perceive the barriers that keep them from growing.

Empowerment is like education: once you have it, it can't be taken away. It lives inside you, reinforcing your thoughts, directing you on the path to enlightened thinking and conscious action. You move toward claiming your power, ever more connected to your true self.

Maintenance

Empowerment is a process, not a destination, and it means we must constantly affirm who we are, what we think, the path we have chosen, and the actions that help us along the way. Remember, wisdom comes from combining what you know intellectually and what you feel in your gut. Always keep negative people from sitting in the front row seats of your life and refuse to let negative thoughts direct your inner and outer traffic.

It's important not to get complacent or think you've "arrived"—or revert to old behaviors that don't support your new commitments. Instead, stop and ask: *Is this good for me? Am I still on my path? Am I listening to my inner voice?*

Become courageous enough to confront your fears because they are often the sources of great power. As you become a more enlightened person your power and love will spread and influence others around you.

In the words of Byllye Avery, *"This is your life, and you deserve to live it as powerfully as possible!"*

AFTERWORD

Over the past five years I have had the honor to represent the Black Women's Health Imperative in advancing change for Black women—from how we are defined, portrayed, and documented to what we need as essential health benefits in the new health reform bill. As I reflect on my 30 years of being intimately involved in the Imperative since the very beginning, I am particularly mindful of the critical role that the Imperative has played in the lives of thousands of women, families, and communities. There is no doubt that we are fulfilling our mission—to work toward optimal health for all Black women across the life span. But we have done more—we have changed lives. Thousands of women and some men give testimony to the way we helped them gain a sense of confidence and purpose. Others speak proudly of our "sister circles" that provided a safe space to speak their truths in the company of other Black women. And there are many who made the decision to change—to begin a journey toward wellness.

Change is coming. And it begins with you. *Health First!* is about who we are and some of the things we need to know in order to bring about change. We hope this book, *Health First!*, will become your personal passport to giving yourself permission to be well.

We'll leave you with one more woman's story—this one from a woman who helped bring this book into being, who, after many of years of telling herself she was well when she wasn't, really did find the courage to put her health first and change her life.

—Eleanor Hinton Hoytt,
President & CEO
Black Women's Health Imperative

I had a chemical exposure during a recent renovation in the office where I work. I was a hacking, coughing mess. It took me a week to see a doctor, and then it was only because my colleagues kept pressing me and because I couldn't draw breath. I had to stop breathing before I would see a doctor about my lungs.

The first time I went to the emergency room, they didn't even pay attention to my lungs. It was all about my elevated blood pressure. I had to go back a second day to get them to take a look at my lungs. And then it was only after some prayers and a "script" given to me by the editor of this book that I was able to tell the doctors what my real problem was. It was only at this time that I felt that I got the attention I deserved.

This entire scenario prompted me to delve more deeply into the book Health First!

Why did it take me a week to see the doctor? Because I don't trust them. I have had a number of negative experiences where doctors are concerned. In my family, we never went to the doctor unless it was really serious—a broken bone or stitches. Maybe I can't always trust the doctors. Maybe they do have prejudices against fat people. Maybe they do not know how to really treat Black women, but that is NO EXCUSE for me not to advocate for MY HEALTH.

My mother was mistrustful of doctors. When I was 12, Mom had a job that included medical benefits, so she took me to have a dental checkup. The dentist took one look at us and told my mother that nearly every tooth in my mouth needed filling. Everyone in my family had healthy teeth and was cavity-free. It was later implied that perhaps the dentist took advantage of us.

When I was 23, I had a corporate job with benefits, so I went to see a therapist for the first time. She specialized in eating disorders, which I was told I had since I was more than 60 pounds overweight at the time. The therapist listened to my story and told me the reason I ate the way I did was because I "hated my mother." That was the last time I ever saw her.

The final straw came when I was 24 during my first gynecological visit. I was still a virgin— but I had missing and spotty periods, so I figured I'd get checked by this renowned doctor and she would help me out. She consulted with me one time. Told me I had PCOS (polycystic ovary syndrome) and recommended birth-control pills. There were no tests. She just told me that I would probably have trouble conceiving and would need fertility treatments if I ever decided to become a mother. Turns out the birth-control pills were the worst thing I could have taken, because I was pre-hypertensive.

Later I found a general practitioner who snatched me off of the birth-control pills fast and put me on hypertensive medications. The medications were the worst. One made my stomach hurt so bad, I would get sweats and feel faint. The other had my heart beating in my ears and I started having palpitations. This was the straw that broke the camel's back.

I cared about my health, but I'd been receiving care that didn't care about me. Now I knew why my mother had always avoided doctors. I used to think it was because she was poor and uninsured, but I came to recognize that she knew more about healing than I did, growing up in the Deep South, in northern Louisiana. Plus, my mother did more with her herbs, potions, tinctures, salves, ointments, and poultices to keep us healthy than any of my experience with doctors did. So I decided then that I would find out about my body.

I started working with my mother's herbs and "holistic" practitioners, taking the potions and tinctures plus changing my diet. I lost more than 60 pounds. And apparently I was able to reverse my condition of PCOS, because I became pregnant.

At age 34, being hypertensive and 100 pounds overweight made me a prime candidate for a high-risk-pregnancy doctor. I spent 10 weeks in the hospital and ended up having a cesarean.

I am currently taking blood pressure medication, and I weigh 327 pounds. I figured that, since I could still walk and climb up and down stairs, I was "healthy." But after reading Health First! *I realize what a lie that is. How can I weight nearly 330 pounds—I am not a sumo wrestler—and consider myself healthy? How can I walk around with a resting blood pressure of 140/90 and be healthy?*

How can I blame doctors for my health, thinking that they are not really out to help me because of some previous bad experiences, and use that as an excuse to not know what's going on right here, right now with my body?

The truth is, having a bp this high can damage my kidneys. I don't want to be on dialysis, and no amount of bad doctoring is going to change the fact that a bp this high is detrimental not only to my health but to my life. Fortunately, my recent tests have confirmed that I'm still in the "safe zone" as far as my kidneys and other major organs are concerned, but for how long?

How can I be too busy to take care of my health? No amount of single parenting, 9-to-5-ing, and school is going to make me successful, if I don't make time for my health. I watched my mother work herself into poor health. I saw her avoid doctors, because they would tell her to lose weight before they would see her for legitimate conditions. I saw her limping around, taking blood thinners to avoid clots. I saw her being hospitalized off and on for a year because she became too tired to fight or care, because she'd been fighting and caring for everyone else but herself.

I used to get angry at my mother for ignoring her medical problems that only grew worse over time; now I find myself in the same circumstances. It wasn't until I read Health First! *that I could see that I have been in major denial about my health.*

I am unhealthy. I am unwell. Thing is, I don't feel *unwell, but if I don't do something now, I will soon enough.*

Even after watching my mother's deterioration, I was in denial. I watched her go from mobility to immobile, I saw her go from obese but moving and grooving to morbidly obese and unable to do anything but sit and watch the world go by.

Denial is something.

I take care of my son's health better than I do my own. He sees the doctor regularly. Mostly because of the requirements of school, but if he's out of balance or if I see or hear something that isn't quite right, I'm making sure everything is in order.

I don't and haven't done the same for myself. Like the book says, like too many Black women, I put more time and care into what goes on my body than what goes in my body.

I've known that I needed to lose weight, but I've had to really get clear on the fact that just because I'm cute and big and modeled when I was younger, that doesn't make me healthy. I have avoided doctors because of their clear prejudice and discrimination and mistreatment, but that is no reason for me not to take better care of myself.

I see Black women all the time carrying more burdens than a mule. In Their Eyes Were Watching God, *Janie, the main character, has a conversation with her grandmother, who schools her on the hierarchy of the world and the Black woman's place in it as she sees it:*

> *Honey, de white man is de ruler of everything as fur as Ah been able tuh find out. Maybe it's some place off in de ocean where de black man is in power, but we don't know nothin' but we see. So de white man throw down de load and tell de nigger man tuh pick it up. He pick it up because he have to, but he don't tote it. He hand it to his womenfolks. De nigger woman is de mule uh de world so far as Ah can see.*

Obviously, the mule is the bearer of heavy loads and burdens. Even for the modern Black woman, this is still true. She is carrying everyone on her back: her man, if she has one, her children, her children's children, her parents, and maybe some sister's or brother's children too.

But the mule also represents a stubborn resistance that has served us. It's time to be mule-ish for ourselves. It is unlikely that Black women will throw down the burdens of taking care of everyone, but we must resist putting ourselves last. We must stubbornly resist seeing our self-care as selfish. We must stubbornly resist thinking that suffering somehow makes us stronger, better, more worthy. We cannot continue to put our health last until crisis forces us to put it first.

We MUST make our health a priority. Not weight loss because we want to be cute—weight loss because it's better for our daily quality of life. We must make our mental health a priority, not considering it because we are about to go DMX on folks, losing our mind up in here, up in here. Our mental health has to come first because we don't HAVE to live in despair —we CAN feel better. We must put our health first because suffering from chronic illness and being unwell doesn't make life worth living.

It is unlikely that I can change the medical profession, but I can change my mind. I have changed it and there's no going back. I'm putting my Health First!

—Kirsten, age 39

RESOURCES

ARTHRITIS

Arthritis Foundation
PO Box 7669
Atlanta, GA 30357-0669
(800) 283-7800
www.arthritis.org

AUTOIMMUNE DISEASES

American Autoimmune Related Disease Association
22100 Gratiot Avenue
East Detroit, MI 48021
(586) 776-3900
www.aarda.org

BACTERIAL VAGINOSIS

(See Sexually Transmitted Diseases)

BIPOLAR DISORDER

Depression and Bipolar Support Alliance (DBSA)
730 North Franklin Street, Suite 501
Chicago, IL 60654
(800) 826-3632
www.dbsalliance.org

BREAST CANCER

African American Breast Cancer Alliance
PO Box 8981
Minneapolis, MN 55408
(612) 825-3675
www.aabcainc.org

Avon Foundation for Women
1345 Avenue of the Americas
New York, NY 10105
(866) 505-AVON
www.avonfoundation.org

National Alliance of Breast Cancer Organizations
9 East 37th Street, 10th Floor
New York, NY 10016
(888) 806-2226
www.nabco.org

National Breast Cancer Coalition
1101 17th Street, NW, Suite 1300
Washington, DC 20036
(800) 622-2838
or (202) 296-7477

Sisters Network, Inc.
2922 Rosedale Street
Houston, TX 77004
(713) 781-0255
(866) 781-1808
www.sistersnetworkinc.org

Susan G. Komen for the Cure
5005 LBJ Freeway, Suite 250
Dallas, TX 75244
(877) 465-6636
www.komen.org

Tigerlily Foundation
11654 Plaza America Drive, #725
Reston, VA 20190
(888) 580-6253
www.tigerlilyfoundation.org

BRONCHITIS

American Association for Respiratory Care
9425 North MacArthur Boulevard, Suite 100
Irving, TX 75063
(972) 243-2272
www.aarc.org

American Lung Association
1301 Pennsylvania Avenue, NW, Suite 800
Washington, DC 20004
(800) 586-4872
www.lungusa.org

CERVICAL CANCER

Gynecologic Cancer Foundation
230 West Monroe Street, Suite 2528
Chicago, IL 60606
(312) 578-1439
www.wcn.org

National Cervical Cancer Coalition (NCCC)
6520 Platt Avenue, #693
West Hills, CA 91307
(800) 685-5531
www.nccc-online.org

National Cervical Cancer Public Education Campaign
230 West Monroe Street, Suite 2528
Chicago, IL 60606
(312) 578-1439
www.cervicalcancercampaign.org

Tamika and Friends
PO Box 2942
Upper Marlboro, MD 20773
(866) 595-2448
www.tamikaandfriends.org

CHLAMYDIA

(See Sexually Transmitted Diseases)

CHRONIC FATIGUE SYNDROME

The Chronic Fatigue and Immune Dysfunction Syndrome Association of America
PO Box 220398
Charlotte, NC 28222
(704) 365-2343
www.cfids.org

The National Chronic Fatigue and Immune Dysfunction Syndrome Foundation
103 Aletha Road
Needham, MA 02492
(781) 449-3535
www.ncf-net.org

National Chronic Fatigue Syndrome and Fibromyalgia Association
PO Box 18426
Kansas City, MO 64133
(816) 737-1343
www.ncfsfa.org

CHRONIC KIDNEY DISEASE

American Association of Kidney Patients
3505 East Frontage Road, Suite 315
Tampa, FL 33607
(800) 749-2257
www.aakp.org

National Kidney Foundation
30 East 33rd Street
New York, NY 10016
(800) 622-9010
www.kidney.org

PKD Foundation
8330 Ward Parkway, Suite 510
Kansas City, MO 64114
(800) 753-2873
(816) 931-2600
www.pkdcure.org

CHRONIC OBSTRUCTIVE PULMONARY DISEASE (COPD)

American Association for Respiratory Care
9425 North MacArthur Boulevard,
Suite 100
Irving, TX 75063
(972) 243-2272
www.aarc.org

American Lung Association
1301 Pennsylvania Avenue, NW,
Suite 800
Washington, DC 20004
(800) 586-4872
www.lungusa.org

COLORECTAL CANCER

American College of Gastroenterology
PO Box 342260
Bethesda, MD 20827
(301) 263-9000
www.acg.gi.org

American Society of Colon and Rectal Surgeons
85 West Algonquin Road, Suite 550
Arlington Heights, IL 60005
(847) 290-9184
www.fascrs.org

Colon Cancer Alliance
1025 Vermont Avenue, NW, Suite 1066
Washington, DC 20005
(877) 422-2030
www.ccalliance.org

Colorectal Cancer Coalition
1414 Prince Street, Suite 204
Alexandria, VA 22314
(703) 548-1225
or (877) 427-2111
www.fightcolorectalcancer.org

S.H.E Circle
1875 Connecticut Avenue, NW,
Suite 710
Washington, DC 20009
(866) 628-8637
www.shecircle.org

DEPRESSION

Emotions Anonymous
PO Box 4245
St. Paul, MN 55104
(651) 647-9712
www.emotionsanonymous.org

Mental Health America
2000 North Beauregard Street, 6th Floor
Alexandria, VA 22311
(800) 969-6642
www.nmha.org

National Alliance on Mental Illness
3803 North Fairfax Drive, Suite 100
Arlington, VA 22203
(703) 524-7600
www.nami.org

National Foundation for Depressive Illness, Inc. (NAFDI)
PO Box 17598
Baltimore, MD 21297-1598
(443) 782-0739
www.ifred.org

DIABETES

American Diabetes Association
National Service Center
1701 North Beauregard Street
Alexandria, VA 22311
(800)342-2383
www.diabetes.org

Juvenile Diabetes Research Foundation International
26 Broadway, 14th Floor
New York, NY 10004
(800) 533-2873
www.jdrf.org

National Diabetes Education Program
1 Diabetes Way
Bethesda, MD 20814
(888) 693-6337
(866) 569-1162
www.ndep.nih.gov

DIVERTICULAR DISEASE

American Society of Colon and Rectal Surgeons
85 West Algonquin Road, Suite 550
Arlington Heights, IL 60005
(847) 290-9184
www.fascrs.org

International Foundation for Functional Gastrointestinal Disorders
PO Box 170864
Milwaukee, WI 53217
(888) 964-2001
(414) 964-1799
www.iffgd.org

EMPHYSEMA

American Association for Respiratory Care
9425 North MacArthur Boulevard, Suite 100
Irving, TX 75063
(972) 243-2272
www.aarc.org

FIBROMYALGIA

National Fibromyalgia Association
2121 South Towne Centre Place, Suite 300
Anaheim, CA 92806
(714) 921-0150
www.fmaware.org

FIBROIDS

Brigham and Women's Hospital Center for Uterine Fibroids
77 Avenue Louis Pasteur
New Research Building
Boston, MA 02115
(800) 722-5520
www.fibroids.net

National Uterine Fibroids Foundation
PO Box 9688
Colorado Springs, CO 80932
(719) 633-3454
www.nuff.org

GONORRHEA

(See Sexually Transmitted Diseases)

HEART DISEASE

American Heart Association
7272 Greenville Avenue
Dallas, TX 75231
(800) 242-8721
www.heart.org

The Heart Truth Campaign
NHLBI Health Information Center
PO Box 30105
Bethesda, MD 20824
(301) 592-8573
http://www.nhlbi.nih.gov/health/heart-truth/index.htm

WomenHeart: The National Coalition for Women with Heart Disease
818 18th Street, NW, Suite 1000
Washington, DC 20006
(877) 771-0030
(202) 728-7199
www.womenheart.org

HEPATITIS (VIRAL)

Hepatitis Foundation International
504 Blick Drive
Silver Spring, MD 20904
(800) 891-0707
www.hepfi.org

Hepatitis Prevention Programs
444 North Capitol Street, NW, Suite 339
Washington, DC 20001
(202) 434-8090
www.hepprograms.org

HERPES (GENITAL)

(See Sexually Transmitted Diseases)

HIV /HUMAN IMMUNODEFICIENCY VIRUS

Balm in Gilead
701 East Franklin Street, Suite 1000
Richmond, VA 23219
(888) 225-6243
(804) 644-2256
www.balmingilead.org

Black AIDS Institute
1833 West 8th Street, Suite 200
Los Angeles, CA 90057
(213) 353-3610
www.blackaids.org

Black Women's Health Imperative
1726 M Street, NW, Suite 300
Washington, DC 20036
(202) 548-4000
www.BlackWomensHealth.org
www.ElevateConversation.org

HIV Law Project
15 Maiden Lane, 18th Floor
New York, NY 10038
(212) 577-3001
www.hivlawproject.org

National Association of People with AIDS (NAPWA)
8401 Colesville Road, Suite 505
Silver Spring, MD 20910
(866) 846-9366
(240) 247-0880
www.napwa.org

National Black Leadership Commission on AIDS
120 Wall Street, Suite 2303
New York, NY 10005
(800) 992-6531
www.nblca.org

National Minority AIDS Council
1931 13th Street, NW,
Washington, DC 20009
(202) 483-6622
www.nmac.org

SisterLove
PO Box 10558
Atlanta, GA 30310
(866) 750-7733
www.sisterlove.org

TheBody.com
250 West 57th Street
New York, NY 10107
(212) 541-8500
www.thebody.com

The Well Project
(888) 616-9355
www.thewellproject.org

The Women's Collective
1331 Rhode Island Avenue, NE
Washington, DC 20018
(202) 483-7003
www.womenscollective.org

Women Alive
1566 South Burnside Avenue
Los Angeles, CA 90019
(323) 965-1564
www.women-alive.org

Women Organized to Respond to Life-threatening Disease
449 15th Street, Suite 303
Oakland, CA 94612
(510) 986-0340
www.womenhiv.org

HPV HUMAN PAPILLOMAVIRUS

(See Sexually Transmitted Diseases)

HYPERTENSION

American Heart Association
7272 Greenville Avenue
Dallas, TX 75231
(800) 242-8721
www.heart.org

National Coalition for Women with Heart Disease
818 18th Street, NW, Suite 1000
Washington, DC 20006
Main (202) 728-7199
(877) 771-0030
www.womenheart.org

The Heart Truth Campaign NHLBI Health Information Center
PO Box 30105
Bethesda, MD 20824
(301) 592-8573
www.nhlbi.nih.gov/health/hearttruth/
index.htm

LUNG CANCER

American Lung Association
1301 Pennsylvania Avenue, NW,
Suite 800
Washington, DC 20004
(800) 586-4872
www.lungusa.org

Lung Cancer Alliance
888 16th Street, NW, Suite 150
Washington, DC 20006
(202) 463-2080
www.lungcanceralliance.org

National Cancer Institute Smoking Quitline
(877) 784-8669
www.women.smokefree.gov

LUPUS

Alliance for Lupus Research
28 West 44th Street, Suite 501
New York, NY 10036
(212) 218-2840
www.lupusresearch.org

Lupus Foundation of America, Inc.
2000 L Street, NW, Suite 410
Washington, DC 20036
(202) 349-1155
www.lupus.org

The Lupus Support Network
PO Box 17841
Pensacola, FL 32522-7841
(800) 458-8211
www.thelupussupportnetwork.org

MIGRAINE

American Headache Society
19 Mantua Road
Mount Royal, NJ 08061
(856) 423-0043
www.achenet.org

National Headache Foundation
820 North Orleans, Suite 411
Chicago, Illinois 60610
(888) 643-5552
www.headaches.org

The National Migraine Association
100 North Union Street, Suite B
Alexandria, VA 22314
(703) 349-1929
www.migraines.org

MULTIPLE SCLEROSIS

National MS Society
1100 New York Avenue, NW, Suite 660
Washington, DC 20005
(800) 344-4867
www.nationalmssociety.org

OBESITY

Obesity Action Coalition
4511 North Himes Avenue, Suite 250
Tampa, Florida 33614
(800) 717-3117
www.obesityaction.org

The Obesity Society
8757 Georgia Avenue, Suite 1320
Silver Spring, MD 20910
(301) 563-6526
www.obesity.org

Weight Control Information Network (WIN)
1 WIN Way
Bethesda, MD 20892
(877) 946-4627
www.win.niddk.nih.gov

OSTEOPOROSIS

National Osteoporosis Foundation
1150 17th Street, NW, Suite 850
Washington, DC 20036
(800) 231-4222
www.nof.org

OVARIAN CANCER

American Society for Reproductive Medicine
1209 Montgomery Highway
Birmingham, Alabama 35216
(205) 978-5000
www.asrm.org

FORCE: Facing Our Risk of Cancer Empowered
16057 Tampa Palms Boulevard West, PMB #373
Tampa, FL 33647
(866) 288-7475
www.facingourrisk.org

Gynecologic Cancer Foundation
230 West Monroe Street, Suite 2528
Chicago, IL 60606
(312) 578-1439
www.wcn.org

National Ovarian Cancer Coalition
2501 Oak Lawn Avenue, Suite 435
Dallas, TX 75219
(214) 273-4200
www.ovarian.org

Ovarian Cancer National Alliance
901 E Street, NW, Suite 405
Washington, DC 20004
(866) 399-6262
www.ovariancancer.org

PELVIC INFLAMMATORY DISEASE

(See Sexually Transmitted Diseases)

PNEUMONIA

American Association for Respiratory Care
9425 North MacArthur Boulevard, Suite 100
Irving, TX 75063
(972) 243-2272
www.aarc.org

American Lung Association
1301 Pennsylvania Avenue, NW, Suite 800
Washington, DC 20004
(800) 586-4872
www.lungusa.org

POST-TRAUMATIC STRESS DISORDER

Freedom From Fear
308 Seaview Avenue
Staten Island, NY 10305
(718) 351-1717
www.freedomfromfear.org

National Center for Post-Traumatic Stress Disorder
U.S Department of Veteran Affairs
810 Vermont Avenue, NW
Washington, DC 20420
(802) 296-6300
www.ptsd.va.gov

SCHIZOPHRENIA

National Alliance for Research on Schizophrenia and Depression
60 Cutter Mill Road, Suite 404
Great Neck, New York 11021
(516) 829-0091
www.narsad.org

SEXUALLY TRANSMITTED DISEASES

American Social Health Association
PO Box 13827
Research Triangle Park, NC 27709
(919) 361-8400
www.ashastd.org

Herpes Resource Center
American Social Health Association
PO Box 13827
Research Triangle Park, NC 27709
(919) 361-8488
www.ashastd.org/herpes/herpes_over-
view.cfm

SICKLE CELL

**American Sickle Cell Anemia
Association**
DD Building at the Cleveland Clinic,
Suite DD1-201
10900 Carnegie Avenue
Cleveland, OH 44106
(216) 229-8600
www.accaa.org

**Sickle Cell Disease Association of
America**
231 East Baltimore Street, Suite 800
Baltimore, MD 21202
(800) 421-8453
www.sicklecelldisease.org

The Sickle Cell Information Center
Grady Memorial Hospital
80 Jesse Hill Jr. Drive, SE
Atlanta, GA 30303
(404) 616-3572
www.scinfo.org

STROKE

American Stroke Association
7272 Greenville Avenue
Dallas, TX 75231
(888) 478-7653
www.strokeassociation.org

National Stroke Association
9707 East Easter Lane, Suite B
Centennial, CO 80112
(800) 787-6537
www.stroke.org

SYPHILIS

(See Sexually Transmitted Diseases)

THYROID DISORDERS

American Thyroid Association
6066 Leesburg Pike, Suite 550
Falls Church, Virginia 22041
(703) 998-8890
www.thyroid.org

The Hormone Foundation
8401 Connecticut Avenue, Suite 900
Chevy Chase, MD 20815-5817
(800) 467-6663
www.hormone.org

**Thyroid Cancer Survivors'
Association, Inc.**
PO Box 1545
New York, NY 10159
(877) 588-7904
www.thyca.org

TRICHOMONIASIS

(See Sexually Transmitted Diseases)

URINARY INCONTINENCE

American Urogynecologic Society
2025 M Street, NW, Suite 800
Washington, DC 20036
(202) 367-1167
www.augs.org

American Urological Association Foundation
1000 Corporate Boulevard
Linthicum, MD 21090
(866) 746-4282
www.urologyhealth.org

National Association for Continence
PO Box 1019
Charleston, SC 29402
(800) 252-3337
www.nafc.org

URINARY TRACT INFECTIONS

American College of Obstetricians and Gynecologists
PO Box 96920
Washington, DC 20090
(202) 638-5577
www.acog.org

American Urogynecologic Society
2025 M Street, NW, Suite 800
Washington, DC 20036
(202) 367-1167
www.augs.org

American Urological Association Foundation
1000 Corporate Boulevard
Linthicum, MD 21090
(866) 828-7866
www.urologyhealth.org

UTERINE CANCER

Gynecologic Cancer Foundation
230 West Monroe Street, Suite 2528
Chicago, IL 60606
(312) 578-1439
www.thegcf.org

Society of Gynecologic Oncologists
230 West Monroe Street, Suite 710
Chicago, IL 60606
(312) 235-4060
www.sgo.org

BLACK HEALTH AND MEDICAL ASSOCIATIONS

Association of Black Cardiologists
2400 N Street, NW, Suite 604
Washington DC 20037
(202) 375-6618
www.abcardio.org

Association of Black Psychologists
7119 Allentown Road, Suite 203
Fort Washington, MD 20744
(202) 722-0808
www.abpsi.org

Black Psychiatrists of America
2020 Pennsylvania Avenue, NW, #725
Washington, DC 20006
(877) 272-1967
www.blackpsych.org

National Association of Black Social Workers, Inc.
2305 Martin Luther King Avenue, SE
Washington, DC 20020
(202) 678-4570
www.nabsw.org

National Black Nurses Association
8653 Fenton Street, Suite 330
Silver Spring, MD 20910
(202) 393-6870
www.nbna.org

National Dental Association
3517 16th Street, NW
Washington, DC 20010
(202) 588-1697
www.ndaonline.org

National Medical Association
8403 Colesville Road, Suite 920
Silver Spring, Maryland 20910
(202) 347-1895
www.nmanet.org

NATIONAL ASSOCIATIONS, CENTERS, AND ORGANIZATIONS

American Association of Retired Persons (AARP)
Women's Initiative
601 E Street, NW
Washington, DC 20049
(202) 434-2400
www.aarp.org

Association of Reproductive Health Professionals
1901 L Street, NW, Suite 300
Washington, DC 20036
(202) 466-3825
www.arhp.org

Boston Black Women's Health Institute
43 Wolcott Street
Dorchester, MA 02121
(617) 297-5274
bbwhi@bbwhi.org.

Center for Black Women's Wellness
477 Windsor Street, Suite 309
Atlanta, GA 30312
(404) 688-9202
www.cbww.org

Center for Young Women's Health
333 Longwood Avenue, 5th Floor
Boston, MA 02115 USA
(617) 355-2994
www.youngwomenshealth.org

California Black Women's Health Project
101 N LaBrea, Suite 610
Inglewood, CA 90301
(310)412-1828
www.cabwhp.org

International Center for Traditional Childbearing
841 North Lombard Street
Portland, OR 97217
(503) 460-0932
www.ictcmidwives.org

National Women's Health Network
1413 K Street, NW, 4th Floor
Washington DC 20005
(202) 682-2640
www.nwhn.org

Philadelphia Black Women's Health Alliance
3801 Market Street, Suite 202
Philadelphia, PA 19104
(215)382-3292
www.blackwomenshealthproject.org

Planned Parenthood Federation of America
434 West 33rd Street
New York, NY 10001
(212) 541-7800
www.plannedparenthood.org

United Lesbians of African Heritage
1125 McCadden Place
Los Angeles, CA 90038
(323) 860-7355
www.uloah.com

GOVERNMENTAL AGENCIES

Centers for Disease Control and Prevention
1600 Clifton Road
Atlanta, GA 30333
(800) 232-4636
www.cdc.gov

National Center for Complementary and Alternative Medicine
NCCAM Clearinghouse
9000 Rockville Pike
Bethesda, MD 20892
www.nccam.nih.gov

National Committee for Quality Assurance
2000 L Street, NW, Suite 500
Washington, DC 20036
(202) 955-3500

National Food and Nutrition Information Center
National Agricultural Library
10301 Baltimore Ave
Beltsville, MD 20705
www.nutrition.gov

National Heart Lung and Blood
Institute Health Information Center
PO Box 30105
Bethesda, MD 20824
(301) 592-8573
www.nhlbi.nih.gov/index.htm

National Institute of Allergy and
Infectious Diseases
6610 Rockledge Drive, MSC 6612
Bethesda, MD 20892
(866) 284-4107
www.niaid.nih.gov

National Institute of Arthritis and
Musculoskeletal and Skin Diseases
(NIAMS)
1 AMS Circle
Bethesda, MD 20892
(877) 226-4267
(301) 495-4484
www.niams.nih.gov

National Institutes of Health
9000 Rockville Pike
Bethesda, Maryland 20892
(301) 496-4000
www.nih.gov

NIH National Institute of Neurological
Disorders and Stroke
PO Box 5801
Bethesda, MD 20824
(800) 352-9424
www.ninds.nih.gov

National Kidney and Urologic Diseases
Information Clearinghouse
Three Information Way
Bethesda, MD 20892
(800) 891-5390
www.kidney.niddk.nih.gov

National Mental Health Information
Center, SAMHSA, HHS
1 Choke Cherry Road
Rockville, MD 20852
(800) 789-2647
www.mentalhealth.samhsa.gov

Office of Research on Women's Health
6707 Democracy Blvd. Suite 400
Bethesda, MD 20892
(301) 402-1770
orwh.od.nih.gov/about/contact.html

Office on Women's Health
Department of Health and Human
Services
200 Independence Avenue, SW,
Room 712E
Washington, DC 20201
(202) 690-7650
www.womenshealth.gov

U.S. Department of Health and
Human Services
200 Independence Avenue, SW
Washington, DC 20201
(800) 232-4636
www.hhs.gov

ENDNOTES

Chapter 1

1. Faye Z. Belgrave, *African American Girls: Reframing Perceptions and Changing Experiences* (New York, NY: 2009), 10.
2. Belgrave, *African American Girls*, 4.
3. Belgrave, *African American Girls*, 4.
4. Belgrave, *African American Girls*, 4.
5. Avis A. Jones-DeWeever, *Black Girls in New York City: Untold Strength and Resilience* (Washington, DC: Institute for Women's Policy Research, 2009), 19.
6. U.S. Census Bureau, "Black Americans: A Profile, Statistical Brief," *U.S. Department of Commerce*, http://www.census.gov/apsd/www/statbrief/sb93_2.pdf (accessed November 4, 2011).
7. U.S. Census Bureau, "America's Families and Living Arrangements," *U.S. Census Bureau, Housing and Household Economic Statistics Division, Fertility and Family Statistics Branch*, http://www.census.gov/population/www/socdemo/hh-fam/cps2010.html (accessed November 2, 2011).
8. Jones-DeWeever, *Black Girls in New York City*, 37.
9. Belgrave, *African American Girls*, 41.
10. Belgrave, *African American Girls*, 42.
11. Holly Kearl, *Stop Street Harassment: Making Public Places Safe and Welcoming for Women* (Santa Barbara, CA: Praeger, 2010), 46.
12. Kearl, *Stop Street Harassment*, 19.
13. Tiffany Townsend et al., "I'm No Jezebel; I am Young, Gifted, and Black: Identity, Sexuality, and Black Girls," *Psychology of Women's Quarterly* 34 (2010): 273-85.
14. Aalece O. Pugh-Lilly, Helen A. Neville, and Karen L. Poulin "In Protection of Ourselves: Black Girls' Perceptions of Self-Reported Delinquent Behaviors." *Psychology of Women's Quarterly* 25 (2001): 145.
15. Rachel Pfeffer, "In Post Racial America Prisons Feast on Black Girls," New America Media EthnoBlog, http://ethnoblog.newamericamedia.org/2011/03/in-post-racial-america-prisons-feast-on-black-girls-1.php (accessed March 15, 2011).
16. Pfeffer, "In Post Racial America Prisons."
17. Mark Penn and E. Kinney Zalesne, *Microtrends: The Small Forces Behind Tomorrow's Big Changes* (New York, NY: Twelve, 2007).
18. Penn and Zalesne, *Microtrends*, 17.
19. Judy Schoenberg, Kimberlee Salmond, and Paula Fleshman, *The New Normal: What Girls Say About Healthy Living*, (New York, NY: Girl Scouts of the USA, 2006), 8.
20. Schoenberg, Salmond, and Fleshman, *The New Normal*, 6.
21. Centers for Disease Control and Prevention, "Youth Risk Behavior Surveillance – United States, 2009," *Morbidity and Mortality Weekly Report: Surveillance Summaries* 59 (2010): 59, http://www.cdc.gov/mmwr/pdf/ss/ss5905.pdf (accessed November 2, 2011).
22. Ronald L. Brathwaite, Sandra E. Taylor, Henrie M. Treadwell, eds., *Health Issues in the Black Community* (San Francisco, CA: Jossey-Bass, 2001), 39.
23. Brathwaite, Taylor, and Treadwell, *Health Issues in the Black Community*, 112.
24. Brathwaite, Taylor, and Treadwell, *Health Issues in the Black Community*, 112.
25. Schoenberg, Salmond, and Fleshman, *The New Normal: What Girls Say About Healthy Living*, 24.
26. Critics argue that Blacks are more likely to get STD-tested in public health clinics and other health facilities that mandate testing, whereas, higher-income people go to private doctors who are not required to report all STDs. This is a valid argument, but it doesn't change the reality that STDs are epidemic in Black America.

27. Bob LaMendola, "1 in 4 Girls Has an STD, Study Says," *The Seattle Times*, March 12, 2008, http://seattle-times.nwsource.com/html/health/2004276232_std12.html (accessed November 2, 2011

28. Centers for Disease Control and Prevention, "CDC Report Finds Adolescent Girls Continue To Bear a Major Burden of Common Sexually Transmitted Diseases," *Press Release*, http://www.cdc.gov/nchhstp/newsroom/STDsurveillancepressrelease.html (accessed November 8, 2011).

29. Kaiser Family Foundation, "Fact Sheet: Black Americans and HIV/AIDS, August 2011," http://www.kff.org/hivaids/upload/6089-07.pdf (accessed November 3, 2011).

30. Brathwaite, Taylor, and Treadwell, *Health Issues in the Black Community*, 40.

31. Susan Lamontagne, "1 in 4 Callers to the National Domestic Violence Hotline Report Birth Control Sabotage and Pregnancy Coercion," National Domestic Violence Hotline, http://www.thehotline.org/2011/02/1-in-4-callers-to-the-national-domestic-violence-hotline-report-birth-control-sabotage-and-pregnancy-coercion/ (accessed November 2, 2011).

32. "Domestic Violence and Birth Control Sabotage: A Report From The Teen Parent Project," Center for Impact Research, http://www.impactresearch.org/documents/birthcontrolexecutive.pdf (accessed November 2, 2011).

33. Lamontagne, "1 in 4 Callers to the National Domestic Violence Hotline."

34. Tufts University, "Africana Voices Against Violence," *Statistics: 2002*, www.ase.tufts.edu/womenscenter/peace/africana/newsite/statistics.htm (accessed November 2, 2011).

35. Centers for Disease Control and Prevention, "Youth Risk Behavior Surveillance," 6-7.

36. Centers for Disease Control and Prevention, "Youth Risk Behavior Surveillance," 6.

37. Centers for Disease Control and Prevention, "Youth Risk Behavior Surveillance," 9.

38. Centers for Disease Control and Prevention, "Youth Risk Behavior Surveillance," 10-13.

39. Centers for Disease Control and Prevention, "Youth Risk Behavior Surveillance," 13-14.

40. Centers for Disease Control and Prevention, "Youth Risk Behavior Surveillance," 14-17.

Chapter 2

1. Michele Chandler, "African American Women Are Moving Ahead Rapidly." *Stanford Graduate School of Business*, http://gsb.stanford.edu/news/headlines/2011-african-american-women.html (accessed July 21, 2011).

2. Adam Isen and Betsey Stevenson, "Women's Education and Family Behavior: Trends in Marriage, Divorce and Fertility," *University of Pennsylvania Center for Economic Studies* 2940 (2010), http://bpp.wharton.upenn.edu/betseys/papers/Marriage_divorce_education.pdf (accessed November 2, 2011).

3. Chandler, "African American Women are Moving Ahead Rapidly."

4. Isen and Stevenson, "Women's Education and Family Behavior."

5. Pew Research Center, "Millennials: A Portrait of Generation Next," http://pewsocialtrends.org/files/2010/10/millennials-confident-connected-open-to-change.pdf (accessed November 2, 2011).

6. Tina Rosenberg, *Join the Club: How Peer Pressure Can Transform the World* (New York, NY: W. W. Norton & Company, 2011), 182.

7. Rosenberg, *Join the Club*, 45.

8. Rakesh Kochhar, "Two Years of Economic Recovery: Women Lose Jobs, Men Find Them." *Pew Research Center*, http://www.pewsocialtrends.org/2011/07/06/two-years-of-economic-recovery-women-lose-jobs-men-find-them/ (accessed July 6, 2011).

9. Women of Color Policy Network, "Wage Disparities and Women of Color," http://wagner.nyu.edu/wocpn/publications/files/Pay_Equity_Policy_Brief.pdf (accessed November 2, 2011).

10. Michelle Miller, "African-American unemployment at 16 percent." *CBS News*, http://www.cbsnews.com/stories/2011/06/19/eveningnews/main20072425.shtml (accessed June 19, 20110).

11. Mariko Chang, "Lifting as we Climb: Women of Color, Wealth, and America," *Insight Center for Community Economic Development* (2010): 10, http://www.mariko-chang.com/LiftingAsWeClimb.pdf (accessed July 21, 2011).

12. Ariane Hegewisch and Claudia Williams, "The Gender Wage Gap: 2010 (Fact Sheet #C350)," *Institute for Women's Policy Research*, http://www.iwpr.org/publications/pubs/the-gender-wage-gap-2010 (accessed November 2, 2011).

13. U.S. Department of Health and Human Services, Health resources and Services Administration, "Women's Health USA: 2009." *Maternal and Child Health Bureau*, http://mchb.hrsa.gov/whusa09/ (accessed November 2, 2011).

14. Wang and Taylor, "For Millennials, Parenthood Trumps Marriage," 7.

15. Wang and Taylor, "For Millennials, Parenthood Trumps Marriage," 2.

16. Wang and Taylor, "For Millennials, Parenthood Trumps Marriage," 1.

17. Wang and Taylor, "For Millennials, Parenthood Trumps Marriage," 2.

18. U.S. Department of Health and Human Services, Health Resources and Services Administration, "Women's Health USA: 2009."

19. See CBS News (2009). *CBS Reports: Children of the Recession.* This poll was conducted among a random sample of 1,874 adults nationwide, interviewed by telephone May 6 – May 12, 2009.

20. U.S. Department of Health and Human Services, Health Resources and Services Administration, "Women's Health USA: 2009," 23.

21. Hegewisch and Williams, "The Gender Wage Gap: 2010 (Fact Sheet #C350)."

22. Black Women's Health Imperative, "Lifecycle Memo," Eleanor Hinton Hoyt, 2011.

23. U.S. Department of Health and Human Services, "Women's Health USA: 2009," 22.

24. U.S. Department of Health and Human Services, Substance Abuse and Mental Health Services Administration, "National Survey on Drug Use and Health: 2010," http://www.samhsa.gov/data/NSDUH/2k10Results/Web/HTML/2k10Results.htm (accessed November 8, 2011).

25. Bureau of Justice Statistics, "Intimate Partner Violence Declined Between 1993 and 2004," http://www.ojp.usdoj.gov/newsroom/pressreleases/2006/BJS07007.htm (accessed November 2, 2011).

26. Susan A. Cohen, "Abortion and Women of Color: The Bigger Picture," *Guttmacher Policy Review* 11 (2008), http://www.guttmacher.org/pubs/gpr/11/3/pbr110302.html (accessed November 2, 2011).

27. Centers for Disease Control and Prevention, "Unintended Pregnancy," http://www.cdc.gov/reproductivehealth/unintendedpregnancy/ (accessed November 2, 2011).

28. Medline Plus, "Preconception Care," *National Center for Birth Defects and Developmental Disabilities*, http://www.nlm.nih.gov/medlineplus/preconceptioncare.html (accessed November 2, 2011).

29. Heather D. Boonstra, "The Challenge in Helping Young Adults Better Manage Their Reproductive Lives," *Guttmacher Policy Review* 12 (2009): 13, http://www.guttamcher.org/pubs/gpr/12/2/gpr120213.html (accessed November 2, 2011).

30. Boonstra, "The Challenge in Helping Young Adults."

31. Boonstra, "The Challenge in Helping Young Adults."

32. Cohen, "Abortion and Women of Color."

33. Hillard Weinstock, Stuart Berman, and Willard Cates Jr., "Sexually Transmitted Diseases Among American Youth: Incidence and Prevalence Estimates, 2000," *Guttmacher Policy Review* 36(2004): 6–10, http://www.guttmacher.org/pubs/journals/3600604.html (accessed November 8, 2011).

34. Centers for Disease Control and Prevention, "Sexually Transmitted Disease in the United States, 2008," http://www.cdc.gov/std/stats08/trends.htm (accessed November 2, 2011).

35. Centers for Disease Control and Prevention, Division of STD Prevention, "Consultation to Address STD Disparities in African American Communities: Meeting report," http://www,cdc.gov/std/general/STDHealthDisparitiesConsultationJune2007.pdf (accessed November 2, 2011).

36. National Organization for Women, "Violence against Women in the United States: Statistics," http://www.now.org/issues/violence/stats.html (accessed November 2, 2011).

37. National Organization for Women, "Violence against Women in the United States."

38. Patricia Tjaden and Nancy Thoennes, "Extent, Nature, and Consequences of Intimate Partner Violence: Findings from the National Violence against Women Survey," *U.S. Department of Justice* (2000): 1-57, https://www.ncjrs.gov/pdffiles1/nij/181867.pdf (accessed November 2, 2011).
39. Bureau of Justice Statistics, "Intimate Partner Violence Declined."
40. National Organization for Women, "Violence against Women in the United States."
41. Melonie Heron, "Deaths: Leading Causes for 2004," *Centers for Disease Control and Prevention National Vital Statistics Report* 56 (2007), http://www.cdc.gov/nchs/data/nvsr/nvsr56/nvsr56_05.pdf (accessed November 2, 2011).
42. National Organization for Women, "Violence against Women in the United States."
43. Rape, Abuse & Incest National Network, "Who are the Victims?" http://rainn.org/get-information/statistics/sexual-assault-victims (accessed November 2, 2011).
44. American Psychological Association, Task Force on the Sexualization of Girls, "Report of the APA Task Force on the Sexualization of Girls," http://www.apa.org/pi/women/programs/girls/report-full.pdf (accessed November 2, 2011).
45. National Adolescent Health Information Center, "2008 Fact Sheet on Health-Care Access and Utilization: Adolescents and Young Adults," http://nahic.ucsf.edu/downloads/Demographics08.pdf (accessed November 2, 2011).
46. Phil Galewitz, "At Least 600,000 Young Adults Join Parents' Health Plans Under New Law," *Kaiser Health News*, http://www.kaiserhealthnews.org/Stories/2011/May/01/young-adult-health-insurance-coverage.aspx (accessed November 2, 2011).

Chapter 3

1. JoAnn E. Manson, "Estrogen." Healthy Women, http://www.healthywomen.org/condition/estrogen (accessed November 2, 2011).
2. Black Women's Health Imperative, "Health Attitudes and Behaviors of Black Women," *Online Health Survey* by Harris Interactive, 2007.
3. National Council of Negro Women, "African American Women as We Age," http://www.ncnw.org/centers/age.htm (accessed November 8, 2011).
4. Derek Kravitz and Christopher S. Rugaber, "Americans' equity in their homes near a record low," *Associated Press*, June 10, 2011, http://articles.boston.com/2011-06-09/business/29639313_1_home-equity-mortgage-rates-mortgage-lenders (accessed November 2, 2011).
5. National Women's Law Center, "Employment Crisis Worsens for Black Women During Recovery," http://www.nwlc.org/resource/employment-crisis-worsens-black-women-during-recovery (accessed November 2, 2011).
6. Tatjana Meschede et al., "Severe Financial Insecurity Among African-American and Latino Seniors," *Institute on Assets and Social Policy* 3 (2010), http://iasp.brandeis.edu/pdfs/SFSI.pdf (accessed November 2, 2011).
7. National Committee on Pay Equity, "Women of Color in the Workplace," http://www.pay-equity.org/info-race.html (accessed November 2, 2011).
8. Paul Fronstin and Craig Copeland, "Notes: Debt of the Elderly and Near Elderly, 1992–2007, and the Relationship between Union Status and Employment-Based Health Benefits," *Employee Benefit Research Institute* 30 (2009): 2-3, http://www.ebri.org/pdf/notespdf/EBRI_Notes_10-Oct09.DebtEldly.pdf (accessed November 2, 2011).
9. Avis Jones-DeWeever, "Losing Ground: Women and the Foreclosure Crisis," *National Council of Jewish Women Journal* (2008): 21-22, http://www.ncjw.org/content_1441.cfm (accessed November 2, 2011).
10. Michele Chandler, "African American Women Are Moving Ahead Rapidly," *Stanford Graduate School of Business: Center for Social Innovation*, http://gsb.stanford.edu/news/headlines/2011-african-american-women.html (November 2, 2011).

11. Orlando Patterson, "Progress or Peril?" *Washington Post* 7 (2007), http://www.washingtonpost.com/wp-dyn/content/article/2007/01/05/AR2007010501611.html (accessed November 2, 2011).

12. U.S. Department of Health and Human Services, Health Resources and Services Administration, "Women's Health USA: 2009," 12.

13. Jones-DeWeever, "Losing Ground: Women and the Foreclosure Crisis."

14. John Leland, "Baltimore Finds Subprime Crisis Snags Women," *New York Times*, January 15, 2008, http://www.nytimes.com/2008/01/15/us/15mortgage.html?pagewanted=all (accessed November 2, 2011).

15. Leland, "Baltimore Finds Subprime Crisis Snags Women."

16. Ron Carmichael Manuel, "African American Women as We Age and Successful Aging: A Report of the Research Findings from a Secondary Analysis of Nationally Representative Data," *Howard University Department of Sociology and Anthropology*, September 20, 2004.

17. Black Women's Health Imperative, "Health Attitudes and Behaviors of Black Women."

18. Monique Burns, "A sexual time bomb: the declining fertility rate of the black middle class," *Ebony*, http://findarticles.com/p/articles/mi_m1077/is_n7_v50/ai_16878134/ (accessed October 23, 2011).

19. Centers for Disease Control and Prevention, National Center for Health Statistics, "National Health Interview Survey, 2008," http://www.cdc.gov/nchs/nhis.htm (accessed November 8, 2011).

20. U.S. Department of Health and Human Services, Centers for Disease Control and Prevention, National Center for Chronic Disease Prevention and Health Promotion, Office on Smoking and Health, "The Health Consequences of Smoking: A Report of the Surgeon General," http://www.cdc.gov/tobacco/data_statistics/sgr/2004/complete_report/index.htm (accessed November 3, 2011).

21. U.S. Department of Health and Human Services, Centers for Disease Control and Prevention, National Center for Chronic Disease Prevention and Health Promotion, Office on Smoking and Health, "Tobacco Use Among U.S. Racial/Ethnic Minority Groups — African Americans, American Indians and Alaska Natives, Asian Americans and Pacific Islanders, and Hispanics: A Report of the Surgeon General," http://www.cdc.gov/tobacco/data_statistics/sgr/1998/complete_report/pdfs/complete_report.pdf (accessed November 3, 2011).

22. R. Lorraine Collins and Lily D. McNair, "Minority Women and Alcohol Use," *National Institute on Alcohol Abuse and Alcoholism*, http://pubs.niaaa.nih.gov/publications/arh26-4/251-256.htm (accessed November 2, 2011).

Chapter 4

1. Dr. Dorothy Height, Fannie Lou Hamer and James Baldwin fall outside of the Silent Generation demographic; they are members of the Greatest Generation.

2. Employee Benefit research Institute, "Chapter 6: Income Statistics of the Population Aged 55 and Over," in *EBRI Databook on Employee Benefits*, http://www.ebri.org/pdf/publications/books/databook/DB.Chapter%2006.pdf (accessed November 4, 2011).

3. Tatjana Meschede et al., "Severe Financial Insecurity among African-American and Latino Seniors," *Institute on Assets and Social Policy* 3 (2010): 3, http://iasp.brandeis.edu/pdfs/SFSI.pdf (accessed November 2, 2011).

4. Meschede et al., "Severe Financial Insecurity among African-American and Latino Seniors," 3.

5. Meschede et al., "Severe Financial Insecurity among African-American Latino Seniors," 3.

6. Chang, "Lifting as we Climb," 8.

7. U.S. Department of Health and Human Services, Administration on Aging, "A Statistical Profile of Black Older Americans, Aged 65+," http://www.aoa.gov/aoaroot/aging_statistics/minority_aging/Facts-on-Black-Elderly-plain_format.aspx (accessed November 4, 2011).

8. U.S. Department of Health and Human Services, Administration on Aging, "A Statistical Profile of Black Older Americans."

9. Centers for Disease Control and Prevention, "National Diabetes Prevention Program," http://www.cdc.gov/diabetes/projects/prevention_program.htm (accessed November 2, 2011).

10. U.S. Department of Health and Human Services, Office on Women's Health, "Minority Women's Health," *Womenshealth.gov*, http://www.womenshealth.gov/minorit-health/african-americans/smoking.cfm (accessed November 2, 2011).

11. National Institutes of Health, National Institute on Drug Abuse, "Drugs of Abuse Information: Drugs of Abuse/Related Topics," http://www.drugabuse.gov/drugpages.html (accessed November 2, 2011).

12. Kristen Robinson, "Trends in Health Status and Health-Care Use Among Older Women," U.S. Department of Health and Human Services, Centers for Disease Control and Prevention, National Center for Health Statistics, *Aging Trends* 1 (2007), http://www.cdc.gov/nchs/data/ahcd/agingintrends/07olderwomen.pdf (accessed November 3, 2011).

Chapter 5

Cancer

1. National Cancer Institute, "Common Cancer Types," http://www.cancer.gov/cancertopics/types/commoncancers (accessed August 28, 2011).

2. National Cancer Institute, "Cancer Health Disparities."

3. Black Women's Health Imperative, "Moving Beyond Pink to End Breast Cancer Disparities Issue Brief," (Washington, DC, 2010).

4. American Cancer Society, "Breast Cancer: Early Detection," http://www.cancer.org/Cancer/BreastCancer/MoreInformation/BreastCancerEarlyDetection/index (accessed August 28, 2011).

5. American Cancer Society, "How to Control Your Cancer Risk," http://www.cancer.org/Cancer/news/Features/how-to-control-your-cancer-risk (accessed August 28, 2011).

6. Black Women's Health Imperative, "Breast Self-Exam Fact Sheet," October 2011.

7. Centers for Disease Control and Prevention, "Cervical Cancer Fact Sheet," *Inside Knowledge*, http://www.cdc.gov/cancer/cervical/pdf/Cervical_FS_0510.pdf (accessed August 28, 2011).

8. Centers for Disease Control and Prevention, "Cervical Cancer Fact Sheet."

9. National Institutes of Health, National Cancer Institute, "Cervical Cancer Treatment Option Overview," http://www.cancer.gov/cancertopics/pdq/treatment/cervical/Patient/page4 (accessed August 28, 2011).

10. Centers for Disease Control and Prevention, "Colorectal Cancer Incidence Rates," http://www.cdc.gov/Features/dsColorectalCancer/ (accessed August 28, 2011).

11. Colon Cancer Alliance, "Prevention and Screening," http://www.ccalliance.org/colorectal_cancer/overview.html (accessed August 28, 2011)

12. National Institutes of Health, National Cancer Institute, "Colon Cancer Treatment," http://www.cancer.gov/cancertopics/pdq/treatment/colon/Patient/page5 (accessed August 28, 2011)

13. American Cancer Society, "Cancer Facts and Figures for African Americans, 2005-2006," http://www.cancer.org/acs/groups/content/@nho/documents/document/caff2005aacorrpwsecuredpdf.pdf (accessed August 28, 2011).

14. American Lung Association, "What's in a Cigarette?" http://www.lungusa.org/stop-smoking/about-smoking/facts-figures/whats-in-a-cigarette.html (accessed August 28, 2011).

15. American Cancer Society, "Cancer Facts and Figures for African Americans."

16. American Cancer Society, "Cancer Facts and Figures for African Americans."

17. Centers for Disease Control and Prevention, "Gynecological Cancers: Ovarian Cancer Treatment," http://www.cdc.gov/cancer/ovarian/basic_info/treatment.htm (accessed October 25, 2011).

18. Centers for Disease Control and Prevention, "Uterine Cancer," *Inside Knowledge*, http://www.cdc.gov/cancer/uterine/pdf/Uterine_FS_0308.pdf (accessed, October 25, 2011).

19. Centers for Disease Control and Prevention, "Gynecological Cancers: Uterine Cancer Treatment Options," http://www.cdc.gov/cancer/uterine/basic_info/treatment.htm (accessed October 25, 2011).

Depression

20. James S. Jackson et al., The National Survey of American Life: A Study of Racial, Ethnic and Cultural Influences on Mental Disorders and Mental Health, *International Journal of Methods in Psychiatric Research* 13 (2004): 196-207.
21. Terrie M. Williams, *Black Pain: It Just Looks Like We're Not Hurting* (New York, NY: Scribner, 2008).
22. "Depression." *Mental Health*. World Health Organization, 2011. Online. Accessed. 30 Sept. 2011.
23. Allen, Daree. "When the Blues Don't Move, Part 1: The Stigma and the Shame." *For Harriet | Celebrating the Fullness of Black Womanhood*. 01 Nov. 2010. Online. Accessed. 30 Sept. 2011.
24. "Mental Health America: Depression and African Americans." *Mental Health America: Welcome*. 2011. Accessed. Sept. 2011.
25. "DALYs (Disability Adjusted Life Years)." *Mental Health*. World Health Organization, 2011. Online. Accessed. 30 Sept. 2011.
26. "Mental Health in the African American Community." *Depression and Bipolar*. Depression and Bipolar Support Alliance, 2007. Web. 30 Sept. 2011.Online. Accessed, Sept. 2011.
27. "Suicide Among Black Americans." *Suicide Prevention Resource Center*. Substance Abuse and Mental Health Services Administration (SAMHSA). Web. 30 Sept. 2011.

Diabetes

28. American Diabetes Association, "National Diabetes Fact Sheet, 2011," http://www.diabetes.org/in-my-community/local-offices/miami-florida/assets/files/national-diabetes-fact-sheet.pdf (accessed November 9, 2011).
29. National Institute of Diabetes and Digestive and Kidney Disorders, "National Diabetes Statistics, 2011," http://diabetes.niddk.nih.gov/dm/pubs/statistics/index.aspx (accessed November 9, 2011).
30. American Diabetes Association, "African Americans & Complications Fact Sheet," http://www.diabetes.org/living-with-diabetes/complications/african-americans-and-complications.html (accessed November 9, 2011).
31. American Diabetes Association, "Treatment and Care," http://www.diabetes.org/living-with-diabetes/treatment-and-care/?loc=DropDownLWD-treatment. (accessed November 9, 2011).

Heart Disease

32. Black Women's Health Imperative, "Heart Disease and Black Women: The Silent Killer That Speaks Volumes," http://www.blackwomenshealth.org/issues-and-resources/heart-disease-and-black-women-the-silent-killer-that-speaks-volumes/ (accessed November 10, 2011)
33. The National Coalition for Women with Heart Disease, "Why Women of Color May Face Higher Risk of Heart Disease," http://www.womenheart.org/supportForWomen/heartsmart101/mieresarticle.cfm (accessed October 9, 2011).
34. National Institute of Health, "Subtle and Dangerous: Symptoms of Heart Disease in Women," publication number: 06-6079.
35. The National Coalition for Women with Heart Disease, "Heart Smart 101," http://www.womenheart.org/supportForWomen/heartsmart101/index.cfm (accessed November 9, 2011).
36. National Institute of Health, "Your Guide to Living Well," publication number: 06-5270.

HIV/AIDS

37. Black Women's Health Imperative, "Health Attitudes and Behaviors of Black Women," *Online Health Survey by Harris Interactive*, 2007.
38. Kaiser Family Foundation, "Fact Sheet: Women and HIV/AIDS in the United States, August 2011," http://www.kff.org/hivaids/upload/6092-09.pdf (accessed September 9, 2011).
39. Centers for Disease Control and Prevention, "Morbidity and Mortality Weekly Report, Vol. 60, No. 21; 2011," http://www.cdc.gov/mmwr/mmwr_wk/wk_cvol.html (accessed September 9, 2011).

40. National Institute of Allergy and Infectious Disease, "HIV/AIDS: HIV Risk Factors," http://www.niaid.nih.gov/topics/HIVAIDS/Understanding/Pages/riskFactors.aspx (accessed September 9, 2011).

41. Adaora A. Adimora, Victor J. Schoenbach, and Michelle A. Floris-Moore, "Ending the Epidemic of Heterosexual HIV Transmission Among African Americans," *American Journal of Preventive Medicine article* (2009): 469, http://www.americanbar.org/content/dam/aba/migrated/AIDS/docs/AMEPRE_2570.authcheckdam.pdf (accessed August 3, 2011).

42. Centers for Disease Control and Prevention, "HIV among African Americans," http://www.cdc.gov/hiv/topics/aa/ (accessed November 9, 2011).

43. Centers for Disease Control and Prevention, "Sexually Transmitted Diseases in the United States, 2008," http://www.cdc.gov/std/stats08/trends.htm (accessed November 9, 2011).

44. Kaiser Family Foundation, "Views and Experiences with HIV Testing Among African Americans in the U.S., June 2009," *Kaiser Public Opinion Survey*, http://www.kff.org/hivaids/upload/7927.pdf (accessed November 9, 2011).

Kidney Disease

45. American Kidney Fund, "Kidney Disease," http://www.kidneyfund.org/ (accessed September 5, 2011).

46. National Kidney Foundation, "Ten Facts about African Americans and Kidney Disease," http://www.kidney.org/news/newsroom/fs_new/10factsabtaframerkd.cfm (accessed September 5, 2011).

47. National Kidney Disease Education Program, "Testing for Kidney Disease," http://nkdep.nih.gov/patients/kidney_disease_testing.htm

48. National Kidney Foundation, "Donations & Transplant," http://www.kidney.org/transplantation/ (accessed September 5, 2011).

49. National Kidney and Urologic Disease Information Clearinghouse, "NKUDIC Home" http://kidney.niddk.nih.gov/index.aspx (accessed September 5, 2011).

Obesity

50. Angela Odoms-Young, PhD, *and Focus Group Report for the National Black Women's Health Imperative Topic: Obesity and Overweight Prevention and Treatment* (Washington, DC: Black Women's Health Imperative, 2007).

51. U.S. National Library of Medicine, "Obesity," http://www.ncbi.nlm.nih.gov/pubmedhealth/PMH0004552/ (accessed November 9, 2011).

52. Larry Cohen, Daniel P. Perales, and Catherine Steadman, "The O Word: Why the Focus on Obesity is Harmful to Community Health," Californian Journal of Health Promotion 3 (2005): 154-161.

STDs

53. Centers for Disease Control and Prevention, "2009 Sexually Transmitted Disease Surveillance," http://www.cdc.gov/std/stats09/default.htm. (accessed September 9, 2011).

54. Centers for Disease Control and Prevention, "Trends in Sexually Transmitted Diseases in the United States: 2009 National Data for Gonorrhea, Chlamydia and Syphilis," http://www.cdc.gov/std/stats07/trends.htm (accessed September 9, 2011).

55. Centers for Disease Control and Prevention, "Trends in Sexually Transmitted Diseases in the United States."

56. Centers for Disease Control and Prevention, Hepatitis Information for the Public, http://www.cdc.gov/hepatitis/C/index.htm. (accessed August 29, 2011).

57. Centers for Disease Control and Prevention. Genital Herpes: CDC Fact Sheet. http://www.cdc.gov/std/Herpes/STDFact-Herpes.htm

58. Eileen F. Dunne et al., "Prevalence of HPV Infection among Females in the United States," Journal of American Medical Association 297 (2007): 813-819.

59. Centers for Disease Control and Prevention, "Trends in Sexually Transmitted Diseases in the United States: 2009 National Data for Gonorrhea, Chlamydia and Syphilis."

60. M. Sutton et al., "The Prevalence of Trichomonas Vaginalis Infection among Reproductive-age Women in the United States, 2001-2004," *Clinical Infectious Diseases* 15 (2007): 1319-26.

Stroke
61. National Institute of Neurological Disorders and Stroke, "Brain Basics," http://www.ninds.nih.gov/disorders/brain_basics/know_your_brain.htm . (accessed September 9, 2011).
62. National Stroke Association, "Fact Sheets," http://www.stroke.org/site/PageServer?pagename=factsheets. (accessed September 9, 2011.
63. National Stroke Association, "Fact Sheet," http://www.stroke.org/site/PageServer?pagename=WOMSYMP. (accessed September 9, 2011).
64. National Stroke Association, "FAST," http://www.stroke.org/site/PageServer?pagename=symp. (accessed September 9, 2011).
65. National Institute of Neurological Disorders and Stroke, "Brain Basics," http://stroke.nih.gov/materials/brainbasics.htm.)accessed September 9, 2011).

Violence
66. L. Y. Marlowe, *Color Me Butterfly* (New York, NY: Three Rivers Press, 2007).
67. Between Friends, "Fact Sheet," http://www.betweenfriendschicago.org/index.html (accessed November 9, 2011).
68. Futures Without Violence, "Fact Sheet online," http://www.futureswithoutviolence.org/ (accessed November 9, 2011).
69. Violence Policy Center, "When Men Murder Women: An Analysis of 2008 Homicide Data," http://www.vpc.org/studies/wmmw2011.pdf (accessed November 9, 2011).
70. Federal Bureau of Investigation, "Uniform Crime Reports," http://www.fbi.gov/about-us/cjis/ucr/ucr (accessed November 9, 2011).
71. University of California Davis Health System, "Reproductive coercion often is accompanied by physical or sexual violence, study finds," EurekAlert!, http://www.eurekalert.org/pub_releases/2010-01/uoc--rco012010.php (accessed November 9, 2011).
72. Scott Beach and Richard Schulz, "Financial Exploitation and Psychological Mistreatment Among Older Adults: Differences Between African Americans and Non-African Americans in a Population-Based Survey," *The Gerontologist* (2010).

Chapter 6

1. National Alliance for Nutrition and Activity, "National Health Priorities: Reducing Obesity, Heart Disease, Cancer, Diabetes, and Other Diet- and Inactivity-Related Diseases, Costs, and Disabilities," http://cspinet.org/new/pdf/cdc_briefing_book_fy10.pdf. (accessed November 3, 2011).
2. Environmental Working Group, "Farm Subsidy Primer," *2011 Farm Subsidy Database*, http://farm.ewg.org/subsidyprimer.php (accessed November 3, 2011).
3. U.S. Department of Agriculture, "America's Diverse Family Farms: 2010 Edition," 6, http://www.ers.usda.gov/Publications/EIB67/EIB67.pdf (accessed November 3, 2011).
4. Michael Pollan, *The Omnivore's Dilemma: A Natural History of Four Meals* (New York, NY: Penguin Press, 2007), 41.
5. Mayo Clinic, "Nutrition and Healthy Eating: Calorie Calculator," http://www.mayoclinic.com/health/calorie-calculator/NU00598 (accessed November 3, 2011).
6. Marion Nestle, *Food Politics: How the Food Industry Influences Nutrition and Health* (Berkeley, CA: University of California Press, 2003), 11.

7. National Cancer Institute, "Fact Sheet: Obesity and Cancer Questions and Answers," http://www.cancer.gov/cancertopics/factsheet/Risk/obesity (accessed November 3, 2011).

8. Nestle, *Food Politics*, viii.

9. Nelson Media Research, "African-American Audience: Weekly TV Usage," http://www.nielsenmedia.com/ethnicmeasure/african-american/AAweeklyusage.html (accessed November 3, 2011).

10. Kaiser Family Foundation, "Generation M2: Media in the Lives of 8 to 18 Year Olds," http://www.kff.org/entmedia/upload/8010.pdf (accessed November 3, 2011).

11. Sonya A. Grier and Shiriki Kumanyika, Targeted Marketing and Public Health, Annual Review of Public Health 31 (2010): 349-69.

12. Nestle, *Food Politics*, 20.

13. Marion Nestle, *What to Eat* (New York, NY: North Point Press, 2006), 46.

14. Harvard School of Public Health, "The Nutrition Source, New Dietary Guidelines: Progress, Not Perfection," http://www.hsph.harvard.edu/nutritionsource/what-should-you-eat/dietary-guidelines-2010/index.html (accessed November 3, 2011).

15. U.S. Department of Agriculture and the U.S. Department of Health and Human Services, "Dietary Guidelines for Americans: 2010," (Washington, DC: U.S. Government Printing Office, 2010), 20.

16. Sarah Treuhaft and Allison Karpyn, "The Grocery Gap: Who Has Access to Healthy Food and Why it Matters," *PolicyLink and the Food Trust*, http://www.policylink.org/atf/cf/%7B97C6D565-BB43-406D-A6D5-ECA3BBF35AF0%7D/FINALGroceryGap.pdf (accessed November 3, 2011). TKTK.

17. Treuhaft and Karpyn, "The Grocery Gap," 14.

18. Feeding America, "Hunger and Poverty Statistics: Feeding the World," http://feedingamerica.org/hunger-in-america/hunger-facts/hunger-and-poverty-statistics.aspx (accessed November 3, 2011).

19. U.S. Department of Health and Human Services Office of Minority Health, "Obesity and African Americans," http://minorityhealth.hhs.gov/templates/content.aspx?ID=6456 (accessed November 3, 2011).

20. Centers for Disease Control and Prevention, "Overweight and Obesity: Defining Overweight and Obesity," http://www.cdc.gov/obesity/defining.html (accessed November 3, 2011).

21. Shiriki Kumanyika, "Obesity, Health Disparities, and Prevention Paradigms: Hard Questions and Hard Choices," *Preventing Chronic Disease: Public Health Research, Practice, and Policy* 2 (2005), http://www.cdc.gov/pcd/issues/2005/oct/05_0025.htm (accessed November 4, 2011).

22. Kristie J. Lancaster, "Diet & Culture in African Americans" (a PowerPoint presentation, September 12, 2008).

23. Shiriki Kumanyiki, "Overweight and Obesity — 'It's Not About Weight, It's About Our Health'" (presentation at Black Women's Health Imperative Celebration, June 2008).

24. Craig Freudenrich, "How the Obesity Paradox Works," http://health.howstuffworks.com/human-body/bodily-feats/obesity-paradox1.htm (accessed November 4, 2011).

25. Kerry S. O'Brien et al., "Reducing Anti-Fat Prejudice in Preservice Health Students: A Randomized Trial," *Obesity* 18 (2010): 2138-44.

26. Yale News, "Pervasive Weight Discrimination a Serious Health Risk," http://opac.yale.edu/news/article.aspx?id=7578 (accessed November 3, 2011).

27. Yale News, "Pervasive Weight Discrimination a Serious Health Risk."

28. Gary Taubes, "Is Sugar Toxic?" *New York Times*, April 13, 2011, http://www.nytimes.com/2011/04/17/magazine/mag-17Sugar-t.html?_r=1&src=me&ref=magazine (accessed November 4, 2011).

29. U.S. Department of Health and Human Services, "Your Guide to Lowering Your Blood Pressure with DASH," http://www.nhlbi.nih.gov/health/public/heart/hbp/dash/new_dash.pdf (accessed November 4, 2011).

30. Michigan Department of Envrionmental Quality, "The Human Body – Water Relationship," http://www.michigan.gov/documents/deq/deq-wb-wws-HumanWaterReqs_267731_7.pdf (accessed November 4, 2011).

31. U.S. Department of Agriculture and the U.S. Department of Health and Human Services, "Dietary Guidelines for Americans: 2010," (Washington, DC: U.S. Government Printing Office, 2010), 20.

32. Gary Taubes, *Why We Get Fat: and What to Do About It* (New York, NY: Knopf, 2010).

33. Harvard School of Public Health, "The Nutrition Source – Fiber: Start Roughing It!" http://www.hsph.harvard.edu/nutritionsource/what-should-you-eat/fiber-full-story/index.html (accessed November 4, 2011).

34. World Cancer Research Fund, American Institute for Cancer Research, "Food, Nutrition, Physical Activity, and the Prevention of Cancer: a Global Perspective – Online," http://www.dietandcancerreport.org/ (accessed November 4, 2011).

35. Natural Resources Defense Council, "Consumer Guide to Mercury in Fish," http://www.nrdc.org/health/effects/mercury/guide.asp (accessed November 4, 2011).

36. Toni Yancey, *Instant Recess: Building a Fit Nation 10 Minutes at a Time*, (University of California, 2010), 55

37. William J. Strawbriege, "Physical Activity Reduces the Risk of Subsequent Depression for Older Adults," *American Journal of Epidemiology* 156 (2002): 328-334, http://aje.oxfordjournals.org/content/156/4/328.full.pdf+html (accessed November 4, 2011).

38. The Free Dictionary by Farlex, "Weight-Bearing," http://medical-dictionary.thefreedictionary.com/weight-bearing (accessed November 4, 2011).

39. Lee Woodard, "Range of Motion Exercises for the Elderly," *Livestrong.com*, http://www.livestrong.com/exercises-for-the-elderly (accessed November 4, 2011).

40. U.S. Department of Health and Human Services, National Heart, Lung, and Blood Institute, "About the Heart Truth," http://www.nhlbi.nih.gov/educational/hearttruth/about/index.htm (accessed November 8, 2011).

41. Centers for Disease Control and Prevention, "National Health Interview Survey," http://www.cdc.gov/nchs/nhis.htm (accessed November 4, 2011).

42. National Heart, Lung, and Blood Institute, "What is Physical Activity?" http://www.nhlbi.nih.gov/health/dci/Diseases/phys/phys_what.html (accessed November 4, 2011).

43. Centers for Disease Control and Prevention, "Physical Activity for Everyone: How Much Physical Activity Do Adults Need?" http://www.cdc.gov/physicalactivity/everyone/guidelines/adults.html#Aerobic (accessed November 4, 2011).

44. National Heart, Lung, and Blood Institute, "What is Physical Activity?"

45. Centers for Disease Control and Prevention, "Physical Activity for Everyone."

46. Gary Taubes, "Why We Get Fat."

47. Nelson Media Research, "African-American Audience: Weekly TV Usage," http://www.nielsenmedia.com/ethnicmeasure/african-american/AAweeklyusage.html (accessed November 3, 2011).

48. John R. Little and Doug McGuff, Body by Science: *A Research-Based Program for Strength Training, Body Building, and Complete Fitness in 12 Minutes a Week* (New York, NY: McGraw-Hill, 2008), 4.

49. Elizabeth Quinn, "The Best Core Exercises," *About.com Guide*, http://sportsmedicine.about.com/od/abdominalcorestrength1/a/NewCore.htm (accessed November 4, 2011).

Chapter 7

1. U.S. Department of Health and Human Services, Substance Abuse and Mental Health Services Administration, Center for Mental Health Services, "Mental Health: A Report of the Surgeon General—Executive Summary," http://www.surgeongeneral.gov/library/mentalhealth/home.html (accessed November 3, 2011).

2. Raising the bar even higher, we could also consider the idea that no one in their right mind would consume the planet faster than the planet can regenerate itself. Some people might call this the very definition of "suicidal", yet that's how most Americans live. We'll leave that conversation to be led by the people who have expertise in that lane.

3. Ron Carmichael Manuel, "African American Women as We Age and Successful Aging: A Report of the Research Findings from a Secondary Analysis of Nationally Representative Data," NCNW, September 20, 2004.

4. U.S. Department of Health and Human Services Office on Women's Health, "Good Mental Health," http://www.womenshealth.gov/mental-health/good/ (accessed November 4, 2011).

5. Sarah Gehlert, et al., Targeting Health Disparities: A Model Linking Upstream Determinants to Downstream Interventions," *Health Affairs* 27 (2008): 339-349. Knowing about the interaction of societal factors and disease can enable targeted interventions to reduce health disparities.

6. National Association on Mental Illness, "What Is Mental Illness: Mental Illness Facts," http://www.nami.org/template.cfm?section=about_mental_illness (accessed November 4, 2011).

7. Charisse Jones and Kumea Shorter-Gooden, *Shifting the Double Lives of Black Women in America* (New York, NY: HarperCollins, 2004), 11.

8. U.S. Department of Health and Human Services, "Mental Health: A Report of the Surgeon General," http://www.surgeongeneral.gov/library/mentalhealth/ (accessed November 3, 2011).

9. Harvard Medical School, Harvard Health Publications, "Dysthymia," http://www.health.harvard.edu/newsweek/Dysthymia.htm (accessed November 4, 2011).

10. The Common Wealth Fund, "Performance Snapshots," http://www.commonwealthfund.org/Maps-and-Data/Performance-Snapshots.aspx (accessed November 8, 2011).

11. Kristin Blank, "Mental Illness & African Americans: Initiative Raises Awareness," Substance Abuse and Mental Health Services Administration, http://www.samhsa.gov/samhsanewsletter/Volume_18_Number_2/MentalIllnessAfricanAmericans.aspx (accessed November 4, 2011).

12. National Institute of Mental Health, "Prevalence of Serious Mental Illness Among U.S. Adults by Age, Sex, and Race," http://www.nimh.nih.gov/statistics/SMI_AASR.shtml (accessed November 4, 2011).

13. National Institute of Mental Health, "Major Depressive Disorder Among Adults," http://www.nimh.nih.gov/statistics/1MDD_ADULT.shtml (accessed November 4, 2011).

14. Michele T. Pato, "Psychiatric News," http://pn.psychiatryonline.org/content/43/15/11.full?etoc (accessed November 4, 2011).

15. Braithwaite, Taylor, and Treadwell, *Health Issues in the Black Community*, 128.

16. U.S. Department of Health and Human Services Substance Abuse and Mental Health Services Administration Office of Applied Sciences, "Results from the 2006 National Survey on Drug Use and Health: National Findings," http://www.oas.samhsa.gov/NSDUH/2k6NSDUH/2k6results.cfm#8.1.1 (accessed November 3, 2011).

17. Braithwaite, Taylor, and Treadwell, *Health Issues in the Black Community*, 119.

18. Braithwaite, Taylor, and Treadwell, *Health Issues in the Black Community*, 127.

19. Peter J. Cunningham, "Beyond Parity: Primary Care Physicians' Perspectives on Access to Mental Health-Care," *Health Affairs Web Exclusive* (2009): w490–w500, http://www.commonwealthfund.org/Content/Publications/In-the-Literature/2009/Apr/Beyond-Parity-Primary-Care-Physicians-Perspectives-on-Access.aspx (accessed November 4, 2011).

20. Aaron Levin, "Depression Care for Black Women May Hinge on Cultural Factors," *Psychiatric News* 43 (2008), 11, http://pn.psychiatryonline.org/content/43/15/11.full?etoc (accessed November 4, 2011).

21. U.S. Department of Health and Human Services Office on Women's Health, "Good Mental Health."

22. John M. Grohol, "Psychotherapy," http://psychcentral.com/psychotherapy/ (accessed November 3, 2011).

23. William Lawson, "Eat Right to Fight Stress," *Psychology Today*, http://www.psychologytoday.com/articles/200302/eat-right-fight-stress (accessed November 3, 2011).

24. Mayo Clinic, "Water: How Much Should You Drink Every Day?" http://www.mayoclinic.com/health/water/NU00283 (accessed November 3, 2011).

25. Harvard Health Publications, Harvard Medical School, "Importance of Sleep: Six Reasons Not to Scrimp on Sleep," http://www.health.harvard.edu/press_releases/importance_of_sleep_and_health (accessed November 3, 2011).

26. Joshua Rubinstein and David Meyer, "Is Multitasking more Efficient? Shifting Mental Gears Costs Time, Especially when Shifting to Less Familiar Tasks," *American Psychological Association*, http://www.apa.org/news/press/releases/2001/08/multitasking.aspx (accessed November 3, 2011).

Chapter 8

1. Gloria Wade-Gayles ed., My Soul is a Witness: African-American Women's Spirituality (Boston, MA: Beacon Press, 1995), 6.
2. Pew Forum on Religion & Public Life, "U.S. Religious Landscape Survey," 40, http://religions.pewforum.org/ (accessed November 8, 2011).
3. Iyanla Vanzant, "Saying Yes to Your Life," in *Tomorrow Begins Today: African American As We Age*, National Council of Negro Women (Washington, DC: National Council of Negro Women, 2005), 236-243.

Chapter 9

1. American Academy of Nurse Practitioners, "Frequently Asked Questions: Why Choose a Nurse Practitioner as Your Healthcare Provider?" http://www.aanp.org/NR/rdonlyres/A1D9B4BD-AC5E-45BF-9EB0-DEFCA1123 204/4710/2011FAQswhatisanNPupdated.pdf (accessed November 8, 2011).
2. Healthcare.gov, "Patient Protection and Affordable Care Act," http://www.healthcare.gov/law/index.html (accessed November 8, 2011).
3. Andrew Gottschalk and Susan A. Flocke, "Time Spent in Face-to-Face Patient Care and Work Outside Examination Room," *Annals of Family Medicine* 3 (2005): 488-493, http://www.ncbi.nlm.nih.gov/pmc/articles/PMC1466945/ (accessed November 8, 2011).
4. Black Women's Health Imperative, "Focus Group – Let's Talk" Initiative: Patient/Provider Group Discussions Final Report," prepared by Branch Associates (Washington, DC, 2008).

INDEX

Page numbers followed by b represents boxes; f, figures.

American Association of Retired Persons, 362

American Autoimmune Related Diseases Association, Inc., 351

American College of Gastroenterology, 130, 353

American College of Obstetricians and Gynecologists, 361

American Diabetes Association, 165, 354

American Headache Society, 358

American Heart Association, 170, 173, 355, 357

American Lung Association, 79, 135, 352, 353, 357, 359

American Sickle Cell Anemia Association, 360

American Social Health Association, 223, 359

American Society for Reproductive Medicine, 358

American Society of Colon and Rectal Surgeons, 130, 353, 354

American Stroke Association, 234, 360

American Thyroid Association, 360

American Urogynecologic Society, 361

American Urological Association Foundation, 361

Amputations, diabetes/diet and, 163, 255

Angelou, Maya, 260

Anger and aggression, 56, 308

Angina, 169

Angioplasty, 172

Angry Black woman syndrome, 146

Anxiety disorders, 290

Arthritis
    in mature adults, 90, 91b, 97, 99
    obesity and, 198b
    resources on, 351, 364

Arthritis Foundation, 351

Asbestos, lung cancer and, 133

Asking for help, 297–298, 303, 309

Asking questions of doctor, 339–340

Assault. *See* Violence/abuse.

Assessment, self-. *See* Self-care/assessment.

Association of Black Cardiologists, 361

Association of Black Psychologists, 153, 361

Association of Reproductive Health Professionals, 223, 362

Atherosclerosis, 170

Atrial fibrillation and stroke, 231

Autoimmune disease, 161, 351. *See also* Immune system response

Avery, Byllye, 344–345

Avon Foundation for Women, 122, 351

Awareness of self, 302–303, 343

B

Baby Boomers, 92–93

Back pain, low, physical activity and, 271, 277

Balance, improving, 271

Balm in Gilead, 183, 356

Battering. *See* Violence/abuse.

Beauty industry and weight, 255

Belgrave, Faye Z., 16, 18, 25, 29, 38, 41, 59

Beverages, 265, 267

Bible study, 322–324

Big Food, 249–250

Bipolar disorder, 291, 351

Birth control. *See* Contraceptive methods.

Birth control sabotage, 45, 239

Birth defects, obesity and, 198b

Black AIDS Institute, 183, 356

Black Girls in New York City: Untold Strength and Resilience (IWPR), 17

Black Mental Health Alliance for Education and Consultation, 153

Black Pain: It Just Looks Like We're Not Hurting (Williams), 148b, 150

Black Psychiatrists of America, 362

"Black superwoman," 93, 297

Black Women's Health Imperative (Imperative), 356
    on adolescent issues, 28, 30
    on AIDS, 177, 183
    breast cancer campaign by, 122
    on depression in women, 240
    on foods and weight, 253, 256
    on Health Wise Woman, 331
    on mature adult issues, 93, 97, 99
    on midlife adult issues, 67, 72, 74–75, 80
    on obesity, 196
    on physical activity, 273
    on wellness, 343
    on young adult issues, 41–42

Blacks in Gerontology, 95–98

BlackWomensHealth.org, 338

Bleeding disorders, stroke and, 228

Blindness and diabetes, 163

Blood pressure, high. *See* Hypertension.

Blood pressure test
    diabetes and, 164
    heart disease and, 171
    kidney disease and, 190
    for mature adults, 107

for midlife adults, 85, 87

monitoring, 333, 333b

obesity bias and, 259

physical activity and, 271

stroke and, 231

for young adults, 62

Blood spills and hepatitis, 215

Blood sugar. *See* Glucose test, blood.

Body, healthy. *See* Physical wellness.

Body mass index (BMI), 197, 256–258, 257f, 333, 333b

Body shapes, 258

TheBody.com, 184, 356

Body-mind-spirit connection, 285–286, 314

Bone density screening, 85, 87, 107, 271

Boston Black Women's Health Institute, 362

Bra for exercise, sports, 279

Brain cancer, 114

Breast cancer

in Black women, 116–118

case example of, 115–116

in midlife adults, 73

obesity and, 119, 199b

reducing risk of, 120–121

resources on, 122–123, 351–352

signs of/diagnosing, 119–120

treatment for, 121–122

Breast exam, clinical/self

breast cancer and, 120–121

for mature adults, 107

for midlife adults, 85, 87

for young adults, 62

Breastfeeding support, insurance to cover, 338

Breasts, dense, 118

Brigham and Women's Hospital, 355

Bronchitis, 79, 352

Brown-Riggs, Constance, 255–256, 263–265, 266

Butter intake, 266

Bypass surgery, coronary artery, 172

C

CA 125 blood test, 138

Calcium in a healthy diet, 268

California Black Women's Health Project, 363

Calorie counting, efficacy of, 263

Cancer

diagnosing, 114–115

life enjoyment versus, 316b

in mature adults, 97

in midlife adults, 73

obesity and, 199b

physical activity and, 271

reducing risk of, 141–142

resource on, 224

types of, 113–114

See also types of cancer

Carbohydrates, healthy, 266

Carcinoma, 114

Cardiovascular disease (CVD). *See* Heart disease.

Caregiving/caregivers

of children and parents, 81

financial abuse and, 240

women conditioned for, 315b

Carpal tunnel syndrome (CTS), obesity and, 200b

CD4 count, 181

Celebration

eating habits and, 262

spiritual health and, 329

Center for Black Women's Wellness, 362

Center for Social Justice and Policy (Georgetown Univ.), 313

Center for Young Women's Health, 362

Centers for Disease Control and Prevention (CDC), 363

on adolescent health, 25–26, 29

on genital herpes, 216

on human papillomavirus (HPV) vaccine, 127, 220

on mammography sites, 122

on midlife adult health, 79

on physical activity, 274

on young adult health, 42f, 46, 56

Cervical cancer

about, 124–127

in adolescents, 28

HPV-associated, 219

resources on, 352

in young adults, 46

Cervical cap contraceptive, 47

Chancre, 221

Change and health habits, 259–263

"Change of life," 77–78

Charity, spiritual health and, 327

Chemotherapy, seek second opinion for, 341

Chesney-Lind, Meda, 22

diabetes and, 162, 164
difficulty in changing, 259–263
healthy tips to change, 264–268
heart disease and, 171
kidney disease and, 190–191, 190b
of mature adults, 98, 99–100
mental health and, 304–305
of midlife adults, 74
reasons for, 196, 248–249
spiritual fasting/cleansing and, 324–325
Echocardiogram, 171
Economic security. *See* Employment; Home owner
    ship; Income.
Education
in adolescence, 22–23, 22f
and mature adulthood, 94
in midlife adulthood, 68–70
in young adulthood, 37–38
Education, patient
insurance to cover, 338
process of, and eating habits, 261
eGFR. *See* Glomerular filtration rate test (eGFR),
    estimated.
Electrocardiogram (ECG/EKG), 171
Electronic technology
multitasking and, 306–307
spiritual health and, 325
Emergency contraception (EC), 48
Emotional abuse, 238
Emotional stressors
in adolescence, 31–32
Black women and, 286, 288–289
in mature adulthood, 104–105
in midlife adulthood, 80–82
in young adulthood, 59–60
See also Mental health screening; Mental illness/
    distress/disorder
Emotional wellness
overview of, 283–285
Black women and, 286, 288–289, 297–298
mind-body-spirit connection in, 285–286
signs of, 284, 300–304
strategies for, 304–309
Emotions, listen selectively to own, 308
Emotions Anonymous, 354
Emphysema, 79, 102, 355
Employment
in midlife adulthood, 68–70

physical activity and, 272
retirement of mature adults and, 93
as a spiritual "call," 313
in young adulthood, 38–39
Empowerment, strategic steps to self-, 343–345
End stage renal disease (ESRD), 188–189, 201b
Endometrial biopsy, 140
Endometrial cancer (EC), 139, 199b
Energy levels, uniqueness of, 274–275
English, Allesa, 292
Environmental factors and health, 248, 275
Esophageal cancer, obesity and, 199b
Estrogen and uterine cancer, 140
Ethnic marketing, 252
Exams, physical health. *See* Health exams/screening.
Exercise. *See* Activity, physical.
Eye exam, comprehensive, 63, 86, 88, 108
Eye problems and diabetes, 162

F

Family "health" tree, 332
Family history. *See* Genes/genetic predisposition;
    History, personal/family health.
Family nurse practitioner (FNP), 335b
Family planning, 52. *See also* Contraceptive methods
Family structure
in adolescence, 17b
changing habits and, 261
of mature adults, 95–96
in midlife adulthood, 70–71, 70–71f
in young adulthood, 40–41
FAST acronym for stroke victim, 231, 232
Fasting/cleansing, 324–325
Fat bias, 198, 258–259
Fat intake, saturated
kidney disease and, 190, 190b
recommendations for, 266
stroke and, 232
Fat metabolism, energy and, 275
Fatigue
depression and, 149, 292
eating habits and, 304
mental health and, 290, 291b
obesity and, 99, 260
Fats, tests for blood.
    See Cholesterol test; Triglycerides test.

Fears
    facing, for empowerment, 344
    of failure/rejection/regret, 309
    of public/self stigma, 294–295
Fecal occult blood test, 86, 88, 108
Feelings, awareness of, 302–303
Fellowship, 329
Fertility, compromised, 46, 56, 76–77
Fiber in a healthy diet, 267
Fibroids, resources on uterine, 355
Fibromyalgia, resources on, 352–353, 355
Financial abuse, 239–240
Financial giving, 327
Fish in a healthy diet, 267
Fitness, aerobic, 276–277. *See also* Activity, physical
Flexibility, improving, 271, 276
Food industry/legislation, 251–252, 268
Food insecure, 254
Food Politics: How the Food Industry Influences Nutrition and Health (Nestle), 251–252
Food supply facts, 249–250
Foods
    availability of, 253–254
    changing choices of, 259–263
    conflicting messages about, 251–253
    disease and, 255
    effects of, 248
    healthy choices in, 264–268
    processed, choosing, 250–251, 263
    spiritual fasting/cleansing and, 324–325
    See also Eating habits; Nutrition
For Colored Girls Who Have Considered Suicide When the Rainbow is Enuf (Shange), 145, 152
FORCE: Facing Our Risk of Cancer Empowered, 138, 359
Foreclosure crisis, 67, 71
Freedom From Fear, 359
Freeman, Pamela, 40–41, 81, 291, 302, 306–307
Fruit juice, 264b, 265, 267
Fruits in a healthy diet, 267
Futures Without Violence, 243

G

Gallbladder disease, obesity and, 201b
Gastric cardia cancer, obesity and, 199b
Gatekeeper health care provider, 335b
Gayles, Gloria Wade, 311–312

Genes/genetic predisposition
    breast cancer and, 118
    caregiving and, 315b
    health history and, 332
    kidney disease and, 189
    lung cancer and, 134
    ovarian cancer and, 137
    physical health and, 260, 275
    stroke and, 228
    weight and, 197
Genital sores, 217
Geriatric nurse practitioner (GNP), 335b
Gestational diabetes, 162
Giving financially, 327
Glomerular filtration rate test (eGFR), estimated, 190
Glucose, types of dietary, 264–265, 264b
Glucose metabolism, 161, 275
Glucose test, blood
    diabetes and, 164
    heart disease and, 171
    for mature adults, 107
    for midlife adults, 85, 87
    monitoring, 333, 333b
    for young adults, 62
Gonorrhea, 29, 55, 211–213
Gout, 201b, 271
Governmental agencies, 363–364
Gowns, exam, 341–342
Graduation rates (high school), 22f
Grandchildren, caring for, 81–82
Grease, use of cooking, 266
Grier, Sonia, 252
Growth hormones, chronic stress and, 286
Gynecologic Cancer Foundation, 127, 138, 141, 352, 359, 361
Gynecology. *See* OB/GYN doctor/visit; Reproductive health.

H

Hair styles and exercise, 280–281
Harassment, physical activity and, 272
Harris Interactive surveys
    on AIDS, 177
    on midlife adult health, 72, 74
    on young adult health, 41–42
Harvard School of Public Health, 98, 252
Head injury, stroke and, 228

P

Pain, chest/low back
    depression and, 292
    heart disease and, 169–170
    obesity and, 203b
Pancreatitis, obesity and, 204b
Pap test
    for adolescents, 33
    cervical cancer and, 125–126
    for mature adults, 107
    for midlife adults, 85, 87
    sexually transmitted disease and, 209, 219
    for young adults, 62
Paradox of plenty, 254
Parenthood. *See* Childbirth.
Partner abuse. *See* Intimate partner violence (IPV).
Patch, birth control, 46f, 49
A Path to Healing: A Guide to Wellness for Body, Mind, and Soul (Sullivan), 284
Patient Protection and Affordable Care Act (2010), 54, 61, 337
Patient rights, 336–337
Patient-information websites, 338–339
Patients, responsibilities/role of, 337–343
Patterson, Orlando, 70
Pediatric nurse practitioner (PNP), 335b
Pedometer, 276
Pelvic exam
    for adolescents, 33
    for mature adults, 107
    for midlife adults, 85, 87
    sexually transmitted disease and, 209
    for young adults, 62
Philadelphia Black Women's Health Alliance, 363
Phillips, Kathleen, 69–70
Phosphorus intake, kidney disease and, 191
Physical activity. *See* Activity, physical.
Physical wellness
    overview of, 247–248
    concepts of weight and, 255–259
    eating habits and, 248–249
    foods/food supply and, 249–255
    healthy eating for, 264–268
    making changes for, 259–263
    physical activity and. *See* Activity, physical
    self-care/assessment of own. *See* Self-care/assessment
    summary of, 281

Physician assistant (PA), 335b, 336
Physicians. *See* Health care providers.
Pill, the (birth control), 46f, 49, 228
PKD Foundation, 192, 353
Planned Parenthood Federation of America (PPFA), 53, 59, 363
Pneumococcal vaccine, 108
Pneumonia, resources on, 359
Pollution, lung cancer and air, 133
Polycystic Kidney Disease (PKD), 185–188, 189, 192
Population statistics
    on adolescents (10-19), 17b
    on mature adults, 91b
    on midlife adults (40-64), 66b
    on young adults (20-39), 36b
Post Traumatic Slave Syndrome: America's Legacy of Enduring Injury and Healing (DeGruy), 288–289
Post traumatic slavery syndrome (PTSS), 288–289
Post traumatic stress disorder (PTSD), 289, 359
Potassium intake, kidney disease and, 191
Poverty rate for Black women, 288
Prayer, mental/spiritual health and, 296–297, 321
Pregnancy, intended/unintended
    in adolescence, 28–29, 32
    fish in diet during, 267
    gestational diabetes and, 162
    in young adulthood, 45–46, 52–53, 58–59
Prevention
    information network on, 224
    lifestyle and, 281
    See also Health exams/screening
Prevention Institute, 198
Primary care providers (PCP), 335b
Primm, Annelle, 289–290, 293, 311, 328
Problem-solving for mental health, 308
Protective order, 241
Protein in a healthy diet, 267–268
Psychiatrist/psychologist. *See* Health care providers.
Psychotherapy, 298–300
Public health authorities, STDs and, 221
Puhl, Rebecca M., 259

Q

Quality assurance, committee on, 363
Quality of life
    aging and, 90, 96

ACKNOWLEDGMENTS

We acknowledge this book as a gift from the many, many people whose expertise and faith helped bring our vision to reality.

The concept of a health resource guide for Black women was born out of many conversations four years ago with the president and associate publisher of SmileyBooks, Cheryl Woodruff, who never wavered in her wise publishing counsel, guiding editorial hand, and insistence that this be the book that shares the Imperative's mission with Black woman everywhere. There is no doubt that this book could not have happened without Cheryl's support.

SmileyBooks' publisher Tavis Smiley and Reid Tracy, CEO of Hay House, both took a leap of faith with the Black Women's Health Imperative and bought into the idea that this book could help make Black women's health *matter*. For that, we are deeply grateful.

Most of all, this book is a reflection of the women who shared their personal stories so that we all could benefit. Thank you for your voices—both identified and anonymous—and for making such a special contribution to our work.

To our issue experts, a wonderful group of women with limitless wisdom and experience and care for Black women, we thank you for your love and support through the countless hours of interviews, e-mails, phone calls, meetings, and writings, all given to bring this health resource to life.

We acknowledge the following subject-matter experts who willingly agreed to our interviews and questions with patience and understanding of the task at hand: M. Natalie Achong, M.D.; Argie Allen, Ph.D., M.F.T.; Tomika Anderson; Catrisse L. Austin, D.D.S.; Faye Z. Belgrave, Ph.D.; Mia Byrd; Tamara Carey, L.S.W., C.C.; Rev. Monica A. Coleman, Ph.D.; Emily Cooper, M.D.; Vanessa Cullins, M.D., M.P.H., M.B.A.; Joy DeGruy, M.A., M.S.W., Ph.D.; Roni DeLuz, R.N., N.D., Ph.D.; Goulda Downer, Ph.D., R.D., L.N., C.N.S.; Rev. Marcia L. Dyson; Pamela Freeman, M.S.W.; Sonia Grier, Ph.D., M.B.A.; Nikki Henderson; Ruth King, M.A.; Kristie Lancaster, M.S., R.D., Ph.D.; Shiriki Kumanyiki, Ph.D., M.P.H.; Debra Powell-Wright; Annelle Primm, M.D., M.P.H.; Constance Brown Riggs, M.S.Ed., R.D., C.D.E.; Aishah Shahidah Simmons; Robin Smith, Ph.D.; Carla Stokes, Ph.D.; Shani Asantewaa Strothers; Andrea Sullivan, Ph.D., N.D.; Latham Thomas, H.H.C., A.A.D.P., R.Y.T.; Emilie Townes, D.Min., Ph.D.; Melicia Whitt-Glover, Ph.D.; Gail E. Wyatt, Ph.D.; Antronette Yancey, M.D., M.P.H., and Aisha Young, M.A.

The steady hand during the final editorial phase was Anne Barthel, an editor extraordinaire, whose determination and kindness gently guided us across the finish line—we are most grateful that you too were committed to the end. The SmileyBooks editorial team, Kirsten Melvey and Thomas Louie, cheered us on as well as providing ongoing editorial and production assistance. Chaz Kyser also provided editorial assistance when we needed it most.

With any project, there have to be exceptional staff, research, and production teams who are behind the scenes but ever contributing and ensuring that you get it right. We had that in the staff and interns of the Imperative and the editorial team at SmileyBooks, who were always able to go with the flow and do what needed to be done.

A special appreciation to Sade Adeeyo and Valerie Rochester, both of whom gave many early mornings, late evenings, and weekends—taking our calls, keeping us on task, organizing, monitoring, tracking our progress checklists, and sharing their thoughts when it was needed most—and to Marisa Spalding, the newest member of the Imperative team, who was always willing to lend a hand and sort through pages of charts, data, and words, all to ensure we put forth the most beneficial health resource possible for Black women.

Thank you to Ronneal Mathews, whose research skills proved invaluable when sorting through mountains of data, and to Samantha Griffin, Zakiya Tanks, Dionne Otey, Veronica Womack, Laura Harker, and Tanise Louden—Imperative staff and interns who played an important role in getting the facts, researching organizations, diseases, and the latest trends, and developing charts and graphs.

With our two readers, Vera Whisenton, a friend, and Sacheen Carr-Ellis, M.D.—our medical advisor and a member of the board of the Black Women's Health Imperative—we were provided swift and honest feedback that we quickly heeded.

Our founder, Byllye Avery, provided invaluable advice and critical feedback and was able to put us back on the right track when we strayed.

Juan Roberts of CreativeLunacy is the genius behind our extraordinary cover. Juan's vision was brought to life through the generous participation of our cover models Shawn Bouyer-Crum, LaVelda Bailey, Chezere Brathwaite, Kimberly Brown, Tatiana Dean, Leigh Dupree, Anna Fuson, Amaechina Doreen (Doreen Haywood), Theresa Kirk, Kamili Mitchell, Cherise Pierce, Yolanda Roberts, Shuronda Robinson, Felicia Sanders, and LaVada Woods. Thank you all so much for helping us let Black women's beauty shine through you.

Without the inspiring talent and extraordinary professionalism of Cindy Shaw of CreativeDetails.net, you would have no book in your hands. Many thanks, Cindy!

ABOUT THE AUTHORS

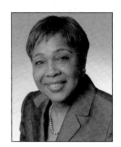

Eleanor Hinton Hoytt, a tireless advocate for eliminating health disparities among women and communities of color, serves as the president and CEO of the Black Women's Health Imperative. Hinton Hoytt produced the groundbreaking book *Tomorrow Begins Today: African American Women As We Age,* for the National Council of Negro Women. She is the proud recipient of the NAACP's Thurgood Marshall Legacy Award and the Keystone Award for Women's Research Advocacy from the NIH Office on Women's Research.

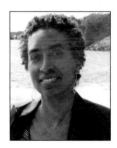

Hilary Beard is an award-winning health journalist specializing in health, healthy lifestyle, and personal development. Beard is the *New York Times* best-selling author of *Friends: A Love Story, 21 Pounds in 21 Days: The Martha's Vineyard Diet/Detox, and Venus and Serena: Serving from the Hip.* She has been editor-in-chief of the *Black AIDS Weekly, Real Health,* and the National Medical Association's *Healthy Living* and *HealthQuest* magazines, and she contributes frequently to *Ebony, Essence,* and *Heart & Soul.*

ABOUT THE BLACK WOMEN'S HEALTH IMPERATIVE

The Black Women's Health Imperative (Imperative) is the leading national organization advancing the health and wellness of our nation's 20 million Black women and girls. Founded as the National Black Women's Health Project in 1983 by internationally recognized health activist and MacArthur Genius Byllye Y. Avery, the Imperative works to promote optimum health for Black women across the life span—physically, emotionally, mentally, and spiritually.

Through advocacy, education, and leadership development, the Imperative works to deepen Black women's resolve in becoming savvy decision makers about our health, achieving optimum health and wellness, and eliminating racial and gender disparities in health. Our aim is to deepen the public's investment in moving health and wellness to the top of every Black woman's life agenda, as well as making it a top priority on the nation's policy and research agenda.

Our *advocacy efforts* move us beyond documenting the enormous health disparities that exist for Black women to focusing on actionable steps for eliminating the undue health burdens Black women face. We believe that prevention is the key to change.

Our *educational initiatives* provide Black women with the information, tools, and resources that help us become informed and empowered health-care consumers and caregivers so we can get the most from our health-care system and build strong partnerships with our health-care providers.

Our *leadership development* programs help strengthen the competencies and skills of Black women so we can become a part of a network of health leaders who work together to champion our causes about the preventable chronic health conditions plaguing Black families and communities.

From organizing the first national Black women's health conference at Spelman College in 1983 to publishing the groundbreaking *Our Bodies, Our Voices, Our Choices: A Black Woman's Primer on Reproductive Health and Rights* in 1991 to launching the most promising campaign to end breast cancer disparities, *Moving Beyond Pink*, in 2010, our commitment to Black women has always been and will continue to be "your health is our #1 priority!"

With headquarters in the District of Columbia, the Imperative works in collaboration with a network of over 50 affiliated organizations, partners, and collaborators across the country with an outreach to more than three million women, a growing constituency base of over 160,000, and five community-based affiliated partners with offices in Atlanta, Boston, Chicago, Los Angeles, and Philadelphia. This expansive network includes a rich blend of national, faith, and grassroots organizations that share a vision for working together to support the improved health and well-being of healthy families in healthy communities.

For more information about the Imperative, visit our award-winning website acclaimed by *Essence* magazine as "the leading virtual destination for Black women's health news and resources": www.BlackWomensHealth.org, follow us on Twitter @blkwomenshealth and become our friend on Facebook at http://facebook.com/blackwomenshealth.

SMILEYBOOKS TITLES
OF RELATED INTEREST

BOOKS

THE COVENANT In Action
Compiled by Tavis Smiley

AMERICA I AM LEGENDS:
Rare Moments and Inspiring Words
Edited by SmileyBooks
Introduction by Tavis Smiley

NEVER MIND SUCCESS…GO FOR GREATNESS!
The Best Advice I've Ever Received
by Tavis Smiley

HOPE ON A TIGHTROPE
Words & Wisdom
by Cornel West

PEACE FROM BROKEN PIECES:
How To Get Through What You're Going Through
by Iyanla Vanzant

BLACK BUSINESS SECRETS:
500 Tips, Strategies and Resources for
African American Entrepreneurs
by Dante Lee

BRAINWASHED:
Challenging the Myth of Black Inferiority
by Tom Burrell

DVDs/CDs

STAND: a film by Tavis Smiley

All of the above are available at your local bookstore, or may be
ordered online through Hay House, at www.hayhouse.com®